S0-BIN-270

Tools for
advancing
tobacco
control in the
21st century

Building blocks for tobacco control

A handbook

WHO Library Cataloguing-in-Publication Data

WHO Tobacco Free Initiative.
Building blocks for tobacco control : a handbook.

(Tools for advancing tobacco control in the 21st century)

1. Smoking – prevention and control. 2. Tobacco – adverse effects 3. Tobacco industry – legislation 4. National health programs – organization and administration 5. Manuals I. Title.

ISBN 92 4 154658 1   (LC/NLM classification: HV 5763)

© World Health Organization 2004

All rights reserved. Publications of the World Health Organization can be obtained from Marketing and Dissemination, World Health Organization, 20 Avenue Appia, 1211 Geneva 27, Switzerland (tel: +41 22 791 2476; fax: +41 22 791 4857; e-mail: bookorders@who.int). Requests for permission to reproduce or translate WHO publications – whether for sale or for noncommercial distribution – should be addressed to Publications, at the above address (fax: +41 22 791 4806; e-mail: permissions@who.int).

The designations employed and the presentation of the material in this publication do not imply the expression of any opinion whatsoever on the part of the World Health Organization concerning the legal status of any country, territory, city or area or of its authorities, or concerning the delimitation of its frontiers or boundaries. Dotted lines on maps represent approximate border lines for which there may not yet be full agreement.

The mention of specific companies or of certain manufacturers' products does not imply that they are endorsed or recommended by the World Health Organization in preference to others of a similar nature that are not mentioned. Errors and omissions excepted, the names of proprietary products are distinguished by initial capital letters.

The World Health Organization does not warrant that the information contained in this publication is complete and correct and shall not be liable for any damages incurred as a result of its use.

This publication contains the collective views of an international group of experts and does not necessarily represent the decisions or the stated policy of the World Health Organization.

Design, layout and editing assistance by Inís – *www.inis.ie*

Printed in France

Contents

PART II:
PUTTING THEORY INTO PRACTICE

Abbreviations

IDRC .... International Development Research Centre
ACS .... American Cancer Society
AFTA .... American Free Trade Area
AIDS .... Acquired Immunodeficiency Syndrome
APACT .... Asia Pacific Association for the Control of Tobacco
ASEAN .... Association of Southeast Asian Nations
ASH Thailand .. Action on Smoking and Health/Thailand
BAT .... British American Tobacco
CDC .... Centers for Disease Control and Prevention, Atlanta
CD-ROM .... Compact Disc Read-Only Memory
CEFTA .... Cental European Free Trade Association
CIG(s) .... Cigarettes
CLO .... Country Liaison Officer
CNCT .... Comité National Contre le Tabagisme
CPI .... Consumer Price Index
CSR .... Corporate Social Responsiblity
C-TOB .... Clearinghouse for Tobacco
DALY .... Disability Adjusted Life Year
DOH .... Department of Health
ECU .... European Currency Unit
EDA .... Environmental Protection Agency
EFTA .... European Fair Trade Association
EIU .... Economics Intelligence Unit
ERC .... ERC Group PLC
ETS .... Environmental Tobacco Smoke
EU .... European Union
EURO .... Regional Office for Europe
FAO .... Food and Agriculture Organization
FCTC .... Framework Convention on Tobacco Control
FIFA .... International Federation of Football Associations
GATT .... General Agreement on Tariffs and Trade
GCC .... Gulf Cooperation Council
GPG .... Global Public Good
GTZ .... Die Deutsche Gesellschaft für Technische Zusammenarbeit
                  (GTZ) GmbH
GYTS .... Global Youth Tobacco Survey
HIS .... Health Information Systems
HIV .... Human Immunodeficiency Virus
HSC .... Health Sponsorship Council
IARC .... International Agency for Research on Cancer
IATH .... International Agency on Tobacco and Health
ICD .... International Classification of Diseases
ICT .... Information Communication Technology
IDRC .... International Development Research Centre
IEC .... Information, Education, Communication
ILO .... International Labour Organization
IMF .... International Monetary Fund
INCA .... Instituto Nacional de Cancer (Brazil)/National Cancer Institute

INFOTAB .... International Tobacco Information Centre
JTI .... Japanese Tobacco International
LCU .... Local Currency Unit
LDC .... Less Developed Country(ies)
MFN .... Most Favored Nation
MSA .... Master Settlement Agreement
NAFTA .... North American Free Trade Agreement
NCD .... Noncommunicable Disease
NGO .... Nongovernmental Organization
NRT .... Nicotine Replacement Therapy
NTCP .... National Tobacco Control Programme
PM .... Philip Morris
POA .... Plan of Action
POS .... Point-of-Sale
PPE .... Probability Proportional to Enrolment
PR .... Public Relations
PSA .... Public Service Announcement
PX .... Post Exchange
RC .... Research Coordinator
RITC .... Research for International Tobacco Control
RP .... Retail Price
RR .... Relative Risk
SARS .... Severe Acute Respiratory Syndrome
SDR .... Standardized Death Rate
SIDS .... Sudden Infant Death Syndrome
STEPS .... STEPwise Approach to Surveillance
TB .... Tuberculosis
TC .... Tobacco Control
TFI .... Tobacco Free Initiative
TMA .... Tobacco Merchants' Association
TNA .... Training Needs Assessment
TOT .... Training-of-Trainers
TTC .... Transnational Tobacco Company
TV .... Television
UICC .... International Union Against Cancer
UNDP .... United Nations Development Programme
UNEP .... United Nations Environment Programme
UNF .... United Nations Foundation
UNICEF .... United Nations Children's Fund
USD .... United States Dollar
USDA .... United States Department of Agriculture
USM .... Universiti Sains Malaysia
VAT .... Value Added Tax
VCR .... Video Cassette Recorder
VicHealth .... Victorian Health Promotion Foundation
VIP .... Very Important Person
WHA .... World Health Assembly
WHO .... World Health Organization
WHS .... World Health Survey
WNTD .... World No Tobacco Day
WR .... WHO Representative
WTO .... World Trade Organization

Acknowledgements

We thank the Regional Advisers of the Tobacco Free Initiative for their participation in the planning of this handbook and assistance in identifying experts with practical experience in tobacco control to contribute to this handbook.

The following individuals served as the editors and primary contributors of this handbook:

da Costa e Silva, Vera Luiza
Director, Tobacco Free Initiative,
World Health Organization, Geneva

David, Annette
Former Regional Adviser,
Tobacco Free Initiative,
World Health Organization,
Regional Office for the Western Pacific
Department of Mental Health and
Substance Abuse, Guam

The following individuals are the primary contributors to Part I (Setting the theoretical foundation for tobacco control) of this handbook:

Bettcher, Douglas
Tobacco Free Initiative,
World Health Organization, Geneva

Bialous, Stella Aguinaga
Tobacco Policy International, USA

Mackay, Judith
Asian Consultancy on Tobacco Control,
Hong Kong SAR

Szilagyi, Tibor
Health 21 Hungarian Foundation,
Hungary

The following individuals are the primary contributors to Part II (Putting theory into practice) of this handbook:

Akaleephan, Chutima
International Health Policy Program, Thailand

Akinsete, Annette
Federal Ministry of Health, Abuja, Nigeria

Awang, Rahmat
Clearinghouse for Tobacco Control, National Poison Center, Universiti Sains Malaysia, Malaysia

Bialous, Stella Aguinaga
Tobacco Policy International, USA

Goldfarb, Luisa
Coordination for Prevention and Surveillance (CONPREV), Ministry of Health, Brazil

Hachey, Dawn
Office of Prevention, Cessation and Education, Tobacco Control Programme, Health Canada, Ottawa, Canada

Hamzeh, Muna
Health Education and Information Department, Ministry of Health, Jordan

Morrow, Martha
Australian International Health Institute, University of Melbourne, Australia

Riseley, Kerryn
South East Asia Tobacco Control Alliance, Thailand

Saloojee, Yussuf
International Non Governmental Coalition Against Tobacco (INGCAT), South Africa

Samarasinghe, Diyanath
Department of Psychological Medicine, Faculty of Medicine, University of Colombo, Sri Lanka

Szilagyi, Tibor
Health 21 Hungarian Foundation, Hungary

Tanghcharoensathein, Viroj
International Health Policy Program, Thailand

Vilain, Claude
Tobacco Free Initiative, World Health Organization, Regional Office for Europe, Copenhagen, Denmark

We thank the following individuals for reviewing and contributing to drafts of this handbook:

Armstrong, Timothy
World Health Organization, Geneva

Asma, Samira
Centers for Disease Control and Prevention, USA

Yurekli, Ayda
World Bank, USA

Bendib, Lydia
World Health Organization, Geneva

Bianco, Eduardo
Director of Tobacco Control, InterAmerican Heart Foundation, Uruguay

Bonita, Ruth
World Health Organization, Geneva

Brigden, Linda
International Development Research Centre (IDRC), Canada

Chapman, Simon
School of Public Health, University of Sydney, Australia

Guha, Snigdha
Indo-German Technical Cooperation for Health, German Technical Cooperation (GTZ), India

Henry, Melinda
World Health Organization, Geneva

Israel, Ruben
Globalink, Switzerland

Latif, Ehsan
Network for Consumer Protection, Islamabad, Pakistan

Ottmani, Salah-Eddine
World Health Organization, Geneva

Simpson, David
International Agency on Tobacco and Health, England

Van Zyl, Greer
World Health Organization, South Africa

Warren, Wick
Centers for Disease Control and Prevention, USA

We thank the following individuals at the Tobacco Free Initiative for reviewing the drafts and providing technical inputs:

Audera-López, Carmen   Onzivu, William   Seoane, Marta

Dhavan, Poonam   Perucic, Ann Marie   Vestal, Gemma

Demeuron, Jean-Yves   Reinders, Lina

Mamniashvili, Lia   Richter-Airijoki, Heide

Poonam Dhavan at the Tobacco Free Initiative provided editorial assistance and managed the overall production with administrative support from Sonia Huang. We thank Maria Cardines and Mary Falvey for copy-editing the handbook and the designing team at Inís for their creative expertise.

Foreword

WE ARE ENTERING A NEW ERA in tobacco control. The World Health Organization Framework Convention on Tobacco Control (WHO FCTC) represents a major leap forward in the effort to curb the toll of death and lost healthy years of life due to tobacco consumption. Through the WHO FCTC, efforts to reduce tobacco use are strategically coordinated for an effective global response to one of the most significant risk factors for premature death and disease.

Member States are in the process of signing and ratifying the Convention. Once the WHO FCTC enters into force, it will provide countries with a powerful means to address the epidemic of tobacco use. However, the WHO FCTC is only part of the solution to this major public health problem.

While the WHO FCTC provides the framework for action against tobacco, the actual work to combat tobacco use must necessarily occur at country level. The success of the WHO FCTC will depend almost entirely on the ability of countries to implement and enforce its provisions. Thus, building and enhancing national capacity for tobacco control in every country are critical if the WHO FCTC is to succeed.

This handbook addresses the need to provide practical guidance for governments and ministries of health in developing their ability to effectively confront the tobacco epidemic. All WHO Regions are represented, and every effort was made to use actual country examples and experiences. The structure and language are intentionally simple and straightforward, to enable as many end-users as possible to benefit.

While the handbook is primarily intended for staff at the national level, programme staff at the subnational and local levels and those in the private sector may benefit from this handbook.

Through resources such as this, WHO aims to continue to support its Member States in building their national tobacco control capacity as a complement to the WHO FCTC. The combination will provide the world with its best hope to control effectively one of the most devastating and prevalent causes of poor health today.

The success of the WHO FCTC as a tool for public health will depend on the energy and political commitment that we devote to implementing it, in countries, in the coming years. A successful result will be global public health gains for all.

Jong-wook Lee, Director-General
World Health Organization

Executive summary

THE TOBACCO EPIDEMIC IS A GLOBAL CHALLENGE demanding concerted global and national action. Recognizing that globalization is accelerating the epidemic's spread and perceiving the limits of national action to contain a public health problem with transnational dimensions, Member States of the World Health Organization (WHO) negotiated and adopted a unique public health treaty for tobacco control. Today, the WHO FCTC contains the blueprint for coordinated global action to address one of the most significant risks to health.

However, national action is critical in order to attain the vision embodied in the WHO FCTC. Building national capacity to carry out effective and sustainable national tobacco control programmes is an urgent priority, and one of the most significant measures required to combat the tobacco epidemic.

The idea for this handbook arose from the awareness that while various official WHO documents called for developing national capacity for tobacco control, there was no comprehensive publication for the development of such capacity. Conceived as a 'how to' manual, the approach is intentionally pragmatic, addressing 'real world' issues and providing practical advice for setting up viable national tobacco control programmes.

OVERVIEW

The handbook contains three main sections. The introduction presents the evolving definition of 'national capacity', identifies the types of capacities needed for effective tobacco control and outlines the key features of building capacity. Part I provides a descriptive overview of the tobacco epidemic, and is further subdivided into four chapters. These chapters address tobacco as a risk factor, with attendant health and economic costs; the global strategies of the tobacco industry; the scientific evidence for effective tobacco control interventions; and the WHO FCTC as a global solution to a health epidemic with prominent politico-legal and sociocultural attributes. Part II focuses on the fundamental capacities necessary to empower countries to take on the tobacco epidemic successfully. The chapters in this section build on early successes in various areas of tobacco control within developed and developing countries that have pioneered the fight against the tobacco epidemic. These chapters apply the lessons learned from the experiences of these countries and offer advice and suggestions to enable Member States to put the theories of tobacco control into practice. This section begins with the development of a national plan of action as the foundation for successful tobacco control at the country level. It addresses the other important elements in national capacity-building, including establishing an effective infrastructure for a national tobacco control programme, training and education, raising public awareness through effective communications and media advocacy, programming specific tobacco control activities, legislating measures for tobacco control and exploring economic interventions and funding initiatives. Chapters on countering the tobacco industry, forming effective partnerships, monitoring and evaluating progress, and exchanging information and research provide valuable insights to augment tobacco control capacity.

SUMMARIES OF THE CHAPTERS

Part I. Setting the Theoretical Foundation for Tobacco Control

Chapter 1. Tobacco as a risk factor: health, social and economic costs

This chapter reviews the global data on the tobacco epidemic. Tobacco is now a major preventable cause of death in developed and developing countries. Every day over 13 000 people worldwide die from tobacco. Assuming constant tobacco use prevalence, WHO projects that from 2000 to 2025 the number of smokers will rise from approximately 1.2 billion to more than 1.7 billion and the annual number of deaths, which is currently estimated at about 5 million, will double in 20 years. Aggressive promotion by the tobacco industry, and permissive environments that make tobacco products readily available and affordable play a major role in inducing young people to take up tobacco use. The addictive nature of nicotine ensures that the majority of tobacco users remain hooked for life. The health and economic costs of tobacco use, however, are borne not only by tobacco users, but by society in general. The chapter examines tobacco consumption trends among adults and youth, presenting cross-country data where available. It illustrates how the costs of tobacco consumption affect tobacco users, non-users, families and communities, businesses, and governments and society, making the tobacco epidemic a concern for everyone.

Chapter 2. The tobacco industry

This chapter offers insights into the nature of the tobacco industry, and the global strategies it uses to maintain the profitability and widespread use of its deadly product. The tobacco industry documents database, made available publicly as a result of the Master Settlement Agreement (MSA) between the tobacco companies and 46 United States territories and states, is a rich source of information on the industry's formerly secret tactics and plans to deter effective measures to control tobacco use. Actual examples in several countries are cited to illustrate how the industry's strategies have been used to impede progress in tobacco control.

Chapter 3. Tobacco control interventions: the scientific basis

The tremendous adverse impact of tobacco use on health and economic indicators worldwide makes tobacco control a public health imperative. This chapter discusses the evidence for effective interventions to reduce tobacco consumption. Both supply- and demand-side interventions are examined. The impact of these strategies on smoking initiation and cessation, and their cost-effectiveness, are discussed. Benefits of tobacco control to individuals, families, communities and governments are enumerated. For tobacco control to succeed, a comprehensive mix of policies and strategies is needed. The chapter concludes by urging governments to act quickly, supporting international efforts through the WHO FCTC and establishing solid national programmes to stem the devastating effects of the tobacco epidemic on current and future generations.

Chapter 4. The WHO Framework Convention on Tobacco Control (WHO FCTC): the political solution

Public health protection has traditionally been viewed mainly as a national concern. With globalization, however, many issues related to health no longer respect the geographical confines of sovereign states, and can no longer be resolved by national policies alone. The WHO FCTC was developed in response to the current globalization of the tobacco epidemic. This effort represented the first time that WHO Member States had exercised their treaty-making powers under Article 19 of the WHO Constitution. The idea behind the WHO FCTC and its future related protocols, is that it will act as a global complement to, not a replacement for, national and local tobacco control actions. The chapter reviews the history of the WHO FCTC, the legal approach selected, utilizing a framework convention and related protocols, and the process for the WHO FCTC to come into force. The various core tobacco control interventions contained in the WHO FCTC are introduced, and the features that are unique to the WHO FCTC are highlighted. Finally, the post-adoption process is reviewed.

Part II. Putting Theory into Practice

Chapter 5. Developing a national plan of action

Creating a national plan of action for tobacco control and establishing the infrastructure and capacity to implement the plan of action are key to the successful mitigation of the tobacco epidemic. This chapter provides an overview of the process of developing a national plan of action, starting with building a national coordinating mechanism for developing a plan of action and doing a situational analysis to determine needs and resources. The steps for setting a strategic direction and drafting a plan of action are discussed, and the elements of a national action plan are identified. The chapter also highlights the importance of ensuring legitimacy by securing official approval of the plan, and lists some of the critical issues that national programme officers must address to ensure that the plan of action is sustained and implemented.

Chapter 6. Establishing an effective infrastructure for national tobacco control programme

As the process of national action plan development unfolds, it is necessary to begin establishing a national infrastructure to carry out the implementation of the national plan of action. This chapter outlines a model for setting up a national network and infrastructure for tobacco control. It discusses the human, logistic and financial resources required to establish a viable national tobacco control programme, and the process of creating and sustaining national networks to support the implementation of tobacco control interventions country wide.

Chapter 7. Training and education

Successful tobacco control depends largely upon having the human resources to develop and implement a range of activities at different levels. This chapter presents an overview of the issues related to training and education of the different groups involved in tobacco control. 'Training' refers to the transfer of skills to build capacity to undertake effective tobacco control. 'Education' means gaining knowledge and understanding about 1) methods of effective tobacco control and 2) dangers of tobacco and methods of cessation. Determining training and education needs of various groups requires an assessment of the current situation. Results of the situational analysis carried out in preparation for developing a national action plan can provide the critical information for this decision. The selection and development of appropriate materials and effective training methods, and the process of conducting effective training workshops are addressed. The chapter also provides examples of curricula from various types of training workshops, taken from actual sessions carried out in several countries.

Chapter 8. Communication and public awareness to build critical mass

The social marketing of tobacco control requires strategic communication. Communication strategies play a key role, not only in ensuring that accurate information is accessible to the population, but also because well-designed communications campaigns can lead to changes in behaviour that are essential for reducing the prevalence of tobacco use. This chapter presents some key strategies and approaches to designing a social marketing and communications campaign for tobacco control. It draws from the experience of several countries, like Australia, Canada, Thailand and the United States of America, where effective social marketing and communications campaigns have curtailed tobacco use.

Chapter 9. Working with the media

The media is a key player in any tobacco control campaign. Mass media is often the most practical means to disseminate information and tobacco control messages rapidly to a large population. Media is the vehicle that shapes public opinion, and influences policy leaders. Often, repeated news coverage of an issue can guide the policy agenda of a government. Thus, developing good working relationships with media professionals is essential. This chapter presents practical advice on cultivating good media relationships and obtaining media coverage for tobacco control, even when resources are limited. Characteristics that make an event newsworthy, and that are required of an effective spokesperson, are identified. Practical tips are provided on how to develop several key pieces for media communication, including letters to the editor, opinion editorials and press releases, with actual examples. The chapter ends with a reminder that media can also become an effective advocate for tobacco control, if properly guided and encouraged.

Chapter 10. Programming selected tobacco control activities

This chapter offers a broad overview of the various programme options that are most often included as part of a comprehensive, integrated tobacco control action plan. It examines the roles of prevention through school-based programmes, cessation and protection of non-smokers through the creation of smoke-free environments within a national action plan for tobacco control, and identifies the key elements that determine the effectiveness of these components in reducing tobacco consumption. A crucial element for success in tobacco control is the engagement of communities in the process of understanding the tobacco epidemic more clearly and responding in an appropriate way to control tobacco use. Pointers on effective community mobilization and tobacco control educational resources for communities are outlined. The need to consider strategies targeting key high-risk population subgroups is discussed.

Chapter 11. Legislative and regulatory measures

Comprehensive tobacco control legislation is a crucial component of a successful tobacco control programme. The aim of this chapter is to build on previous WHO publications on tobacco control legislation – *Tobacco control legislation: an introductory guide,* and *Developing legislation for tobacco control: template and guidelines* – offering practical advice relevant to countries seeking to develop and implement tobacco control legislation. The legislative tobacco control measures that WHO recommends as part of a comprehensive tobacco control programme are summarized, and steps necessary to persuade national decision-makers to support these measures are identified. Legislation should be designed to be self-enforcing and should be supported by a commitment to resource adequately an information, implementation, monitoring and enforcement programme. To this end, tools and strategies to implement and enforce legislation are elucidated. The importance of harnessing the international legislative experience is reinforced, and online databases of tobacco control legislation are provided.

Chapter 12. Exploring economic measures and funding initiatives

The economic aspects of tobacco production and consumption play a critical role in developing strategies for reducing tobacco use. This chapter presents basic information on the key economic issues in tobacco control. It highlights the evidence on price and tobacco consumption, key steps to introduce or increase tobacco taxes and prices, which countries may adapt according to their specific socioeconomic and political situation, and funding initiatives for tobacco control, with examples of successful funding initiatives from Australia, New Zealand and Thailand. Key references from the World Bank, which address these issues in greater detail, are cited.

Chapter 13. Countering the tobacco industry

Tobacco is unique among the risks to health in that it has an entire industry devoted to the promotion of its use, despite the known adverse health impact of tobacco consumption. Predictably, the tobacco industry aggressively blocks any attempt to effectively reduce tobacco use. This chapter focuses on strategies to counter the tobacco industry. Building capacity to face the greatest opponent of successful tobacco control must be a priority for national and local tobacco control officers. In many cases, tobacco control advocates and nongovernmental organizations (NGOs) are more experienced in this area, and much can be learned from them. The chapter stresses the importance of recognizing the true nature of the tobacco industry and offers guidance in searching the tobacco industry database to learn more about the industry's tactics in a specific country. It also discusses strategies to monitor the tobacco industry and neutralize its efforts to impede or delay tobacco control interventions as a necessary element of building national capacity to curb the tobacco epidemic.

Chapter 14. Forming effective partnerships

In every country with successful tobacco control legislation, NGOs have played a major role in promoting change. This chapter focuses on the contribution citizen groupings can make to tobacco control efforts in the legislative field. In particular, it highlights the role and responsibilities of civil society; focuses on how to build and strengthen national tobacco control movements; and provides suggestions for working with the private sector.

Chapter 15. Monitoring, surveillance, evaluation and reporting

Once a tobacco control policy or programme has been launched on the basis of a thorough assessment of the situation, the evaluation process will consist mainly of assessing its relevance and adequacy, reviewing progress in implementation, and assessing impact and effectiveness for the reorientation and formulation of relevant policies and activities. Surveillance and evaluation play a major role in documenting tobacco control policy accountability for policy-makers, health managers and professionals, and for the general public. Therefore, a comprehensive surveillance and evaluation system should be an integral and a major element of all tobacco control policies and programmes. This chapter introduces the key concepts and issues in tobacco control programme monitoring, surveillance, evaluation and reporting. Selected indicators, methodologies and tools are discussed. Because the topic is a comprehensive one, the reader is provided with a list of earlier WHO publications that examine this topic in greater detail.

Chapter 16. Research and exchange of information

The WHO FCTC provides guidance on surveillance, research and exchange of information on tobacco control. Translating research into public information is essential to assist individuals, communities and governments to take action to reduce tobacco consumption. A mechanism to communicate the evidence for tobacco control is necessary to support a national tobacco control programme. This chapter considers the various challenges to research in tobacco control, and offers practical steps to overcome these challenges. The importance of linking research to policy change is emphasized, and the need to communicate information derived from research effectively to target audiences is highlighted. Establishing a mechanism for information exchange is explored, and as an example, an existing web-based information clearinghouse is presented.

Introduction

*Defined as the capacity to influence,
power is therefore the capacity to
make things happen...*
—*M. Scott Peck,* A World Waiting to be Born

*Leadership is the capacity to translate
vision into reality.*
—*Warren G. Bennis*

THE PROBLEM

The tobacco epidemic demands real solutions. Two factors spurred the development of a unique public health treaty for tobacco control by WHO's Member States: the realization that globalization was accelerating the spread of the epidemic and the recognition of the limits of national action to contain what has become a public health problem with transnational dimensions *(1)*. Today, the WHO FCTC contains the roadmap for coordinated global action to tackle one of the most significant risks to health. But attaining the vision embodied in the WHO FCTC remains critically dependent on national action.

Many tobacco control documents allude to the importance of 'national capacity-building' for effective and sustainable tobacco control. What exactly is 'national capacity', and how does one go about 'building' it?

NATIONAL CAPACITY-BUILDING

The developmental perspective

The conventional definition of capacity-building in the public sector had two elements: development of human resources and organizational engineering, or "institution building". The inclusion of the institutional dimension implied that capacity-building extended beyond the development of technical human resources, as it encompassed acquisition of management skills in addition to technical expertise, creation and expansion of a supporting infrastructure and programme efficiency and sustainability *(2)*.

At present, development experts acknowledge that the process of building national capacity needs to go beyond the public sector, because it is inherently influenced by at least two additional factors outside public institutions: the state of governance, and entities in the private sector, which include commercial enterprises and civil society organizations, also known as NGOs *(3)*. The United Nations Development Programme defines capacity as "the ability to perform functions, solve problems and achieve objectives" at three levels: individual, institutional and societal. The third level is deemed vital, as it encompasses those processes that lie at the heart of human development: the "opening and widening of opportunities that enable people to use and expand their capacities to the full" *(4)*. The process of national capacity-building can therefore be viewed as a long-term process for the acquisition of skills and the capabilities to use them effectively to attain specific societal objectives. Appropriate consideration should be given to the development of a supporting infrastructure and the complex influence of the policy environment, political will and leadership, social capital and globalization. Nowhere is this more relevant than in the area of tobacco control.

Defining capacity

Community capacity can be defined as a community's current ability (as opposed to inherent ability) to respond to certain pressures. When looking at the impact of tobacco on communities, one must look not only at tobacco use rates and patterns, but also at the ability of a community to respond to tobacco control comprehensively.

Source: Asian Pacific Partners for Empowerment and Leadership (APPEAL) (http://www.appealforcommunities.org)

The need to build national capacity for tobacco control

Despite the overwhelming evidence of the gravity of the tobacco epidemic, many countries still lack the infrastructure, resources and political will to sustain a basic national programme to control tobacco. Few national governments have staff working full time on tobacco control. A good number of countries still do not have national plans of action to control the tobacco epidemic. Many still need to develop a policy environment that supports tobacco control, while in countries where tobacco control policies and laws exist, enforcement capacity often lags behind policy development, rendering these policy instruments ineffective.

In the WHO European Region, for example, which has 51 Member States, only 27 have a national action plan for tobacco control, and 32 have a national coordinating body for tobacco control *(5)*. In the WHO Eastern Mediterranean Region, of those Member States providing data, a quarter (25%) lack a multisectoral committee for tobacco control, almost half (45%) have no national tobacco control programme at all, and nearly 90% identified lack of human and financial resources as the main obstacles to the implementation of tobacco control activities and programmes *(6)*.

Linking the WHO FCTC to national capacity

While the WHO FCTC addresses global tobacco control interventions and provides a roadmap for country-level tobacco control, specific actions against the tobacco epidemic must be taken at the national level. The success of the WHO FCTC will depend almost entirely on the ability of countries to implement and enforce its provisions. Thus, building national capacity to carry out effective and sustainable national tobacco control programmes is an urgent priority in the fight against the tobacco epidemic. Moreover, understanding the mechanisms that link the WHO FCTC at the international level with work that needs to be carried out at the country level is crucial to counteracting this public health threat.

Member States can use the WHO FCTC as a starting point for building national capacity. The treaty requires countries to establish a tobacco control focal point and infrastructure, and leads them to identify and activate mechanisms for multisectoral coordination of tobacco control efforts. The WHO FCTC also outlines the key elements of a national plan of action for tobacco control, and provides all the current, evidence-based interventions that should guide the development and implementation of national tobacco control activities. Moreover, the WHO FCTC addresses the need for international cooperation, exchange of information and technical assistance to support countries, particularly those in the developing world, as they begin to develop capacity for tobacco control. In addition, the WHO FCTC includes provisions for monitoring and evaluating progress towards control of this epidemic through surveillance and database management. Finally, the WHO FCTC provides a way to prevent and counteract the hazardous strategies of the tobacco industry.

Beyond the WHO Framework Convention on Tobacco Control: practical tobacco control approaches for countries

To take action against tobacco, countries must develop their ability to deal with the following *(3)*:

- **Defining objectives** – This implies an understanding of the national and local contexts based on sound data about the current state of the tobacco epidemic and about current needs. The ability to identify vulnerable groups is also essential for this task.
- **Developing strategies** – This implies the ability to identify the political scenario, to prioritize needs and find ways of meeting them, and to develop meaningful indicators to measure progress.
- **Drawing up action plans** – This is based on agreed strategies, with a detailed listing of required actions, expected outcomes and products, accountable parties and a timetable.
- **Developing and implementing appropriate policies** – This requires the ability to formulate policies and enforcement strategies, as well as methods to assess policy implementation and accountability.
- **Developing regulatory and legal frameworks** – This requires adapting national laws and regulations to comply with the WHO FCTC.
- **Building and managing partnerships** – This calls for full, constructive and ongoing consultation and communication among key stakeholders to secure commitments by the institutions and organizations that are going to be involved in the implementation of the national plan of action.
- **Fostering an enabling environment for civil society** – This calls for effective communication and advocacy, because the success and sustainability of tobacco control activities require the full and informed participation of all relevant stakeholders in the public and private sectors.
- **Mobilizing and managing resources** – This involves quantifying and mobilizing human, financial and other resources that are needed for the implementation of cost-effective and sustainable programmes.
- **Implementing action plans** – Individuals and institutions responsible for carrying out every part of the plan must be properly selected and trained, aware of their responsibilities and accountability, and appropriately mandated.

- **Monitoring progress and applying lessons learned to the process** – This requires resources to measure agreed benchmarks and indicators, and to provide for feedback so that objectives and strategies can be adjusted to achieve consistent and sustainable progress.

Countries are at different stages in their response to the tobacco epidemic. This handbook is intended primarily for those countries that are in the early stages of building a tobacco control capacity. Officers and staff in the public sector are the primary audience, although other tobacco control stakeholders may find this information useful for their own work.

The idea for this handbook arose from the realization that while various official WHO documents called for the development of national capacity for tobacco control, there was no comprehensive publication for the development of national capacity to control tobacco. Conceived as a 'how to' handbook, the approach is intentionally pragmatic, addressing 'real world' issues and providing practical advice for setting up viable national tobacco control programmes. Collaborating authors were chosen because of their experience and technical expertise in the various topic areas. Every effort was made to ensure gender and geopolitical balance during the selection. Thus, all of the WHO regions are represented by authors from both developed and developing countries.

This handbook is not meant to be definitive or prescriptive. It incorporates information from various sources, reflecting the different experiences of Member States, with their diverse sociopolitical and cultural backgrounds. Because tobacco control remains a relatively new field in public health, it is anticipated that new approaches and insights will emerge over time. This manual should therefore be considered a work in progress. It will be periodically updated to reflect the emerging experiences and practices of Member States.

This handbook is divided into two main parts. The first part presents an overview of tobacco control, and sets the theoretical foundation for action to control tobacco use. It begins by introducing tobacco as a risk factor for poor health, with its attendant economic and social costs. This is followed by a review of the global strategies that the tobacco industry employs to maintain high levels of tobacco consumption. The scientific evidence underlying effective interventions to reduce tobacco use is examined, and the WHO Framework Convention on Tobacco Control as a political/legal solution to the tobacco epidemic is presented.

The second part focuses on the fundamental capacities needed to empower countries to successfully take on the tobacco epidemic. Based on early successes in various areas of tobacco control within developed and developing countries, and applying the lessons learned from those societies which have pioneered the fight against the tobacco epidemic, the chapters under this section offer advice and suggestions to enable Member States to put the theories of tobacco control into practice. This section begins with the development of a national plan of action as the foundation for successful tobacco control at country level. It addresses important aspects of national capacity-building such as the establishment of an effective infrastructure for a national tobacco control programme; training and education; awareness-raising through effective communications and media advocacy; planning of specific tobacco control activities; legislative measures for tobacco control; economic interventions and funding initiatives. Chapters on how to prevent and counter hazardous influences of the tobacco industry, form effective partnerships, monitor and evaluate progress, and exchange information and research, provide valuable insights to augment tobacco control capacity.

Key lessons in the capacity-building process

The authors of this handbook were guided by the following lessons in national capacity-building, drawn from a long history of developmental work *(3)*:

- **Capacity development is an endogenous process** – Successful capacity-building is never predominantly driven by external pressures, but is the outcome of self-determination. This handbook is meant to provide national tobacco control officers with assistance in establishing comprehensive tobacco control programmes, as the starting point of a long-term process that these national officers shape and direct. The process of transforming national capacity is conceived as an organic process, building on existing capabilities in a manner that respects continuity and fosters sustainability.

- **Capacity development must be grounded in the local context** – Every country is unique, and interventions to build capacity to control tobacco must be relevant and specific to each country. This implies that there cannot be one standard approach to national capacity-building. While countries cannot expect to replicate exactly the experiences of other nations reflected in some of these chapters, the readers of this handbook are challenged to assess the applicability of the insights and lessons learned, and adapt these to their particular needs.

- **Capacity-building must involve many levels and many sectors** – The development of national capacity for tobacco control concerns a range of different stakeholders in the public, private and civic domains, and at central and local levels. Partnerships and collaboration with these diverse stakeholders are necessary. The complex nature of tobacco control, the variety of interventions that need to be carried out simultaneously, and the formidable influence of the tobacco industry require a united societal response. The ability to seek out appropriate partners and to establish solid networks is as important as developing expertise in the technical areas of tobacco control, and is addressed in several chapters.

- **Capacity-building responds to external stimuli** – Referred to as the "power of the process", much of what is currently happening at country level is directly related to the work carried out over the past 4 years on the WHO FCTC. The momentum gained from the WHO FCTC process should be utilized to drive national tobacco control capacity-building forward, just as the provisions contained within the WHO FCTC should guide national tobacco control interventions. The WHO FCTC also refers to the importance of technical and information exchange, and workable mechanisms to promote intercountry cooperation to enhance capacity-building. This should enable countries in the early stages of capacity development to benefit from the collective wisdom gained by other countries that have faced the exceptional challenges of attempting to control the tobacco epidemic.

- **In capacity-building for tobacco control, enlightened leadership and political will are crucial** – The handbook highlights the importance of finding champions, and targeting key decision-makers, to support tobacco control. Strong and legitimate leadership is fundamental when attempting to fight the tobacco epidemic, and is required to ensure beneficial changes in the policy environment.

- **Capacity-building is a long-term process, requiring commitment and perseverance** – Developing the capacities of individuals, institutions and societies to successfully control the tobacco epidemic takes time. Some countries have already committed years of work and considerable resources to tobacco control. Nevertheless, many of those countries still need to build their capacity to successfully tackle all aspects of tobacco control. The complex nature of tobacco control, the need to remove the social acceptability of tobacco use and the power of the tobacco industry imply that efforts to reduce the health and economic burden of tobacco will require patience, perseverance and steadfast commitment.

Key strategies for strengthening national capacity for tobacco control

- analyse the national tobacco control situation: impact of use, political willingness, public awareness;
- outline national tobacco control strategies considering the national profile, sociopolitical environment and global evidence;
- establish national coordination: a multisectoral committee for tobacco control policy and programme development or a focal point;
- build a comprehensive national plan of action reflecting national priorities and realities;
- establish and implement comprehensive educational, communications, public awareness and training programmes to ensure sustained public support and a shift of attitudes in favour of tobacco control;
- develop consensus and political commitment for tobacco control in the country;
- establish through national regulation sustained funding mechanisms for tobacco control programmes;
- incorporate national tobacco control efforts into existing national, state and district level health structures to ensure sustainability;
- broaden the domestic infrastructure for implementation of tobacco control at national and local levels and guarantee outreach of programme activities;
- develop strategies for monitoring and counteraction of tobacco industry activities in the country;
- establish a system of monitoring and evaluation of tobacco control policies and implementation.

Strategies for developing and strengthening
national capacity for tobacco control

The key strategies for developing and strengthening national capacity for tobacco control refer to the 10 skills and tasks described earlier, which are needed to effectively respond to the tobacco epidemic.

The chapters that follow provide practical advice on how to accomplish these strategies for strengthening national capacity and show how they fit in with the approach established by the WHO FCTC. Capacity-building is a process of transformation, but meaningful change can only happen from within. By sharing lessons learned from countries representing each region, and utilizing numerous examples, it is hoped that this handbook will assist and inspire health professionals and others working within their national governments to take on the challenge of reducing tobacco consumption and its attendant mortality and morbidity.

References

1. Da Costa e Silva V, Nikogossian H. Convenio Marco de la OMS para el control del tabaco: la globalizacion de la salud publica. [WHO Framework Convention on Tobacco Control: the globalization of public health.] *Prevencion del Tabaquismo, [Prevention of tobacco addiction]* 2003, 5(2):71–75.

2. Economic and Social Council (ECOSOC). *United Nations system to support capacity building.* New York, 2002 (E/2002/58).

3. Browne S, ed. *Developing capacity through technical cooperation: country experiences.* London, Earthscan, 2002.

4. Fukuda-Parr S, Lopes C, Malik K, eds. *Capacity for development: new solutions to old problems.* London, Earthscan, 2002.

5. Tobacco Free Initiative/WHO Regional Office for Europe (TFI-EURO). *Cross-country profile,* Geneva, World Health Organization (http://data.euro.who.int/tobacco/); see also *WHO European country profiles on tobacco control.* Copenhagen, WHO Regional Office for Europe, 2003.

6. Tobacco Free Initiative/WHO Regional Office for the Eastern Mediterranean (TFI-EMRO). *Regional tobacco control profile,* Geneva, World Health Organization (http://www.emro.who.int/tfi/countryprofile.htm).

Part I

Setting the theoretical foundation for tobacco control

Part I
Setting the theoretical foundation for tobacco control

1. Tobacco as a risk factor: health, social and economic costs

2. The tobacco industry: global strategies

3. Tobacco control interventions: the scientific basis

4. WHO Framework Convention on Tobacco Control:
   the political solution

1
Tobacco as a risk factor: health, social and economic costs

Tobacco surely was designed to poison,
and destroy mankind.
— *Philip Freneau*

DISEASE BURDEN

Active tobacco use

Tobacco is the major preventable cause of death in many parts of the world today. In developed countries, where the tobacco epidemic took hold much earlier than in the rest of the world, tobacco-related cardiovascular and lung diseases and cancers cause a significant proportion of total deaths and chronic disability. Among countries undergoing the epidemiologic transition, chronic diseases caused by tobacco are rapidly overtaking the more traditional causes of mortality. In fact, current estimates suggest that smoking prematurely kills as many people in the developing as in the developed world. Even in those countries where infectious diseases are the main cause of death, the effects of tobacco use compound the lethality of pulmonary infections such as pneumonia and tuberculosis.

Tobacco use is harmful and addictive. All forms of tobacco cause many fatal and disabling health problems throughout the life cycle.

> **Tuberculosis kills about 1.6 million people each year. A study published in *The Lancet* in 2003 showed that smoking causes half the male tuberculosis deaths in India. Tobacco use also increases the risk of developing clinical TB, which can kill and can easily be spread to others.**
>
> —V Gajalakshm et al., 2003

Scientific evidence has conclusively shown that smokers are more prone to different types of cancer, particularly lung cancer. In addition, smokers are at far greater risk of developing heart disease, stroke, emphysema and many other fatal and non-fatal diseases. If they chew tobacco, they risk cancer of the lip, tongue and mouth. There is no safe way of using tobacco.

Women who smoke run even more risks than men. For example, the adverse effects of oral contraceptive use are markedly increased in women smokers. Osteoporosis is accelerated with tobacco use. Some evidence indicates that fertility is impaired with smoking. Tobacco use is also associated with a higher rate of spontaneous miscarriages. In pregnancy, smoking contributes to perinatal complications such as bleeding, which is dangerous for both mother and fetus, especially in poor countries where health facilities are inadequate. Intrauterine growth retardation and low-birth-weight babies are known outcomes of smoking during pregnancy. The harm from maternal smoking can extend beyond pregnancy, affecting the child's growth and development. This is often compounded by the child's exposure to second-hand smoke from parents and other adults.

Passive smoking

Smoking harms non-smokers, too. The first conclusive evidence of the danger of passive smoking came from a study carried out by Takeshi Hirayama, in 1981, on lung cancer in non-smoking Japanese wives married to men who smoked *(1)*. Surprising at the time, those women showed a significantly increased risk of dying from lung cancer, despite never having smoked a cigarette. Hirayama et al. believed that passive smoking (i.e. breathing in the smoke from their husbands) caused these women's excess cancer risk. About 40 further studies have confirmed this link.

Today, research indicates that passive smoking can also give rise to other potentially fatal diseases such as heart disease and stroke, and new scientific evidence on the adverse effects of second-hand smoke continues to accumulate.

> **An hour a day in a room with a smoker is nearly a hundred times more likely to cause lung cancer in a non-smoker than 20 years spent in a building containing asbestos.**
>
> — Sir Richard Doll, 1985

Table 1. Adverse health effects of smoking

Body system or organ	Established or suspected adverse health effect of cigarette smoking	Body system or organ	Established or suspected adverse health effect of cigarette smoking
Lungs	• Lung cancer • Chronic obstructive pulmonary disease • Increased severity of asthma • Increased risk of developing various respiratory infections	Bones	• Disc degeneration • Osteoporosis • Osteoarthritis • Less successful back surgery • Delayed fracture healing • Muscoloskeletal injury
Heart	• Coronary heart disease • Angina pectoris • Heart attack • Increased risk of repeat heart attack • Arrhythmia • Aortic aneurysm • Cardiomyopathy	Reproduction	• Infertility • Impotence • Decreased sperm motility and density • Miscarriage • Earlier menopause
Blood vessels	• Peripheral vascular disease • Thromboangiitis obliterans (Buerger's disease)	The unborn child	• Fetal growth retardation • Prematurity • Stillbirth • Enhanced transmission of HIV to fetus • Birth defects • Intellectual impairment • Sudden infant death syndrome
Skin	• Earlier wrinkling • Fingernail discoloration • Psoriasis • Palmoplantar pustulosis		
Cancer	• Lung cancer • Esophageal cancer • Laryngeal cancer • Oral cancer • Bladder cancer • Kidney cancer • Stomach cancer • Pancreatic cancer • Vulvular cancer • Cervical cancer • Colorectal cancer	Brain	• Transient ischaemic attack • Stroke • Worsened multiple sclerosis
		Others	• Cataracts • Macular degeneration • Snoring • Periodontal disease • Stomach and duodenal ulcers • Crohn disease • Impaired immunity

Over 60% of children in Argentina, Bulgaria, China (Tianjin), Cuba, India, Indonesia, Jordan, Lebanon, Mali (Bamako), the Philippines, Poland, Uruguay and the West Bank are exposed to passive smoking at home.

— Global Youth Tobacco Survey, 2003

Children are at particular risk from exposure to adults' smoking. Unborn babies can be harmed by their mothers' exposure to other people's smoking. The effects are magnified when combined with further exposure to second-hand smoke after birth. Tobacco use in the home is a risk factor in sudden infant death syndrome (SIDS). Passive smoking can cause pneumonia, bronchitis, coughing and wheezing, and it can aggravate asthma and middle ear disease in young children. Some studies *(2, 3)* appear to link exposure to second-hand smoke in childhood with neuro-behavioural impairment and cardiovascular disease in adulthood. After reviewing the evidence, a WHO consultation on the effects of environmental tobacco smoke (ETS) on children in 1999 concluded that ETS is a real and substantial threat to child health, causing death and suffering throughout the world.

Deaths from tobacco use *(3)*

Of the people alive today, 650 million will eventually be killed by tobacco.

Cigarettes kill half of all lifetime users, and half of those die in middle age (35–69 years). There is no other consumer product on the market that is remotely as dangerous, or kills as many people. Tobacco kills more than AIDS, legal drugs, illegal drugs, road accidents, murder and suicide combined.

Tobacco already kills more men in developing than in industrialized countries, and it is likely that deaths among women will soon be the same.

Every day more than 13 000 people around the world die from tobacco. Assuming constant tobacco use prevalence, the World Health Organization projects that between 2000 and 2025 the number of smokers will rise from approximately 1.2 billion to more than 1.7 billion and the annual number of deaths, which is currently estimated at about 5 million, will almost double in 20 years (see Table 2).

TOBACCO CONSUMPTION

Tobacco use initiation and continuation

Smokers and other tobacco users start and continue for different reasons. Children and young people can start smoking from curiosity, risk taking, rebellion, parental and sibling smoking, peer pressure, the desire for weight control, the desire to look 'grown up', and the perception that tobacco use is normal or 'cool'. Aggressive promotion by the tobacco industry and permissive environments that make tobacco products readily available and affordable play a major role in inducing young people

Table 2. Current and projected estimates of the tobacco epidemic (if tobacco use prevalence stays at the 2003 level)

	Year	
	2000	**2025**
Number of smokers (billions)	1.2[a]	1.7[a]
Males (age 15 years and older, billions)	1.0[a]	1.4[a]
Females (age 15 years and older, billions)	0.2[a]	0.3[a]
Number of smokers in developing countries (billions)	0.9[a]	1.4[a]
Annual tobacco deaths (millions)	4.9[b,c]	10[d,e,f] (2030)
Children exposed to ETS (millions)	700[g]	770[h]
Economic losses (US$ billions)	200[i] (1994)	—
Smokers in developing countries and transitional economy countries	84%[a]	88%[a]

[a] Source: Guindon & Boisclair *(4)*
[b] Source: WHO *(5)*
[c] Source: *Lancet (6)*
[d] Source: Ezzati & Lopez *(7)*
[e] Source: WHO *(8)*
[f] Source: Peto *(9)*
[g] Source: WHO *(10)*
[h] Source: WHO *(11)*
[i] Source: Barnum *(12)*

to take up smoking. In certain cultures, oral tobacco use forms part of the social tradition, and can begin in early childhood.

While tobacco use is prompted by several different factors, the continuation of tobacco use is largely fuelled by addiction. Human and animal studies have shown that nicotine is the substance in tobacco that leads to addiction. Nicotine is readily absorbed from the lungs or mouth, rapidly enters the blood stream, dispersing throughout the body and interacting with specific receptors in the brain *(14)*. Some of these receptors are responsible for the feeling of pleasure – the 'rush' – that smokers and other tobacco users get from tobacco. Other receptors kick in when nicotine levels begin to drop, causing a constellation of symptoms that characterize the 'withdrawal syndrome', similar to what heroin and cocaine addicts experience. People addicted to tobacco need to smoke or chew tobacco regularly and frequently to keep their nicotine levels up, so that they can feel pleasure and avoid the discomfort of withdrawal. Other factors that reinforce tobacco use include social and psychological pressure, lack of knowledge of the risk to health and difficulty in quitting.

Talking points

- In many parts of the world, smokers still do not know about the dangers of tobacco use. For instance, in China, in 1996, 7 out of 10 Chinese smokers thought smoking did them "little or no harm" *(14)*.

- Nicotine addiction is extremely powerful. About 70% of current smokers in high-income countries want to quit, but 80% of those who try to give up smoking fail.

Tobacco consumption patterns *(4, 15)*

Since the mechanization of cigarette manufacturing at the turn of the 20th century, global consumption of cigarettes has been rising steadily. Today, more people are smoking, and consuming more cigarettes per capita, than ever before. At present, about 1070 million males and 230 million females in the world smoke, generating an epidemic of global magnitude. In developed countries, the prevalence of smoking among adult males is decreasing, but the increasing number of adult male smokers in developing countries offsets this. Smoking is still rising among females in developed countries, with the exception of a few countries such as Australia, Canada, the United Kingdom and the United States. With the expansion of the tobacco industry's marketing campaigns into the developing world, more and more people are taking up smoking in countries least able to deal with the grave public health consequences of tobacco use.

Tobacco companies produce approximately 7 million tonnes of tobacco annually. Cigarettes represent the largest share of manufactured tobacco products, accounting for 96% by value of total sales. Every year, cigarette factories produce more than 5.5 trillion cigarettes – enough to provide every individual on the planet with 1000 cigarettes. Asia, Australia and the Far East are by far the largest consumers (2715 billion cigarettes), followed by the Americas (754 billion), eastern Europe and former Soviet economies (631 billion), and western Europe (606 billion).

China produces about a third of all the cigarettes in the world. It is also a major tobacco consumer, since nearly 60% of adult Chinese males smoke, representing one-third of all smokers globally. Currently, it is estimated that one out of every three cigarettes in the world is smoked in China.

Youth

Tobacco use often begins before adulthood. The Global Youth Tobacco Survey (GYTS), the largest database of its kind in the world today, has data from 75 sites in 43 countries and the Gaza Strip/West Bank region. It shows that a disturbingly high number of school children between the ages of 13 and 15 are currently using or have tried tobacco. Nearly a quarter of those young smokers began before the age of 10.

The most serious consequences of tobacco use appear later in adulthood. However, there are immediate adverse health effects of smoking that affect the growing number of young tobacco users. Addiction to nicotine occurs faster in young smokers, and the risks of developing tobacco-related cancer and chronic heart and lung diseases are greater the younger one starts to smoke.

According to the Global Youth Tobacco Survey *(16):*

- The highest youth smoking rates are found in Central and eastern Europe, parts of India, and some of the Western Pacific islands.
- Current use of tobacco products ranges from 62.8% to 3.3%, with high rates of oral tobacco use in certain regions.
- Current cigarette smoking ranges from 39.6% to less than 1%.
- Nearly 25% of students who smoke admit to having smoked their first cigarette before the age of 10.
- Most current smokers want to stop smoking and have already tried to quit, although very few students who currently smoke have ever attended a smoking-cessation programme.
- Exposure to advertising is high (75% of students had seen pro-tobacco adverts).
- Exposure to environmental tobacco smoke is very high in all countries. In Bulgaria, Northern Mariana Islands, and selected cities in Burkina Faso, India, Indonesia and Mali, over 75% of young people surveyed indicated significant exposure to second-hand smoke in public places.
- Only about half of the students reported that they had been taught in school about the dangers of smoking during the year preceding the survey.
- Girls are smoking as much as boys in more than 30% of surveyed countries.

Adult male

Current geographical distribution and rates of tobacco use among men:

- Most of today's smokers are male, and most live in developing countries. Nearly a third – 300 million – live in China.
- The highest rates of tobacco use are found in Cambodia, Djibouti, Indonesia, Myanmar, Papua New Guinea, and Viet Nam.
- Half of all males in developing countries currently smoke as compared to about 35% in developed countries, a proportion that has fallen in recent decades.
- Trends in both developed and developing countries show that smoking rates among males are slowly declining. However, this is an extremely slow process occurring over decades. In the meantime, millions of males are dying because of tobacco.
- Better educated males are tending to give up smoking, so tobacco use is becoming a habit of poorer, less educated males.
- If actual prevalence remains, it is estimated that the number of male smokers worldwide will rise from 1 billion in 2000 to 1.4 billion in 2025.

Adult female

Current geographical distribution and rates of tobacco use among females:
- The tobacco epidemic started later among females. Currently, an estimated 22% of females in developed countries and 9% in developing countries smoke tobacco, totalling about 230 million females.
- In addition, many females in South Asia and the Pacific chew tobacco.
- The highest rates of tobacco use among females are recorded in Guinea, Myanmar, Nauru, Papua New Guinea, Tokelau, and Turkey.
- Cigarette smoking among females is declining in many developed countries, notably Australia, Canada, the United Kingdom, USA, and Australia. But this trend is not found in all developed countries: in several southern, central and eastern European countries cigarette smoking is either still increasing among females or has not shown any decline.
- As social traditions fade and incomes rise, the number of females smoking could double to 460 million by 2030.
- Arguably, the greatest public health challenge in primary prevention in the next 30 years will be to prevent a rise in smoking among girls and women in developing countries, especially in Asia.

THE SOCIAL AND ECONOMIC COSTS OF TOBACCO USE

The costs to individuals and their families

The costs to the individual smoker, and to non-smoking family members, include:
- loss of money spent on buying tobacco;
- loss of income through illness and premature death;
- health care costs induced by tobacco-related illnesses;

Unhealthy choices

- Bangladesh, China, Ghana, Moldova, Pakistan and Papua New Guinea, 2000: 20 imported cigarettes cost more than 50% of daily income.
- China, 1990: farmers near Shanghai spent more on cigarettes and wine than on grains, pork and fruits.
- Minhang, China, 1993: smokers spent on average 60% of their personal income and 17% of household income on cigarettes.
- Panama, 2000: one packet of imported cigarettes costs as much as 12 eggs.

Source: Scientific Committee on Tobacco and Health (2)

- the cost of the time spent by other family members looking after smokers or taking them to hospital (which may sometimes be measured in days in developing countries);
- the cost of illness or death in family members exposed to passive smoke in the home;
- higher health insurance premiums;
- miscellaneous costs, such as increased fire risk.

Smokers clearly perceive some benefit in smoking and are willing to pay for their tobacco. However, smokers' purchases can come at the expense of their families. In developing countries, where families have less available income, money spent on tobacco could be used instead for food, shelter, health care or other basic necessities (see Table 3).

Global evidence shows that smokers may not always be fully aware of the damage to health caused by smoking. Young smokers also tend to underestimate the power of nicotine addiction. When young smokers develop tobacco-related diseases, many often say they regret starting. The chronic diseases caused by tobacco require frequent use of the health care system, and are resource-intensive. The considerable costs of accessing this type of care can be a heavy economic burden on smokers and their families.

Smokers inflict direct costs on non-smokers, who risk several potentially disabling diseases as a result of exposure to tobacco smoke. When health care costs are partially or fully borne by government or private insurance, and the contributions to those institutions are shared by smokers and non-smokers alike, then smokers also impose an economic burden on society. The World Bank estimates that the gross costs of health care attributed to the extra health needs of smokers can range from 0.1% to 1.1% of gross domestic product in the high-income countries. There is less information available on low-income countries, but existing data indicate that the gross health care expenditure may be proportionately as high as in the developed countries.

The cost of tobacco for governments, employers and the environment

The economic burden of tobacco use on governments and societies can be summarized as follows.
- Social, welfare and health care costs: Governments often have to bear the burden of caring for chronically sick and terminally ill smokers, and providing for their spouses and children in the event of social incapacity or premature death.
- Loss of foreign exchange in importing cigarettes: In countries where tobacco is not grown or is insufficient to meet national demand, the importation of cigarettes could lead to a net loss of foreign currency.
- Loss of arable land that could be used to grow food.
- Higher costs for employers due to absence from work, decreased productivity, higher accident rates and higher insurance premiums: Absence from work is often higher among smokers due to illness. Smokers also take smoke breaks during

work, contributing to lower productivity. Some studies reveal a higher accident rate among smokers. Employers generally pay higher fire and accident insurance premiums in buildings where smoking is allowed. They also have to pay higher insurance premiums for health and life insurance policies for their employees who smoke. In addition, cleaning and maintenance cost more for buildings where smoking is permitted, adding to the burden borne by employers.

- The cost of fires and damage to buildings as a result of careless smoking.
- Environmental costs: The wood needed to cure tobacco and the paper used for cigarettes require cutting down large tracts of forest, contributing to deforestation. Cigarettes often start fires, causing massive environmental losses. For example, in 1987, cigarettes sparked off China's worst fire in recent history, causing 300 deaths, destroying 1.3 million hectares of land and making 5000 people homeless *(17, 18)*. It is estimated that every year, 1 million fires are started by children using cigarette lighters. Annual global estimates for 2000 indicate that smoking-related fires contributed to 10% of all fire deaths, and cost US$ 27 billion in damages *(19)*.

Unhealthy choices

- In 1994, Telecom Australia lost AU$ 16.5 million from time off work due to tobacco-related illnesses.

- Workplace smoking costs the USA US$ 47 billion each year.

Source: Mackay & Eriksen *(15)*

Table 3. Estimates of annual health care costs attributable to tobacco use, in US$ (billions) (2002 or latest available estimates, selected countries)

Country	Health care costs (US$ billions)
Australia	6.0
Canada	1.6
China	3.5
Germany	14.7
New Zealand	0.8
The Philippines	0.6
United Kingdom	2.3
USA	76.0

Source: Mackay & Eriksen *(15)*

Everyone pays for tobacco use

While the cost to the individual smoker is often obvious and accepted, in reality tobacco use costs everyone in society. Tobacco use leads to inefficient allocation of resources, justifying the need for government intervention to reduce tobacco consumption. Policy-makers need to become aware of the costs, as the rationale for instituting policies aimed at controlling tobacco use.

References

1. Hirayama T. Non-smoking wives of heavy smokers have a higher risk of lung cancer: a study from Japan. *British Medical Journal,* 1981, 282:183–185.

2. Great Britain Scientific Committee on Tobacco and Health (SCOTH). *Report of the Scientific Committee on Tobacco and Health.* London, The Stationary Office, 1998.

3. *International Consultation on Environmental Tobacco Smoke (ETS) and Child Health: Geneva, 11–14 January 1999.* Geneva,World Health Organization, 1999 (WHO/NCD/TFI/99.10).

4. Guindon GE, Boisclair D. *Past, current and future trends in tobacco use.* Washington, DC, The World Bank, 2003 (Health Nutrition and Population Discussion Paper, Economics of Tobacco Control, paper no. 6).

5. *The world health report 2002: reducing risks, promoting healthy life.* Geneva, World Health Organization, 2002:65.

6. Ezzati M, Lopez AD. Estimates of global mortality attributable to smoking in 2000. *Lancet,* 2003, 362 (9387):847–852 (http://www.thelancet.com/journal/vol362/iss9387/full/llan.362.9387.original_research.27132.1).

7. Ezzati M, Lopez AD. Burden of disease attributable to smoking and oral tobacco use. Global and regional estimates for 2000 (in press).

8. *The world health report 2001.* Geneva, World Health Organization, 2001:31.

9. Peto R. Education and debate – smoking and death: the past 40 years and the next 40. *British Medical Journal,* 1994, 309:937–939.

10. *International Consultation on Environmental Tobacco Smoke (ETS) and Child Health: Geneva, 11–14 January 1999.* Geneva,World Health Organization, 1999 (WHO/NCD/TFI/99.10).

11. *International Consultation on Environmental Tobacco Smoke (ETS) and Child Health: Global estimate of children aged 0–14 years exposed to ETS at home. Calculations by Dr A. Lopez: Geneva, 11–14 January 1999.* Geneva, World Health Organization, 1999.

12. Barnum H. The economic burden of the global trade in tobacco. *Tobacco Control,* 1994, 3(4):358–361.

13. *The health consequences of smoking: nicotine addiction. A report of the US Surgeon General.* Maryland, United States Department of Health and Human Services, 1988.

14. *Smoking and health in China:1996 National Prevalence Survey of Smoking Pattern.* Beijing, China Science and Technology Press, 1996:85.

15. Mackay J, Eriksen M. *The tobacco atlas.* Geneva, World Health Organization, 2002:40–41.

16. The Global Youth Tobacco Survey Collaborative Group. Tobacco use among youth: a cross country comparison. *Tobacco Control,* 2002,11:252–270 (http://www.tobaccocontrol.com/cgi/content/abstract/11/3/252).

17. Reuter. Sacked foreign minister was in the hospital during the blaze. *South China Morning Post,* 8 June 1987.

18. Associated Press. Eleven face court after death fires. *South China Morning Post,* 14 June 1988:8.

19. Leistikow BN, Martin DC, Milano CE. Fire injuries, disasters, and costs from cigarettes and cigarette lights: a global overview. *Preventive Medicine,* 2000, 31:91–99.

2
The tobacco industry

Woe to those
That deal in fraud.
—Surah 83: Al Mutaffifin: 1, 1616

INTRODUCTION

More than 120 companies worldwide produce tobacco products; some of them are local, national or state-owned. However, around 40% of the world's cigarette market is controlled by a handful of transnational tobacco companies (TTCs) *(1)*. The combined net revenue of the three biggest multinationals (Altria Group, Inc, formerly known as Philip Morris (PM), British American Tobacco (BAT) and Japan Tobacco International (JTI)) comes close to US$ 100 billion per year (see Figure 1), surpassing the gross national income of all but the 35 richest countries in the world *(2)*.

Worldwide, the tobacco industry's main goal is to make a profit selling cigarettes. TTCs are economic entities, owned by shareholders (see Box 1 and Figure 2). Their managing directors are responsible for increasing the value of the shareholders' investments. These directors are driven primarily by the need to improve market shares and profitability, and are compensated based on how well they achieve this. Not surprisingly, transnationals are the major driving force for the promotion of tobacco use and the main impediments to preventing the introduction of effective measures to limit the tobacco epidemic. Predictably, the greater the effectiveness of a planned tobacco control measure, the fiercer the reaction of TTCs against the adoption of that measure.

Knowledge of the industry's strategies to promote the continued use of tobacco and to counter effective public health interventions is extremely important for those working to curb tobacco use. Governments and public health professionals and advocates as well as the public can strengthen efforts to reduce tobacco consumption by accessing previously secret tobacco industry internal documents, which provide an improved understanding of industry strategies (see Box 2 and Chapter 13). The approximately 38 million pages of documents include typical business plans to increase sales, profits and market share, along with analyses of the competition's activ-

Figure 1. Transnational tobacco companies – revenue/year (US$ billions)

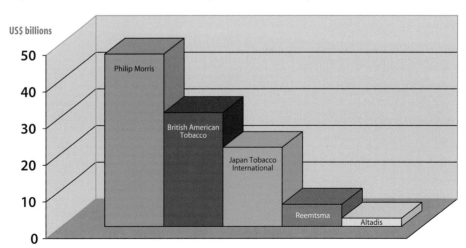

Source: *The tobacco atlas (1)*

Box 1. What motivates the tobacco industry?

- the need to make a profit
- the fear of litigation
- the need to protect tobacco from regulation
- the desire to promote an image that is socially responsible and reformed.

---

ities. They also include several thousand pages of industry-financed research on topics such as nicotine addiction and the health effects of tobacco use and efforts to dismiss scientific evidence on the harmful effects of exposure to tobacco smoke. Of greater relevance are documents detailing corporate and public affairs strategies. They reveal much about the industry's lobbying and public relations to thwart tobacco control efforts. The documents highlight the considerable difference between public declarations of industry officials and their internal discussions.

The first significant set of internal tobacco industry documents became available in the early 1990s, when an industry whistleblower sent several boxes of documents to a university professor in the United States, resulting in the publication of several articles and a book *(3)*.

In the late 1990s, litigation by several states in the United States against the tobacco companies to recover the costs of treating tobacco-related illnesses resulted in a much larger set of documents becoming available. With the Minnesota case settlement, and later, in November 1998, the MSA between 46 United States territories and states and the tobacco companies, industry documents that were and continued to be produced during legal proceedings were made public. They were placed in a document depository in the state of Minnesota and in the United Kingdom as well as on industry-maintained web sites. The exception is that BAT, being based in the United Kingdom, is not obligated to place its documents on a web site; it only has to maintain them at the Guildford Depository. However, BAT's United States subsidiary, Brown & Williamson, must follow the same legal requirements as the other United States-based companies *(4)*.

These documents will be maintained by the tobacco industry until 2008, and there are several efforts under way to ensure that their public availability and academic analysis continue after this date *(5)*.

Tobacco industry global strategies

TTCs use their considerable economic and political influence to create an environment that encourages the continued consumption of tobacco, primarily by interfering with the development of tobacco control legislation. Some of these tactics and strategies are reviewed below.

Although strategies are presented here separately, it is important to note that most of the time the tobacco companies use one or more of these strategies concomitantly and they often have a synergistic effect.

Influence the political process

A general strategy of tobacco companies is to use their size and wealth to influence the political process at the local and national levels, focusing on their main goals of opposing taxation and regulation and maintaining marketing freedoms and social acceptability of smoking. Specific approaches include political campaign donations, lobbying, threats of legal action, as well as donations to causes that are universally popular with ruling politicians, such as domestic abuse prevention and childhood immunization *(6–13)*.

These efforts aim to influence the regulatory or legislative process to favour the industry, either through defeating comprehensive tobacco control policies or through introducing industry-friendly amendments, such as inclusion of pre-emption of local level measures *(14)*.

When the industry is unable to stop legislation from passing, it tends to apply its efforts to making implementation and enforcement difficult, leading to a policy failure that favours industry interests *(15–19)*.

The political manipulation strategy is more or less covert depending on the country's own legislation regarding monitoring of private interests' influence on governmental affairs. In the United States, for example, where political campaign contributions

---

Box 2. In the industry's own words

- The International Tobacco Information Centre (INFOTAB) was a tobacco industry-funded consortium. "INFOTAB has been coordinating a lobbying effort in 38 countries where tobacco is economically significant, working through member companies, national tobacco associations and leaf dealers. I am coordinating a similar effort through the International Chamber of Commerce. The aim of these activities is to get national delegates to the WHA (World Health Assembly) to oppose the extreme anti-tobacco recommendations" *(33)*.

- In the United States, the industry aimed to "establish better communication channels between the Washington office and corporate contributions so that these contributions serve the company's political objectives better" *(34)*.

- These tactics have been extended to the rest of the world:

  – "In the GCC (Gulf Cooperation Council) member countries, we have set up a major network of information sources and resources through which to lobby the appropriate officials" *(35)*.

  – Philip Morris has taken a leading role in the Philippine Chamber of Commerce, "... We assisted with the highly successful US visit made by President Aquino. Philip Morris International personnel now occupy key positions in a wide array of international organizations that can assist us in the years to come" *(35, 36)*.

are public information, this knowledge is used by advocates to pressure legislative bodies *(20–25)*.

In Poland, donations by tobacco companies to political parties are banned. The measure eliminates an obvious way of buying supporters in the legislature.

In addition, the tobacco industry also uses its wealth and political clout to influence international policy-making and regulatory bodies *(26–32)*.

These efforts are usually geared toward undermining product regulation and marketing restrictions as well as promoting massive misinformation and denial campaigns that play down the public health and sociodevelopmental impact of tobacco use in developing countries.

Keep tobacco products affordable

Tobacco companies have always acknowledged that cigarette prices are "the most critical variable" influencing sales, brand share and profitability *(37)*. Inversely, price increases, principally by raising the taxes on cigarettes' retail price, are the most effective tobacco control intervention *(38)*. Thus, companies oppose it fiercely. For example, in central and eastern Europe, as elsewhere in the world, Philip Morris sought "to minimize the total tax burden on cigarettes in all instances" *(39)* and to "keep smoking affordable" *(40)*. In Asia, "the government in Hong Kong [Hong Kong SAR] responded to Philip Morris pressure by narrowing the differential between duties on imported leaf and finished cigarettes, significantly benefiting Philip Morris". And in South America, "…in Guatemala, a campaign was begun to prevent changes in the country's existing price/tax structure" *(35)*.

The development of new, low- to middle-priced brands, the rampant use of discounting, and sales of single cigarettes and of small packages, are tactics to ensure that tobacco products remain affordable to consumers. Some companies are willing to narrow their profit margins, generate price wars, or even take a moderate loss per pack of cigarettes in order to gain higher share of market and maintain brand affordability. Simultaneously, tobacco companies have been known to:

- lobby legislators and officials in finance ministries to keep tobacco prices low *(36);*
- threaten governments contemplating tax raises with increased smuggling, unemployment, and a fall in state revenues (studies from the World Bank indicate these are not consequences of tobacco tax increases) *(36);*
- accuse governments of infringing on the rights of poor individuals to smoke, while totally neglecting these individuals' risk to health – in a major *faux pas* in the Czech Republic, Philip Morris even argued that the tobacco industry improves the country's economic balance because smokers die early, thus saving welfare and retirement costs (see Box 3).

Moreover, the industry documents revealed that in its attempt to increase market share the tobacco industry resorted to an exploration of the contraband market, an issue that is currently being considered by several governmental authorities. For example, a note of a meeting between senior BAT and Philip Morris executives with responsibility for Latin America shows "extensive cartel behaviours in seeking market share agreements, price-fixing and attempts to limit market support expenditures.

It shows that BAT and Philip Morris can determine prices in the smuggled and legal markets independently" *(41)*. Despite the documentary evidence, the industry denies any involvement with smuggling of cigarettes *(42–57)*.

Promote tobacco in new and innovative ways

A 1999 World Bank report *(59)* concluded that a comprehensive ban on advertising, promotion and sponsorship reduces tobacco consumption. The tobacco industry strongly opposes such a measure. Countries that have put in place a comprehensive tobacco advertising ban are increasingly finding that the industry still continues to target children, teenagers and women, in less obvious and more creative ways *(60–74)*.

Other 'non-traditional' ways for promoting tobacco products include brand-stretching/brand-sharing, promotional item and sampling distribution, direct mail advertising and sales, coupons, product placements and events sponsorship in sports, music, fashion and the arts, Internet advertising and sales, corporate sponsorships *(9)* and recently, in at least one country, the use of text messaging to promote cigarettes *(75)*. In another country, young men and women dressed in the colours of cigarette brands distribute, sell and promote cigarettes at dance clubs and other venues patronized by youth *(76)*.

Box 3. "They would not dare say that in the United States": The Czech Philip Morris report at a glance

The Czech Republic Prime Minister Milos Zeman, a heavy smoker, once defended tobacco use by arguing that it helps his country's finances, since "smokers die sooner, and the state does not need to look after them in their old age". In 2001, Philip Morris produced and distributed a report to the Czech Republic Parliament, echoing the dark-humoured statement of Zeman, in an attempt to block a new set of anti-smoking measures. The report claimed that tobacco use is beneficial because, by dying early, smokers saved the Czech Republic Government US$ 30 million in 1999 in health care, pensions and housing for the elderly.

When leaked to the media, a leading Czech Republic newspaper called the report "monstrous" and "extremely nasty", adding that "in the United States they [Philip Morris] would not dare say anything like that even under a blanket". Once the outcry erupted, Philip Morris realized that the report had been a big mistake. In late July 2001, the company publicly admitted that the report "exhibited terrible judgement as well as a complete and unacceptable disregard of basic human values". The decision to commission the study was "…not just a terrible mistake. It was wrong. All of us at Philip Morris, no matter where we work, are extremely sorry for this", according to Philip Morris chief executive Geoffrey C Bible.

Matthew L Myers of the Campaign for Tobacco-Free Kids responded that the "apology can only be viewed as a cynical act of damage control … Without action to back up its words, one has to question what Philip Morris really regrets – the report's callous conclusions or the damage done to Philip Morris's efforts to portray itself as a reformed, responsible company" *(58)*.

To dissuade governments from enacting comprehensive advertising bans, tobacco companies offer 'self-regulation' or 'voluntary advertising codes'. However, these protect certain forms of advertising, allegedly to 'respect' the freedom of speech and the companies' ability to 'communicate with consumers'. Experience has shown that tobacco industry-initiated voluntary regulation of advertising and promotion are rarely enforced, and without any legislative imperative tobacco companies can disregard them at any time. This renders them ineffective as tobacco control measures. In addition, partial bans allow the industry to re-distribute marketing expenditures into more diverse and creative product promotion practices *(77–81)*.

WHO advises governments, therefore, to reject industry-initiated voluntary codes, and instead recommends that they stand firmly for a comprehensive ban.

Countries should also consider advertising at the point of sale (POS) with great caution. Other countries, such as Hungary, also shared New Zealand's experience with the post-ban flourishing of POS advertising *(82)*.

The Hungarian advertising regulation left the definition of POS advertising unclear and, as such, open to interpretation. Without delay, TTCs applied their own, liberal interpretation, resulting in advertisements clearly visible from outside shops.

Events sponsorship, corporate citizenship and philanthropy are not only instruments for gaining visibility and media coverage, but also provide legitimacy, and draw supporters, friends and allies to tobacco companies. Organizations openly supportive of tobacco control could be silenced with grants coming from the industry; governments can be misled by industry-sponsored 'youth smoking prevention programmes'.

Figure 2. **Philip Morris profits from tobacco 1988–1998 (domestic versus international, in US$ billions)**

US$ billions

(bar chart: Domestic tobacco profits and International tobacco profits for years 1988, 1990, 1992, 1994, 1996, 1998, y-axis from 0 to 6)

Source: Joosens and Ritthiphakde *(83)*

The industry's youth smoking prevention programmes purport to tell young people not to smoke, but fail to discuss any of the health-related risks of tobacco use and convey the message that smoking is an adult decision. These programmes are often combined with equally ineffective retailer education programmes to minimize the sales of tobacco products to minors. So, while pretending to embrace public health messages, the industry is, in fact, controlling the political and policy agenda, attempting to prevent policy-makers from adopting marketing restrictions to reduce consumption *(62, 82, 84–87)*.

Governments and civil groups should not accept tobacco industry funding. WHO advises governments to avoid any form of partnership with tobacco companies, since such collaboration would inevitably distort public health priorities *(88)*.

Sponsoring Formula-1 and other world sports events provides tobacco companies the opportunity for circumventing advertising bans, allowing their logos to appear on TV screens and newspapers despite such bans. To prevent this, tobacco company sponsorship of sports and other events should be forbidden along with other forms of tobacco promotion.

Change names and improve the tobacco industry's corporate image

After industry documents were made openly available, TTCs launched a new public relations (PR) strategy claiming the start of a new era of ethical behaviour. Since then, no substantial action has backed up the industry's claim, leading tobacco control advocates and researchers to conclude that there is no new, reformed tobacco industry, *(36, 89–90)* only a misleading public relations strategy aimed at offsetting the damage done by exposing the industry's internal documents.

BAT's new initiative – its Corporate Social Responsibility or CSR programme – the 'stakeholder dialogue' and its 'social reporting' are efforts to erase the company's links to its past, and to the dishonest and unethical behaviour of former industry executives. The company invites a wide range of pro- and anti-tobacco stakeholders, purportedly to advise the company on how to transform itself in accordance with the shifting expectation of societies. However, there is no evidence, to date, that any recommendations are being implemented. Furthermore, the 'socially responsible' actions developed by these companies are not uniform and vary from country to country *(89)*. Changing the name "Philip Morris" to "Altria Group, Inc" is a similar attempt to dissociate the company from its past actions *(91)*.

Distort information and generate 'pseudo-science'

The internal tobacco industry documents indicate that the industry intentionally creates controversy over the known health effects of tobacco use. Until recently, the industry publicly denied the association between smoking and lung cancer, and the addictiveness of nicotine. The internal documents, however, reveal that the industry was aware of the causative relationship between smoking and lung cancer, and knew how to manipulate nicotine levels in cigarettes to keep smokers addicted *(92)*. Since the release of these findings, some TTCs now admit that smoking is a "health risk factor" and may cause serious diseases in published statements and on their corporate web sites. At country level, however, this message is not always echoed by TTCs' local

Box 4. Tobacco industry's interference in WHO's research on second-hand tobacco smoke

The existence of a carcinogenic risk from passive smoking adds a new dimension to the debate on health effects of tobacco since, in contrast to the diseases affecting the active smoker, it represents a health damage imposed on people who do not smoke. This difference has great implications in terms of regulation of smoking in public settings, and may, in the long run, be a major factor contributing to the decrease in tobacco consumption. This explains the tobacco industry's keen interest in monitoring and discrediting studies that contribute to establishing the causal link between passive smoking and cancer. This text box highlights an example of the industry's attempts to interfere in a particular study that links second-hand smoke to cancer.

In April 2000, researchers from the University of California at San Francisco reported the results of a review of internal documents from Philip Morris and other tobacco companies in *The Lancet*. The documents provide evidence that the tobacco industry had closely monitored and tried to actively interfere with the conduct of an international epidemiological study on lung cancer in non-smokers following exposure to passive smoking.

The study was coordinated by the International Agency for Research on Cancer (IARC) in Lyon, France, a research institute of WHO. The results were published in the *Journal of the National Cancer Institute (93)* and showed that exposure to passive smoking at the workplace or through a spouse results in an increased relative risk (RR) of 1.16, a small factor when compared to the RR of more than 20-fold associated with active cigarette smoking. However, given the large populations exposed to passive smoking, it has been calculated that each year passive smoking causes 3000 cases of lung cancer in the United States and up to 2500 cases in Europe.

Among the actions undertaken by the tobacco industry to disrupt and discredit this study were the establishment of a task force to react to the publication of the results, the use of consultants to contact the IARC investigators to obtain confidential information on the study, and plans to influence the scientific policy and financing of IARC. In 1998, the IARC study was the object of a strong defamation campaign in the media orchestrated by the tobacco industry through a lead article in London's *Daily Telegraph*.

Although these attacks did not pre-empt the publication of the report in the medical literature, they created confusion and controversy about the interpretation of the results. The documents reviewed in the article in *The Lancet* suggest that this media campaign was part of a broader long-planned tobacco industry strategy on passive smoking.

The industry continues to claim that the "WHO study" did not prove that there was a link between passive smoking and cancer, perpetuating the confusion and attempting to create controversy where none exists *(94)*.

subsidiaries or by their front groups. Much of the communication from the industry at the country level remains ambiguous on smoking and health issues. The industry continues to deny any links between second-hand smoke exposure and health and to actively perpetuate erroneous information about such effects, as well as about the detrimental impact of tobacco control on economies (see Box 4).

Even the academic community has not been spared. While the public has become increasingly sceptical about industry-funded research, companies continue to fund academic institutions, scientists and consultants who are willing to support the industry's case through research funding efforts such as Philip Morris's External Research Program *(95)*.

The latest report claiming that there is no causal relation between environmental tobacco smoke and tobacco-related mortality *(96)* is another example of this ongoing industry practice. These efforts are also part of the industry's strategies to maintain credibility with the public, the media and policy-makers.

Create influential networks and front groups

The tobacco industry also influences policy-making at the local, national and international level by creating influential networks and using front groups and alliances to convey the industry's message. The industry needs influential supporters within governments to counter the development of tobacco control legislation.

Finance and agricultural ministries are often targets of the industry search for 'inside connections'. The tobacco industry bombards them with findings of industry-commissioned research and misleads them with a well-constructed set of myths about its economic importance and the detrimental effect of controlling tobacco. These government officials are usually unaware of the solid evidence base supporting tobacco control policies and may well give the green light to promoting the industry in the mistaken belief that tobacco provides a net benefit to the economy.

The tobacco industry also often targets ministries of education or sports to promote its youth prevention programmes. As discussed previously, the covert aim of these programmes is to avoid comprehensive legislation banning advertising and marketing, restricting sales to minors, and other measures that are effective in curbing smoking among youth (see Box 5).

Box 5. The truth about tobacco and tobacco advertising

- nicotine is a drug
- nicotine is addictive
- second-hand tobacco smoke exposure is harmful to health
- industry attempts to develop less harmful tobacco products have been a failure
- tobacco advertising, promotions and product design target youth
- tobacco advertising aims to increase consumption of tobacco products.

Faced with a growing loss of credibility, the industry uses a variety of groups that it either funds or creates. Such groups present themselves as 'interested parties' and seldom disclose their financial ties with the tobacco industry. Links have been uncovered with groups as diverse as the hospitality industry (restaurants, bars, hotels, etc.), the advertising industry, and citizen interest groups allegedly protesting tax and liability burdens, for example.

The industry also frequently creates and/or funds tobacco-growers associations, most notably the International Tobacco Growers Association, and smokers' rights groups *(26, 97)*.

Another strategy is the funding of think tanks, i.e. research and policy groups that issue reports and opinions that favour the industry without disclosing their financial ties. These groups create pressure with policy-makers, the media and the public, who often believe these are legitimate grass-roots movements, independent of the tobacco interests *(98)*. The representatives of these front groups usually are able to sustain good relationships with decision-makers, and aggressively lobby their contacts in government when tobacco control is on the legislative agenda. With the availability of the industry documents it is possible to identify many front groups to industry funding *(26, 82, 99–101)*.

The media can also be coopted to support the tobacco industry, which works with it in many ways. The tobacco industry conducts training seminars for top media executives in order to ensure that the message is uniform across the board, and promotes media seminars to 'educate' journalists about smoking and health and other issues that are important to the industry's bottom line. The industry's goal is to have the media publish its perspective, which is another way to influence the opinions of decision-makers and the public. In addition to offering seminars to journalists, the industry also donates to media-related groups *(26–82)*.

The tobacco industry will also flex its economic muscle and threaten to withhold advertising placement as a means of pressuring media conglomerates to support industry-friendly positions. In the Philippines, for example, TV stations that were airing the Department of Health's (DOH) anti-smoking campaign "Yosi Kadiri" were pressured by the tobacco companies to stop giving the DOH free air time in exchange for the tobacco companies' continued purchase of advertising time *(102)*.

With a cadre of media contacts, it becomes easier for the industry to communicate its public relations efforts. This was recently apparent in the industry's ongoing CSR programme, through which the industry is trying to convince the public, with the media's help, that the tobacco industry is an integral and essential part of any society. The CSR effort overlaps and complements the industry's other public relations efforts such as donations to social and political causes *(9)*.

GLOBAL EXPANSION OF TTCs – BRINGING THE TOBACCO EPIDEMIC TO THE DEVELOPING WORLD

Countries have much to learn from recent trends emerging from the globalization of tobacco manufacturing and trade. Declining cigarette sales in developed countries have compelled TTCs to expand to new markets in the developing world. The removal of trade barriers under bilateral and multilateral trade agreements has facilitated trade in tobacco and tobacco products, and compliance with the provisions of these trade agreements has enabled the TTCs to gain entrance into markets previously closed to foreign tobacco and tobacco products.

In the past decade, the International Monetary Fund (IMF) has also contributed to opening cigarette markets in countries such as the Republic of Korea, the Republic of Moldova, Thailand (see Box 6) *(103)* and Turkey. It has done so by insisting on privatization of state tobacco monopolies as a precondition for loans *(1)*.

Box 6. Forcing Thailand to open up for foreign cigarette imports

The most important multilateral agreement of the World Trade Organization (WTO) on tobacco trade is the General Agreement on Tariffs and Trade (GATT). One of the principles established by GATT requires that products imported into a country cannot be treated differently from similar products produced within that country.

The agreement, however, provides a limited exception for measures "necessary" to protect public health, which may be adopted and enforced even if such measures violate GATT principles. Thailand thus attempted to prevent the importation of foreign cigarettes by citing cigarettes as a health hazard. However, in 1990, American tobacco companies challenged Thailand's ban on imports of foreign cigarettes on the grounds that Thailand allowed its local tobacco industry to continue to manufacture and sell cigarettes. The United States trade representative referred the matter to GATT, arguing that "no prohibition or restriction shall be maintained by any contracting party on the importation of any product of the territory of any other contracting party".

In its precedent decision, a GATT panel had concluded that Thailand could give priority to human health over trade liberalization as long as the measure taken is "necessary" and there is no alternative measure to provide that level of protection. However, Thailand's practice of permitting the sale of locally manufactured cigarettes and banning cigarette imports was found not justifiable and the country was forced to remove the import ban *(103)*.

POLITICAL AND ECONOMIC CHANGES
AS INCENTIVES FOR EXPANSION

The decline and privatization of former state tobacco monopolies in the 1980s (e.g. in Asia), and the opening of markets previously closed behind ideological walls in the 1990s (e.g. former communist countries) are providing opportunities for TTCs to boost sales and expand their market base. To avoid import taxes and lower production and transportation costs, TTCs are moving their production facilities to countries with less stringent tobacco-related regulation. Research indicates that the post-privatization period, which generally coincides with the entry of TTCs, is usually followed by increased tobacco consumption, which, in turn, leads to increases over time in tobacco-related morbidity and mortality in affected countries *(103–104)*.

ESTABLISHING NEW MARKETS –
INDUSTRY STRATEGIES IN SELECTED COUNTRIES

Around 60 000 formerly state-owned cigarette-manufacturing facilities were opened for privatization after the collapse of communist regimes *(1)*. Usually pressed for economic capital, these countries urgently needed foreign investments, which put TTCs in advantageous negotiating positions.

In many cases, privatization agreements provided TTCs with significant concessions, such as being exempted from profit taxes (e.g. Hungary, Kyrgyzstan and Ukraine) or receiving favourable conditions for the withdrawal of dividends *(104)*.

In Kazakhstan, Kyrgyzstan and Uzbekistan, BAT became the sole cigarette producer, establishing a private monopoly in place of the former state monopoly. "It must be absolutely clear that what we wish to buy is not manufacturing assets or brands but an opportunity to dominate the market", states BAT commenting on the privatization in Uzbekistan *(105)*.

Records indicate that TTCs employed intermediaries whose personal and professional relationships with key government officials in these countries were used to the advantage of the tobacco industry. For example, a former Hungarian citizen, who left the country during the 1956 uprising but still maintained good relationships with friends occupying high positions in the government, was sent back to Hungary by Philip Morris to help secure a licence agreement with conditions favourable to the company.

During the privatization of tobacco production facilities, TTCs reportedly managed to tap officials of the finance and agriculture portfolios to facilitate the takeover process. "The [Hungarian] State Property Agency has received instructions to conclude the proposed transaction as rapidly as possible [from finance and agricultural ministry officials]", announced an internal memo of Philip Morris *(106)*.

Records show that diplomats of countries harbouring TTCs also intervened in the support of their companies in new markets. In Ukraine, the British ambassador and the commercial secretary "were extremely useful" and "valuable allies" *(107)* in obtaining government support for BAT's privatization plans.

CONCLUSION

The globalization of tobacco manufacturing, trade, marketing and industry influence poses a major threat to public health worldwide. Yach and Bettcher characterize the tobacco industry as a "global force" that considers the world as "its operating market by planning, developing and marketing its products on a global scale" *(108)*.

The industry uses a variety of strategies to buy influence and power and penetrate markets, ensuring that the tobacco epidemic continues to propagate and affect the health of millions of people around the world. Governments and tobacco control advocates must familiarize themselves with the common strategies used by the industry, and apply this knowledge when developing effective interventions, at the global and local levels to curb tobacco use.

To date, the tobacco industry's response to increased public awareness is focused on image change, rather than structural change. Structural change would involve sharing the goal of reducing tobacco use worldwide, and working towards a gradual conversion of the tobacco industry to non-lethal areas of business.

References

1. Mackay J, Eriksen M. *The tobacco atlas.* Geneva, World Health Organization, 2002 (http://www.myriadeditions.com/tobacco.html).

2. World Bank. *CIA fact book.* World Bank, 2002 (Nationmaster.com).

3. Glantz S et al. *The cigarette papers.* Berkeley, University of California Press, 1996 (http://www.library.ucsf.edu/tobacco/cigpapers/book/contents.html).

4. Master Settlement Agreement (with Exhibits A–U), National Association of Attorneys-General (NAAG). Washington, DC, NAAG, 1998 (http://www.naag.org/tobac/cigmsa.rtf).

5. Bero L. Implications of the tobacco industry documents for public health and policy. *Annual Review Public Health,* 2003, 24:3.1–3.22 (http://publhealth.annualreviews.org/cgi/content/abstract/24/1/267).

6. Pan American Health Organization. *Profits over People.* Washington, DC, PAHO, November 2002 (www.paho.org).

7. Bialous S, Fox B, Glantz S. Tobacco industry allegations of "illegal lobbying" and state tobacco control. *American Journal of Public Health,* 2001, 91(1):62–67.

8. Philip Morris Companies Inc. Five-Year Plan 1995–1999 Confidential 1994 Strategic Plan. Virginia, USA, Philip Morris. Access Date: 23 September 2001. Bates No. 2031590820/2031591093 (www.pmdocs.com).

9. Rosenberg J, Siegel M. The use of corporate sponsorship as a tobacco marketing tool: a review of tobacco industry sponsorship in the United States, 1995–1999. *Tobacco Control,* 2001, 10(Autumn):239–246 (http://tc.bmjjournals.com/cgi/content/full/10/3/239; http://www.ftc.gov/os/comments/tobaccocomments2/sponsorship.pdf).

10. Anon. BATCo 1996–1998 Company Plan. Minnesota Document Depository. BATCo. Strategic Plan. Access Date: 26 September 2001. Bates No. 800250638/800250704.

11. Chaloupka FJ et al. Tax, price and cigarette smoking: evidence from the tobacco documents and implications for tobacco company marketing strategies. *Tobacco Control,* 2002, 11(Suppl 1):62–72.

12. Neuman M, Bitton A, Glantz S. Tobacco industry strategies for influencing European Community tobacco advertising legislation. *Lancet,* 2002, 359(9314):1323–1330.

13. Yach D, Bettcher D. Globalization of tobacco industry influence and new global responses. *Tobacco Control,* 2000, 9(2):206–216.

14. American Medical Association. *Pre-emption: taking the local out of tobacco control.* American Medical Association, 2002 (http://www.ama-assn.org/ama/pub/category/7323.html).

15. DiFranza J, Rigotti N. Impediments to the enforcement of youth access laws. *Tobacco Control,* 1999, 8(2):152–155.

16. Siegel M et al. Preemption in tobacco control. Review of an emerging public health problem. *Journal of the American Medical Association,* 1997, 278(10):858–863.

17. DiFranza J, Godshall W. Tobacco industry efforts hindering enforcement of the ban on tobacco sales to minors: actions speak louder than words. *Tobacco Control,* 1996, 5(2):127–131.

18. Jacobson P, Wasserman J, Raube K. The politics of antismoking legislation. *Journal of Health Politics, Policy & Law,* 1993, 18(4):787–819.

19. Jacobson P, Wasserman J. The implementation and enforcement of tobacco control laws: policy implications for activists and the industry. *Journal of Health Politics, Policy & Law.* 1999, 24(3):567–598.

20. Begay M, Traynor M, Glantz S. The tobacco industry, state politics, and tobacco education in California. *American Journal of Public Health,* 1993, 83(9):1214–1221.

21. Monardi F, Glantz S. Are tobacco industry campaign contributions influencing state legislative behaviour? *American Journal of Public Health,* 1998, 88(6):918–923.

22. Moore S et al. Epidemiology of failed tobacco control legislation. *Journal of the American Medical Association,* 1994, 272(15):1171–1175.

23. Givel M, Glantz S. Tobacco lobby political influence on US state legislatures in the 1990s. *Tobacco Control,* 2001, 10(2):124–134.

24. Goldstein A, Bearman N. State tobacco lobbyists and organizations in the United States: crossed lines. *American Journal of Public Health,* 1996, 86(8):1137–1142.

25. Lee C, Glantz SA. *The tobacco industry's successful efforts to control tobacco policy making in Switzerland.* San Francisco, CA: Institute for Health Policy Studies, University of California at San Francisco, January 2001 (http://www.library.ucsf.edu/tobacco/swiss).

26. Committee of Experts on Tobacco Industry Documents. *Tobacco company strategies to undermine tobacco control activities at the World Health Organization.* Geneva, World Health Organization, 2000.

27. Saloojee Y, Dagli E. Tobacco industry tactics for resisting public policy on health. *Bulletin of the World Health Organization,* 2000, 78(7):902–910.

28. Bialous S, Yach D. Whose standard is it, anyway? How the tobacco industry determines the International Organization for Standardization (ISO) standards for tobacco and tobacco products. *Tobacco Control,* 2001, 10:96–104.

29. Stinnett A. The Tobacco Industry vs. the World Health Organization. National Health Law Program, Washington, DC, 2000 (http://www.healthlaw.org/pubs/200008tobacco.html).

30. Mongoven C, Biscoe & Duchin. Destroying tobacco control activism from the inside. *Tobacco Control,* 2002, 11(2):112–118.

31. Francey N, Chapman S. "Operation Berkshire": the international tobacco companies' conspiracy. *British Medical Journal,* 2000, 321(7257):371–374.

32. Neuman M, Bitton A, Glantz S. Tobacco industry strategies for influencing European Community tobacco advertising legislation. *Lancet,* 2002, 359(9314):1323–1330.

33. R Marcotullio. *Regarding World Health Organization.* Memo, 17 March 1986. Bates No. 505745424 (http://www.rjrtdocs.com).

34. Philip Morris. *Government affairs objectives,* 7 January 1982. Bates No. 2023200348/0355 (http://www.pmdocs.com/getallimg.asp?if=avpidx&DOCID=2023200348/0355).

35. A. Whist. Memo to Board of Directors, Philip Morris International Corporate Affairs, 17 December 1986. Bates No. 2025431401/1406 (http://www.pmdocs.com/getallimg.asp?DOCID=2025431401/1406).

36. Campaign for Tobacco Free Kids, Action on Smoking and Health UK. *Trust us We're the Tobacco Industry,* United Kingdom, ASH-UK, April 2001.

37. Anon. Marketing Dept. Millbank. Analysis of price and value for money in the cigarette market. PMB, April 1984 (http://tobacco.health.usyd.edu.au/site/gateway/docs/pdf2/pdf/BW538011320_1397).

38. Jha P, Chaloupka FJ. *Tobacco Control in Developing Countries.* Washington, DC, The World Bank, 2000 (http://www1.worldbank.org/tobacco/tcdc.asp).

39. Anon. 1993–1995 Three-Year Plan for the EEMA Region. Situation assessment. Bates No. 2500108232_8304 (http://www.pmdocs.com/getallimg.asp?if=avpidx&DOCID=2500108232/8304).

40. Anon. Three Year Plan 1994–96. Philip Morris (http://www.pmdocs.com/getallimg.asp?if=avpidx&DOCID=2500070154/0218).

41. BAT Meeting with Philip Morris Representatives at PennyHill Park, Bagshot, 5 August 1992. BAT Guildford Depository, Bates No. 301653380-85.

42. *Findings of the International Expert Panel on Cigarette Descriptors. Ministerial Advisory Council on Tobacco Control.* Health Canada, 7 September 7 2001 (http://www.hc-sc.gc.ca/english/pdf/media/cig_discrip_rep2.pdf).

43. European Union alleges U.S. companies sent black-market cigarettes to Iraq. Source: AP, 2002-02-22 (http://www.tobacco.org/news/86642.html).

44. Tobacco Traffic. NOW With Bill Moyers. PBS Television, 19 April 2002 (http://www.pbs.org/now/indepth/041902_smuggling.html; http://www.pbs.org/now/transcript/transcript114_full.html).

45. Tobacco Traffic: Black Market Peso Exchange. NOW With Bill Moyers. PBS Television, 19 April 2002 (http://www.pbs.org/now/indepth/041902_peso.html; http://www.pbs.org/now/transcript/transcript114_full.html).

46. *Action on Smoking and Health. BAT under investigation by DTI: ASH says Imperial Tobacco should be next.* United Kingdom, ASH-UK, 2000 (http://www.ash.org.uk/html/press/001030a.html).

47. *Action on Smoking and Health. BAT and tobacco smuggling.* Submission to the House of Commons Health Select Committee. United Kingdom, ASH-UK, 2000 (http://www.ash.org.uk/html/smuggling/html/submission.html).

48. Beelman M et al. How smuggling helps lure generations of new smokers. *The Guardian.* 31 January 2000 (http://www.guardian.co.uk/bat/article/0,2763,191296,00.html).

49. Beelman M et al. *Major tobacco multinational implicated in cigarette smuggling, tax evasion, documents show.* Washington, DC, International Consortium of Investigative Journalists (ICIJ), Center for Public Integrity, 31 January 31.

50. Campbell D, Maguire K. Clarke company faces new smuggling claims. *The Guardian*/ICIJ, 22 August 2001 (http://www.icij.org/investigate/campbell1.html).

51. International Consortium of Investigative Journalists (ICIJ). *Philip Morris accused of smuggling, money-laundering conspiracy in racketeering lawsuit.* Washington, DC, Center for Public Integrity, 2000.

52. International Consortium of Investigative Journalists (ICIJ). *Tobacco companies linked to criminal organizations in cigarette smuggling: Latin America.* Washington, DC, Center for Public Integrity, 3 March 2001.

53. Joossens L, Raw M. Cigarette smuggling in Europe: who really benefits? *Tobacco Control,* 1998, 7:66–71 (http://tc.bmjjournals.com/cgi/reprint/7/1/66.pdf).

54. Marsden W. Tiny isle is key to illicit trade. *The Gazette,* 5 March 2001.

55. Pan American Health Organization. *Profits over people.* Washington, DC, PAHO, November 2002 (www.paho.org).

56. US District Court. Departments of the Republic of Colombia v. Philip Morris & BAT. New York City, NY, 2000, (http://www.public-i.org/download/AmdendedColombiaSuit.pdf).

57. Bowers S. Imperial rejects smuggling claim. *The Guardian,* 2002 (http://www.guardian.co.uk/Archive/Article/0,4273,4400132,00.html).

58. *Wall Street Journal,* 26 July 2001; *Los Angeles Times,* 5 August 2001.

59. The World Bank. *Curbing the epidemic: governments and the economics of tobacco control.* Series: Development in practice. Washington, DC, The World Bank, 1999 (http://www1.worldbank.org/tobacco/reports.htm).

60. Action on Smoking and Health. *Tobacco Explained: 3. Marketing to children.* London, ASH-UK, 1998 (http://www.ash.org.uk/html/conduct/html/tobexpld3.html).

61. Action on Smoking and Health–UK. *Danger! PR in the playground. Tobacco industry initiatives on youth smoking.* London, ASH-UK, 2001 (http://www.ash.org.uk/html/advspo/pdfs/playgroundreport.pdf).

62. http://www.ash.org.uk/

63. Action on Smoking and Health–UK. *Advertising and sponsorship/sports and cultural sponsorship,* London, ASH-UK, 2001 (http://www.ash.org.uk/html/advspo/html/sportssponsor.html).

64. Bates C. Editorial: Tobacco Sponsorship of Sport. *British Journal of Sports Medicine,* 1999, 33(5):299–300 (http://www.ash.org.uk/html/advspo/html/sport.html).

65. Campaign for Tobacco Free Kids (CTFK*). Special Report: Big Tobacco Still Addicting Kids.* Washington, DC, Campaign for Tobacco Free Kids, 2003 (http://tobaccofreekids.org/reports/addicting/).

66. Hammond R. *Mundo de Marlboro: Big Tobacco smothers Latin America.* Americas.org, 1999 (http://www.americas.org/News/Features/199904_Exporting_Death/tobacco.htm).

67. Ling P, Sepe E, Glantz S. *Tobacco marketing to young adults: tobacco control lessons from industry documents.* Paper presented at 129th Annual Meeting of the American Public Health Association. Atlanta, GA, 21–25 October 2001.

68. Ling P, Landman A, Glantz S. It is time to abandon youth access tobacco programmes. *Tobacco Control,* March 2002, 11:3–6 (http://tc.bmjjournals.com/cgi/content/full/11/1/3).

69. Pierce J et al. Tobacco industry promotion of cigarettes and adolescent smoking. *Journal of the American Medical Association.* 18 February 1998, 279(7):511–515.

70. Pierce J, Gilpin E, Choi W. Sharing the blame: smoking experimentation and future smoking-attributable mortality due to Joe Camel and Marlboro advertising and promotions. *Tobacco Control,* 1999, 8(1):37–44.

71. Pollay R, et al. The last straw: cigarette advertising and realized market shares among youth and adults, 1979–1993. *Journal of Marketing,* 1996, 60:1–16.

72. Pollay R. *How cigarette promotion works: rich imagery and poor information. History of advertising archives, faculty of commerce*: University of British Columbia, 30 October 2000 (http://www.nsra-adnf.ca/DOCUMENTS/PDFs/pollay.pdf, accessed 2002).

73. Pollay R. Targeting youth and concerned smokers: evidence from Canadian tobacco industry documents. *Tobacco Control,* 2000, 9(2):136–147.

74. Samet J, Yoon S. *Women and the tobacco epidemic: challenges for the 21st century,* Geneva, World Health Organization/Institute for Global Tobacco Control, Johns Hopkins School of Public Health, 2001 (http://tobacco.who.int/repository/tpc49/WomenMonograph.pdf).

75. ABC News Online. *Government to review tobacco advertising laws.* 30 August 2003 (http://www.abc.net.au/news/newsitems/s935709.htm).

76. Tobacco makers use 'cigarette girls' to skirt ad ban, Post says, Bloomberg News, 1 October 2003.

77. Richards J, Tye J, Fischer P. The tobacco industry's code of advertising in the United States: myth and reality. *Tobacco Control,* 1996, 5(4):295–311.

78. International Marketing Standards, 2001 (http://www.bat.com/oneweb/sites/uk__3mnfen.nsf/vwPagesWebLive/DO52ADRK?opendocument&TMP=1).

79. Anon. Proposal for a voluntary code for cigarette advertising. Proposal. Guildford Depository. Access Date: 21 September 2001. Bates No. 500899945/500899446.

80. Non-Smokers' Rights Association. *A catalogue of deception: the use and abuse of voluntary regulation of tobacco advertising in Canada.* Ottawa, Non-Smokers' Rights Assocation, 1986.

81. Saloojee Y, Hammond R. *Fatal deception: the tobacco industry's "new" global standards for tobacco marketing,* INB-3 Alliance Bulletin – Framework Convention Alliance, 2001 (http://fctc.org/bulletin/Issue_14.pdf).

82. Pan American Health Organization. *Profits over people.* Washington, DC, PAHO, November 2002 (www.paho.org).

83. Joossens, Ritthiphakde. *Role of multinationals and other private actors: trade and investment practices.* Paper presented at the WHO international conference on global tobacco control law: Towards a WHO Framework Convention on Tobacco Control. New Delhi, India, 2000 (http://www.who.int/tobacco/media/en/LUK2000X.pdf).

84. Action on Smoking and Health–UK. *Danger! PR in the playground. Tobacco industry initiatives on youth smoking.* London, ASH-UK, 2001 (http://www.ash.org.uk/html/advspo/pdfs/playgroundreport.pdf).

85. Anon. Youth Campaigns. Philip Morris, Virginia, USA. 29 November 1996. Table. Access Date: 23 September 2001. Bates No. 2501109037/2501109038 (www.pmdocs.com).

86. British American Tobacco Company Limited. *Youth smoking prevention* (http://www.bat.com/oneweb/sites/uk__3mnfen.nsf/vwPagesWebLive/DO52ANVW?opendocument&TMP=1).

87. Ontario Medical Association (OMA). *More smoke and mirrors: Tobacco industry-sponsored youth prevention programs in the context of comprehensive tobacco control programs in Canada. A position statement.* February 2002, Toronto, OMA (http://www.oma.org/phealth/smokeandmirrors.htm).

88. Statement by the Director-General to the International Negotiating Body on the WHO Framework Convention on Tobacco Control at its Fifty-fifth session, Geneva, 15 October 2002 (http://www.who.int/gb/fctc/PDF/inb5/einb5d7.pdf).

89. Action on Smoking and Health-UK. *BAT Social Report Re-visited: ASH comes to BAT.* London, ASH-UK, October 2002 (http://www.ash.org.uk/).

90. Rowell A. MP's verdict: *tobacco boss is a "liar and a crook."* London, ASH-UK, June 2002 (http://www.andyrowell.com).

91. Myers ML. Philip Morris changes its name, but not its harmful practices. *Tobacco Control,* 2002, 11:169–170

92. Campaign for Tobacco Free Kids, Action on Smoking and Health UK. *Trust us We're the Tobacco Industry,* United Kingdom, ASH-UK, April 2001.

93. Boffetta et al. Multicenter case-control study of exposure to environmental tobacco smoke and lung cancer in Europe. *Journal of the National Cancer Institute,* 1998, 90: 1440–1450.

94. International Agency on Research for Cancer. *Cancer Press Release,* Geneva, Switzerland, World Health Organization, 7 April 2000 (http://www.iarc.fr).

95. Hirschhorn N, Bialous SA, Shatenstein S. Philip Morris' new scientific initiative: an analysis. *Tobacco Control,* 2001, 10:247–252 (http://www.tobaccoscam.ucsf.edu/pdf/9.6-Hirschhorn&Bialous.pdf, accessed 27 May 2003).

96. Enstrom JE, Kabat GC. Environmental tobacco smoke and tobacco related mortality in a prospective study of Californians, 1960–1998. *British Medical Journal,* 17 May 2003, 326:1057 (http://bmj.com/cgi/reprint/326/7398/1057.pdf).

97. Anon. *A smokers' alliance* (Draft). Philip Morris. 9 July 1993. Presentation. Access Date: June 2000. Bates No. 2022839671/2022839727 (www.pmdocs.com).

98. Traynor M, Begay M, Glantz S. New tobacco industry strategy to prevent local tobacco control. *Journal of the American Medical Association,* 1993, 270(4):479–486.

99. Givel M, Glantz S. Tobacco lobby political influence on US state legislatures in the 1990s. *Tobacco Control,* 2001, 10(2):124–134.

100. Mongoven C, Biscoe & Duchin. Destroying tobacco control activism from the inside. *Tobacco Control,* 2002, 11(2):112–118.

101. Tobacco Free Initiative. *The Tobacco Industry and Scientific Groups ILSI: A Case Study.* Geneva, World Health Organization, 2001 (http://www.who.int/genevahearings/inquiry/ilsi.pdf).

102. Personal communication, Senator Juan M. Flavier, 2002.

103. Jha P, Chaloupka FJ. The impact of trade liberalization on tobacco consumption. In: *Tobacco Control in Developing Countries.* Washington, DC, The World Bank, 2000.

104. Beyer J, Yurekli A. Privatization of state-owned tobacco enterprises in Turkey and Ukraine. In: *Economic, social and health issues in tobacco control.* Report of a WHO International Meeting Kobe, Japan, 3–4 December 2001. Geneva, World Health Organization, 2003.

105. Gilmore A. *Great CEE Smokeout: An update on the tobacco epidemic in the former Soviet Union.* Presentation at the CEE Smokeout Seminar in Warsaw, Poland, April 2002, citing a BAT Marketing Report on Uzbekistan. November 1993.

106. Philip Morris. *1991 Revised Forecast.* 6 June 1991. Bates No. 2500058044-90 (http://www.pmdocs.com/getallimg.asp?if=avpidx&DOCID=2500058044/8090).

107. Gilmore A. *Great CEE Smokeout: An update on the tobacco epidemic in the former Soviet Union.* Presentation at the CEE Smokeout Seminar in Warsaw, Poland, April 2002, citing a BAT Report on Schroder's visit to Kiev in October 1992.

108. Yach D and Bettcher D. Globalization of tobacco industry influence and new global responses. *Tobacco Control,* 2000, 9:206–216.

3

Tobacco control interventions: the scientific basis

When an argument is based on evidence there is little need for frequent quotations.
—*Michael Hopkins, on* http://www.talkorigins.org/faqs/quotes/

The TREMENDOUS ADVERSE EFFECTS of tobacco use on health and economic indicators worldwide makes tobacco control a public health imperative. Policy leaders and public health planners need to acknowledge and accept this fact if countries are to develop effective interventions to reduce tobacco use. The interventions must be proportionate in magnitude and scope to the tobacco epidemic.

The World Bank and WHO have considered the relative merits of a number of interventions to curb tobacco consumption. They can be divided into two general categories: those that seek to reduce the demand for tobacco and those that aim to reduce the supply of tobacco (see Table 1). Strategies to reduce demand can be further subdivided into price measures (seeking to increase tobacco prices) and non-price measures. In general, interventions to reduce the demand for tobacco are deemed more likely to succeed.

Ancillary measures include support for research into tobacco control, establishment of surveillance and monitoring systems, systematic exchange of information about tobacco and tobacco control, consideration of litigation to recover costs of tobacco-related health care, counteracting the tobacco industry and creation of funding mechanisms to assist developing countries.

Interventions to reduce demand: price measures

The impact of these measures can be summarized as follows.
- Raising the price of tobacco and tobacco products, primarily through tax increases, is the single most effective measure to reduce short-term consumption.
- More importantly, price has been shown to play a tremendous role in determining how many young people will start smoking, thus profoundly influencing long-term consumption trends.

Table 1. Interventions to reduce tobacco consumption

Interventions that reduce demand	Interventions that reduce supply
• Price measures: increasing prices of tobacco and tobacco products, primarily through taxes on tobacco • Non-price measures: – comprehensive bans on tobacco product advertising and promotion; – legislation to prohibit smoking in public places and workplaces; – use of prominent and strongly worded health warnings on cigarette packets; – information and advocacy campaigns; – cessation programmes to assist those who want to quit smoking	• Control of smuggling • Restricting access of minors to tobacco • Crop substitution for tobacco farms • Elimination of government subsidies for tobacco farming

- There is a clear inverse relationship between tobacco taxes and tobacco consumption. While there may be some differences among countries, overall for every 10% increase in cigarette taxes, there is approximately a 4% reduction in consumption.
- Young people, minorities, and low-income smokers are two to three times more likely to quit or smoke less than other smokers in response to price increases. Hence, raising the prices of tobacco and tobacco products protects those vulnerable segments of the population that are at greatest risk from tobacco.

Interventions to reduce demand: non-price measures

The impact of these measures can be summarized as follows.
- Comprehensive advertising bans: Research from 102 countries show that comprehensive advertising bans reduce cigarette consumption by 6% (1).
- No-smoking policies in public places and workplaces: Data from the USA indicate these policies can reduce tobacco consumption by 4% to 10%.
- Prominent health warnings: Half of the smokers intending to quit or reduce their consumption were motivated to do so by warnings on cigarette packets in Canada.
- Information and advocacy campaigns: In general, available data suggest that awareness of the dangers of smoking is not very high in low- and middle-income countries.
- Cessation programmes: In many countries, a day's supply of nicotine replacement therapy (NRT) costs about the same as the average daily consumption of tobacco. Increasing the use of NRT could persuade an additional 6 million smokers to quit, averting 1 million deaths.

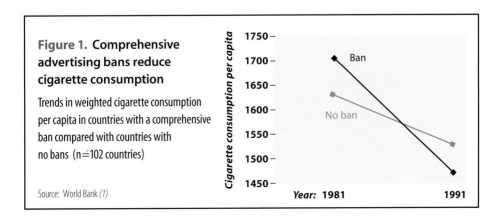

Figure 1. Comprehensive advertising bans reduce cigarette consumption

Trends in weighted cigarette consumption per capita in countries with a comprehensive ban compared with countries with no bans (n=102 countries)

Source: World Bank (1)

Interventions to reduce supply

Current approaches to restrict the supply of tobacco have shown little effect in reducing smoking. One important exception is the control of smuggling. As an immediate measure, national programmes for tobacco control should focus on the control of smuggling as the main intervention to reduce supply.

- Controlling smuggling: It is essential to tackle massive global smuggling *(2)*, which amounts to about one-third of all legally exported cigarettes and 6.5% of all cigarettes sold. Furthermore, cigarette smuggling causes immeasurable harm:
  - top international brands become available at affordable prices to low-income consumers and to image-conscious young people in developing countries;
  - illegal cigarettes evade legal restrictions and health regulations;
  - the industry uses the threat of increased smuggling to persuade governments not to raise tobacco tax;
  - governments lose tax revenue on every pack of smuggled cigarettes;
  - tobacco industry documents indicate that some of the tobacco companies themselves may be involved in smuggling operations.
- Some governments are now suing tobacco companies for the lost revenue associated with smuggling activities the companies are alleged to have condoned.
- Tackling the problem involves monitoring cigarette routes; installing tracking systems; using technologically sophisticated tax-paid markings on tobacco products; printing unique serial numbers on all packages of tobacco products; licensing manufacturers, exporters, importers, wholesalers, warehouses, transporters and retailers; and increasing penalties *(3)*.

Ancillary measures: litigation

Litigation cases now include smokers and non-smokers filing for damage to health; public interest law suits seeking to force the industry or government to comply with legal or constitutional requirements; governments suing for tobacco-attributable health care costs or for taxation lost because of smuggling; and cases brought by the tobacco industry against individuals, organizations or even governments. At the end of 2001, for instance, British American Tobacco faced 4419 lawsuits in the USA alone.

IMPACT OF INTERVENTIONS ON SMOKING INITIATION AND CESSATION

The different interventions have varying degrees of effectiveness. Table 2 shows that price increases are the most effective way of reducing initiation of smoking by youth, with much weaker evidence currently to show the effectiveness of education, advertising bans, or smoking restrictions and reducing youth access to tobacco. Price increases also encourage smokers to quit, as do a combination of other interventions.

Table 2. Impact of interventions on initiation and cessation

Intervention	Initiation	Cessation
10% price increase	3–10% decrease	11–13% shorter duration; 3% higher cessation
Anti-smoking media	Weak evidence	Increased attempts & success
Advertising & promotion bans	Reduces experimenting and initiation, higher effects on women	Complete ban reduces consumption by about 6%
Youth access	Weak evidence	No evidence
Smoking restrictions	Some evidence of lower initiation	Work and household restrictions most effective
Nicotine Replacement Therapy	No evidence	More people decide and attempt to quit

Source: Ross (4)

Key point:

For tobacco control to succeed, a comprehensive mix of policies and strategies is needed. If resources are limited, efforts should focus first on raising tobacco prices through increased taxes.

COST EFFECTIVENESS OF VARIOUS TOBACCO CONTROL INTERVENTIONS

One of the myths perpetuated about tobacco control is that it is neither relevant nor cost effective in developing countries. Table 3 shows that tobacco control interventions are cost effective in low/middle- and high-income countries, and that price increases are the most effective of all.

- In low- and middle-income countries, price measures are the most cost-effective way of reducing consumption, especially among young people, followed by non-price measures such as comprehensive bans on tobacco advertising and promotion; bans on smoking in public places including workplaces; strong warning labels; information and research. Pharmaceutical products are relatively more expensive.

- In high-income countries, price increases are still the most cost-effective measure, followed by pharmaceutical assistance with quitting, and non-price measures.

Table 3. Cost of various tobacco control interventions in low/middle- and high-income countries

Region	Values for various tobacco control interventions (US$ per DALY saved)		
	Price 10%	Non-price measure with 5% effectiveness	NRT with 25% cover
Low/middle-income	4–17	68–272	276–297
High-income	161–645	1 347–5 388	746–1 160

Source: World Bank *(1)*

Around the world, the product is the same or similar, hence the action that needs to be taken is the same, and the obstacles are the same. Interventions are highly cost-effective, but differ from one region to another.

- Many interventions, such as warnings on packages or the creation of smoke-free areas, cost nothing except political will. Some price measures, such as increasing tobacco tax and cracking down on smuggling, will actually increase government tax revenue, while reducing the number of young smokers and encouraging adults to quit.
- Some measures will cost money, but will be cost-effective (e.g. provision of quitting services, including nicotine replacement treatment, and bans on advertising and promotion).

BENEFITS OF TOBACCO CONTROL

Tobacco control makes economic sense to governments, employers and smokers in both rich and poor countries *(1)*. The magnitude of the tobacco epidemic, its pervasive and deadly impact on survival and health, and the significant resources it drains from individuals, families, the business sector and governments make tobacco control an urgent public health priority.

- Benefits to governments include:
  - more land to grow food instead of tobacco
  - reduced loss of foreign exchange to cigarette imports
  - reduced health care costs for smokers' illnesses
  - reduced costs of premature death
  - reduction in costs of fires caused by careless smoking
  - reduced maintenance costs of buildings, etc.

- Benefits to employers include:
  - more productive workforce (less illness, less time off work, no smoke breaks)
  - fewer fires and accidents
  - lower insurance
  - lower cleaning costs
  - reduced risk of being sued.
- Benefits to smokers and their families include:
  - money saved from purchasing cigarettes
  - less time off work
  - lower health care costs
  - less risk of passive smoking for the family
  - quitting is effective at any age and stage.

CONCLUSION

The tobacco epidemic is one of the greatest public health challenges in the history of humankind. No other legal substance is as deadly, or as powerfully addictive. Ironically, tobacco-related deaths and diseases are entirely preventable. The interventions to reduce tobacco consumption are known and well researched. In addition, the cost effectiveness of these interventions is established in both developed and developing countries.

Tobacco control is far from being the prerogative of western nations.

- The first known tobacco control regulation in the world was issued in Bhutan in 1729, banning tobacco use in all religious places, a ban that is still observed today.
- In general, tobacco control is more advanced in developed than in developing countries, though there are exceptions.
- For example, legislation is far stronger in Brazil, Fiji, Hong Kong SAR, Mongolia, Singapore, South Africa, Thailand and Viet Nam than in many western countries, showing that developing countries can tackle the epidemic.
- Singapore banned all advertising 30 years ago, celebrates World No Tobacco Month (not Day) each year, has banned duty free cigarettes, licenses tobacco retailers, and has the lowest prevalence rates in the world.
- Thailand has involved monks in the anti-smoking campaign, has a total advertising ban, requires ingredient disclosure, and has strong health warnings, including direct messages such as "Smoking causes impotence".

Previously, governments and public health planners tended to leave tobacco control in the hands of medical practitioners. The role of the health profession is vital, but we now know that the medical model alone is not enough. Tobacco control requires a comprehensive approach, using a strategic mix of policies, legislation and programme interventions, and the involvement of other partners in society.

The Health Ministry, as the main agency responsible for public health, should assume the leading role in promoting tobacco control at the national level. Governments should act quickly, supporting international efforts through the WHO FCTC and establishing solid national programmes to stem the devastating effects of the tobacco epidemic on current and future generations.

References

1. *Curbing the epidemic: Governments and the economics of tobacco control.* Washington, DC, The World Bank Development in Practice series, 1999.

2. Jha P, Chaloupka FJ. *Tobacco control in developing countries.* Oxford, Oxford University Press, 2000, Table 15.3, p. 373.

3. Joossens L, Raw M. Cigarette smuggling in Europe: who really benefits? *Tobacco control,* 1998, 7:66–71, Joossens L, Tobacco smuggling, *Tobacco Control Fact Sheet,* 21 Feb 2002 (http://www.ash.org.uk/html/factsheets/.html).

4. Ross H. *Economic determinants of smoking initiation and cessation.* Conference on public and private sector partnerships to reduce tobacco dependence, Prague, Czech Republic, 13–14 December 2001. Illinois, USA, International Tobacco Evidence Network, 2002.

Bibliography

Curbing the epidemic: governments and the economics of tobacco control. Washington, DC, The World Bank Development in Practice series, 1999.

International Consultation on Environmental Tobacco Smoke (ETS) and Child Health. 11–14 January 1999. Report. Geneva, World Health Organization, 1999 (WHO/NCD/TFI/99.10).

Jha P, Chaloupka FJ. *Tobacco control in developing countries.* Oxford, Oxford University Press, 2000.

Mackay J, Eriksen M. *The tobacco atlas.* Geneva, World Health Organization, 2002 (http://www.who.int/tobacco).

Samet JM, Yoon SY, eds. *Women and the tobacco epidemic: challenges for the 21st century.* Geneva, World Health Organization, 2001 (WHO/NMH/TFI/01.1).

Selin H, Bolis M. *Developing legislation for tobacco control: template and guidelines.* Washington, DC, Pan American Health Organization, 2002 (http://www.paho.org/Project.asp?SEL=TP&LNG=ENG&CD=SMOKE).

Simpson D. *Doctors and tobacco: medicine's big challenge.* Tobacco Control Resource Centre, British Medical Association, 2000.

The world health report 2002: Reducing risks, promoting healthy life. Geneva, World Health Organization, 2002 (http://www.who.int/whr/2002/en/).

Warner KE. The economics of tobacco: myths and realities. *Tobacco Control,* 2000; 9:78–89.

World Health Organization. The Framework Convention on Tobacco Control. Available in:

Arabic: http://www.who.int/gb/EB_WHA/PDF/WHA56/aa56r1.pdf
Chinese: http://www.who.int/gb/EB_WHA/PDF/WHA56/ca56r1.pdf
English: http://www.who.int/gb/EB_WHA/PDF/WHA56/ea56r1.pdf
French: http://www.who.int/gb/EB_WHA/PDF/WHA56/fa56r1.pdf
Russian: http://www.who.int/gb/EB_WHA/PDF/WHA56/ra56r1.pdf
Spanish: http://www.who.int/gb/EB_WHA/PDF/WHA56/sa56r1.pdf

4

The WHO Framework Convention on Tobacco Control (WHO FCTC): the political solution

The Framework Convention process will activate all those areas of governance that have a direct impact on public health... The challenge for us comes in seeking global and national solutions in tandem for a problem that cuts across national boundaries, cultures, societies and socioeconomic strata.

— *Dr Gro Harlem Brundtland, Director-General Emeritus, World Health Organization*

GLOBALIZATION AND INTERNATIONAL LAW

Globalization is the flow of information, goods, capital and people across political and geographical boundaries *(1)*. As a dynamic force driving countries towards greater economic, political and social interdependence, globalization has significant implications for the health of populations all over the world. For example, the epidemic of Severe Acute Respiratory Syndrome (SARS) demonstrated the contribution of international travel to the rapid global spread of an infectious disease. However, globalization offers great opportunities for the prevention and control of disease as well.

Public health protection has traditionally been viewed as falling within the domain of national concern *(2)*. Because of globalization, however, many issues related to health no longer respect the geographical confines of sovereign states, and can no longer be resolved by national policies alone *(3)*. As domestic and international spheres of health policy become more intertwined *(3),* the opportunity arises to apply international legal instruments to address global public health problems *(4)*. With globalization comes the need for global ethical and scientific norms, standards and commitments in public health that are legally binding *(5),* that deal with global threats to health and that create opportunities for promoting health.

Global integration has produced a paradigm shift: public health is a topic of global concern, and countries are recognizing the global dimension of public health. In this respect, the desired outcomes in public health can be viewed as global public goods (GPGs) for health *(6)*. GPGs can be further subdivided into intermediate GPGs and final GPGs.

- Intermediate GPGs, like international regimes, contribute to providing final GPGs *(7)*.
- Final GPGs are 'outcomes' rather than 'goods' as commonly understood. They may be tangible, like the environment or the common heritage of humankind, or intangible, such as peace or financial stability.

Since there is no supranational authority that can provide global public goods, greater intersectoral action and transnational cooperation and partnerships are needed to attain final GPGs as tangible outcomes. A central component of this cooperation is the expanded use of international instruments, including conventional international law *(8)*. International legal agreements such as the WHO FCTC are among the most important intermediate public health goods that will actively contribute to attaining the final GPG. In the case of the WHO FCTC, this means reducing the burden of disease and death attributable to tobacco *(9)* and thus improving global public health.

THE WHO FCTC AND THE GLOBALIZATION
OF THE TOBACCO EPIDEMIC

The WHO FCTC was developed in response to the current globalization of the tobacco epidemic, which was amplified by a variety of complex factors with cross-border effects, including trade liberalization, foreign direct investment, global marketing, transnational tobacco advertising, promotion and sponsorship, and the international movement of contraband and counterfeit cigarettes. This global epidemic constitutes one of the major public health disasters of the 20th century. Currently, in the 21st century, the epidemic of tobacco addiction, disease and death is rapidly shifting to developing and transitional market countries; the majority of smokers today are in developing countries. If this trend goes unchecked, it has been projected that within the next two or three decades tobacco will not only be the leading cause of premature mortality in industrialized nations, but also the leading cause of premature death worldwide *(10)*. Indeed, in low-mortality developing countries, tobacco is already a leading cause of preventable morbidity and mortality *(11)*.

In order to strengthen and coordinate global responses to the tobacco epidemic, the World Health Assembly adopted, on 24 May 1999, a resolution to pave the way for accelerated multilateral negotiations on a WHO framework convention on tobacco control and possible related protocols. This represented the first time that WHO Member States had exercised their treaty-making powers under Article 19 of the WHO Constitution, which stipulates that "the Health Assembly shall have authority to adopt conventions or agreements with respect to any matter within the competence of the Organization" *(12)*.

The launching of the WHO FCTC negotiations was catalysed by the unique convergence of a number of factors:

- Accumulation of solid scientific evidence over a 50-year period, demonstrating the causal links between tobacco use and over 20 major categories of disease *(13)*, and evidence pointing to the global toll of tobacco-related diseases.
- Strengthening of the evidence pointing to the adverse economic implications of the tobacco epidemic; the work of the World Bank has been crucial in this area *(13)*.
- Strengthening of the evidence that cost-effective tobacco control measures exist *(13)*.
- Release of over 35 million pages of previously secret tobacco industry documents as a result of litigation in the United States, which provided a unique opportunity to better understand the strategies and tactics of the tobacco industry and, in doing so, to advance the public health agenda *(14)*.
- Establishment of a WHO cabinet project, the Tobacco Free Initiative, to focus international attention, resources and action on the global tobacco epidemic. This new initiative provided a platform to push forward the negotiation mandate for WHO's first treaty-making enterprise.
- The examples of various countries with successful tobacco control experiences. These countries have different legislative and political systems, cultural characteristics, stages of development and tobacco production features *(15)*.

- The support of civil society in the form of public pressure on governments for tougher tobacco regulations as the public becomes more aware of the dangers of tobacco *(15)*.

The regulatory approach adopted in drafting the WHO FCTC is a novel one. The regulation of tobacco products has presented a regulatory conundrum. For instance, cigarettes sit in a regulatory no-man's-land, in that they are neither completely regulated as licit products nor treated as illicit ones *(16)*. The WHO FCTC focuses on the global implementation of evidence-based strategies to decrease demand rather than focusing on the supply side of the equation, as is the case with drug control treaties *(14)*. In this respect, the WHO FCTC represents a paradigm shift in developing regulatory strategies for addictive substances: in contrast to previous drug control treaties, the WHO FCTC asserts the importance of reducing demand as well as supply.

The idea behind the WHO FCTC and future related protocols is that it will act as a global complement to, not a replacement for, national and local tobacco control actions. The conclusion of the WHO FCTC negotiations and the opening of the Convention for signature and ratification[1] represent a landmark opportunity for countries to strengthen their national tobacco control capacity and improve the health of the world's population.

THE WHO FCTC PROCESS AND THE LESSONS LEARNED

The framework convention/protocol approach

The legal model chosen to tackle global tobacco control was the framework convention/protocol approach. The term 'framework convention' is used to describe a variety of legal agreements that establish broad commitments and a general system of governance for an issue. Unlike comprehensive treaties[2] which try to address all issues in one document – the Law of the Sea Agreement, for example – a framework convention is accompanied by protocols.[3] A framework convention establishes consensus on the relevant facts and obligations required for an appropriate international response, while protocols supplement, amend or qualify that framework convention and usually establish more specific commitments or additional institutional arrangements *(17, 18)*. Thus, the negotiation of a framework convention is not a complete process but the beginning of one that will include the formulation of one or more protocols.

For the WHO FCTC, two initial protocols were favoured by a number of negotiating States: one on illicit trade in tobacco products, and one on the elimination of

---

[1] Hereinafter, ratification also refers to its legal equivalents, namely acceptance, approval, accession or formal confirmation.

[2] A treaty is an international legal agreement concluded between States in written form, and governed by international law; a convention is a different name for a treaty.

[3] A protocol is also a type of treaty. It typically supplements, clarifies, amends or qualifies an existing international agreement, for example, a framework convention.

cross-border advertising, promotion and sponsorship. It was decided at the World Health Assembly in May 2003 that the decision on the negotiation of future protocols should rest with the Conference of the Parties once the treaty enters into force. This decision is consistent with the text set forth in Article 33 of the treaty, which stipulates that "only Parties to the Convention may be Parties to a protocol".

The history of the WHO FCTC

Just over a decade ago, the idea of something like the WHO FCTC, an international treaty for public health, would have seemed implausible. The courage and leadership of key people such as Celso Amorim, the Foreign Minister of Brazil, Ambassador Seixas Corrêa of Brazil, and Dr Brundtland, the then-Director-General of WHO, helped to make the final text of the WHO FCTC a reality. The negotiation of the treaty was difficult and many challenges were met along the way. The foresight of the Brazilian Chairs of the negotiating body, Minister Amorim and Ambassador Seixas Corrêa, ensured that the negotiating process was kept on track and that the text was adopted according to the timetable set forth in the initial World Health Resolution adopted in May 1999.

The first session of the Intergovernmental Negotiating Body was convened in Geneva from 16 to 21 October 2000. The provisional texts of the proposed draft elements for a WHO framework convention on tobacco control, which were the output of a pre-negotiation working group, were accepted as a sound basis for initiating negotiations. Subsequently, Minister Amorim prepared a chair's text of the Framework Convention; that first draft was released in January 2001 as a basis for further negotiations at the second session.

At the second session of the negotiating body (Geneva, 30 April – 5 May 2001), responsibility for consideration of the proposed draft elements was divided between three working groups. The principal output was the set of three co-chairs' working papers, an inventory of textual proposals made at the session merged with the chair's original text. These working papers became the draft text of the WHO FCTC.

At the third session (Geneva, 22–28 November 2001), two working groups issued revised texts and Working Group One later drafted a text. Those documents were used to further negotiations during the fourth session.

Having taken over as Permanent Representative of Brazil in Geneva, in replacement of Minister Amorim, Ambassador Seixas Corrêa was elected Chair of the Intergovernmental Negotiating Body on the WHO Framework Convention on Tobacco Control during its fourth session (Geneva, 18–23 March 2002).

It was agreed that Ambassador Seixas Corrêa should prepare a new chair's text, which would form the basis of negotiations during the fifth session of the negotiating body (14–25 October 2002). The text was released in July 2002. The first four sessions of the negotiating body had considered numerous textual alternatives. Concerted deliberations at the fifth session narrowed the options, resulting in more focused negotiations.

The sixth and final session of the negotiating body ran from 17 February to 1 March 2003. The negotiations were intense and broad ranging. Important issues such as advertising, promotion and sponsorship, and financial resources were discussed in two informal groups. At the final plenary meeting, the Intergovernmental Negotiating Body agreed to transmit the text to the 56th World Health Assembly to be considered for adoption in accordance with Article 19 of the Constitution. Public health history was made when the text was adopted unanimously by the 56th World Health Assembly on 21 May 2003.

The power of the process

Multisectoral partnerships will play a critical role in the post-adoption stage of the WHO FCTC process. While a lack of multisectoral coordination and collaboration constituted a challenge during negotiations, the process left governments more aware and motivated than ever before to implement comprehensive tobacco control measures. The WHO FCTC also provides a powerful incentive for several ministries to be involved.

The negotiation of the WHO FCTC itself served to galvanize tobacco control measures at national, regional and global levels. Many countries have created multisectoral tobacco control committees to prepare for the WHO FCTC negotiation. The treaty-making process has created the opportunity to broaden the dialogue to ministries of foreign affairs, trade and agriculture as well. The WHO FCTC process has also catalysed national coordinating committees, bringing together different sectors. WHO provided technical briefings and seed grants to countries to encourage this process. For example, as part of its role in strengthening national capacities for tobacco control, WHO provided seed grants to several countries from different regions to initiate or strengthen national tobacco control activities through key intervention areas. WHO also provided technical assistance to those countries through workshops, such as the one held in Rio de Janeiro for the group of Portuguese-speaking countries. The project "Protecting youth against tobacco in five countries" of the United Nations Foundation (UNF) incorporates the national capacity-building framework of WHO. Pilot countries have identified national professional officers for tobacco control, and are developing national plans of action and working on certain key intervention areas in tobacco control. Under this project, key partnerships for tobacco control have been formed within countries, between different ministries, public health institutes, and NGOs as well as other international agencies that would contribute to the sustainability of tobacco control.

The WHO FCTC process also won support from the civil society, particularly among NGOs. When the WHO FCTC negotiation process was being initiated in 1998, only a handful of NGOs were aware and interested in being part of this pioneering public health process. At the end of the negotiations an international alliance of over 200 NGOs had rallied behind the WHO FCTC. These NGOs are in the forefront of efforts to counteract attempts by the tobacco industry to undermine effective tobacco control programmes. In October 2000, before the formal negotiations began,

WHO organized global public hearings, the first in the Organization's history. Those hearings provided an opportunity for all members of civil society, from public health groups to farmers and tobacco industry groups, to express their views on the WHO FCTC negotiations: over 500 submissions were received during this exercise, and over 140 NGOs provided verbal testimonies in Geneva.

At the global level, a United Nations Task Force under the leadership of WHO was established by Secretary-General Kofi Annan to consolidate support for tobacco control within the United Nations system. The Ad Hoc Interagency Task Force on Tobacco Control was established in 1999 to intensify joint United Nations response and to galvanize global support for tobacco control; the Task Force includes agencies such as the Food and Agriculture Organization (FAO), the International Labour Organization (ILO), the IMF, the United Nations Development Programme (UNDP), the United Nations Environment Programme (UNEP), the United Nations Children's Fund (UNICEF), the World Bank (WB) and the WTO.

What is the WHO FCTC?

The WHO FCTC is a delicately balanced package deal. It is essential to be aware of provisions that create obligations for Parties to implement effective legislative, executive, administrative or other measures in response to the need to reduce the prevalence of tobacco use and exposure to tobacco smoke.

The objective of the Convention set forth in Article 3 provides a unique opportunity to improve public health and to reduce death and suffering attributable to tobacco:

> The objective of this Convention and its protocols is to protect present and future generations from the devastating health, social, environmental and economic consequences of tobacco consumption and exposure to tobacco smoke by providing a framework for tobacco control measures to be implemented by the Parties at the national, regional and international levels in order to reduce continually and substantially the prevalence of tobacco use and exposure to tobacco smoke *(19)*.

The growing global consensus on these best practices is now crystallized in the WHO FCTC. After it has entered into force, this important treaty will obligate countries that have become Parties to it to enact legislative or regulatory measures in a number of specific areas. Independently of its formal obligations, however, the treaty identifies the most effective legislative strategies in most areas. In this respect, the WHO FCTC may be used as a truly global framework for action, even in countries that may not become Parties to the treaty.

The WHO FCTC recognizes this logical starting point, and requires each Party, acting in accordance with its capabilities, "[to] establish or reinforce and finance a national coordinating mechanism or focal point for tobacco control..." *(20)* This mechanism may be a centralized office within the ministry of health or similar agency. For example, in 1989 Thailand formally established an interagency committee, consisting, inter alia, of the Ministry of Public Health and the Department of Medical Services *(21)*. This committee is responsible for formulating the country's policy on tobacco control *(21)*. Alternatively, responsibility for different aspects of the programme may be divided among several agencies, as is the case of Brazil, where the national tobacco control programme is directed by an office accountable to the Ministry of Health, while a separate regulatory agency is responsible for product regulation.

From the first preambular paragraph, which states that the "Parties to this Convention [are] determined to give priority to their right to protect public health…", the WHO FCTC is a global trendsetter. As noted above, it has established a new paradigm for regulating the consumption of addictive substances.

The specific provisions concerning the reduction of tobacco demand and supply are contained in articles 6–17 of the WHO FCTC.

On the demand reduction factor of the tobacco control equations, the WHO FCTC calls upon the Parties to enact, update and implement effective legislative, executive, administrative or other measures in the following areas:

- **Price and tax measures to reduce the demand for tobacco (Article 6).** Price and tax measures are an effective and important means of reducing tobacco consumption, especially among young people *(22)* – a fact specifically recognized by the WHO FCTC *(23)*.

- **Protection from exposure to tobacco smoke (Article 8).** The WHO FCTC requires Parties to adopt and implement effective legislative, executive, administrative and/or other measures "providing for protection from exposure to tobacco smoke in indoor workplaces, public transport, indoor public places and, as appropriate, other public places" *(24)*. Where a Party lacks legal jurisdiction to do this at the national level, it is to "actively promote" equivalent measures at the subnational level *(24)*. The scientific evidence leaves little doubt that the way to achieve genuine protection is to require smoke-free environments in these settings.

- **Regulation of the contents of tobacco products (Article 9).** The Conference of the Parties is to develop guidelines that can be used by countries for testing, measuring and regulating contents and emissions. Parties must adopt pertinent measures at the national level.

- **Regulation of tobacco product disclosures (Article 10).** In addition, the WHO FCTC obligates countries to require that manufacturers and importers of tobacco products disclose to governmental authorities information about product contents and emissions. Measures for public disclosure of information must also be adopted.

- **Packaging and labelling of tobacco products (Article 11).** The tobacco package provides a potent vehicle for tobacco promotion, and has increased in importance within the "marketing mix" as other forms of promotion are restricted *(25)*. Aside from the obvious visibility of packages to smokers each time they light a cigarette, tobacco retailers in many countries are paid by tobacco companies to prominently display tobacco packages row upon row near the cash register, providing an attractive promotional display just at the point when consumers are ready to purchase *(26)*.

Conversely, if conspicuous health warnings are required on packages, their display becomes a valuable vehicle for health promotion messages. Seen by every smoker several times a day, packages are one of the most cost-effective communication tools available to governments to educate and inform consumers about the harmful effects of tobacco use *(27)*. Consistent with this, many countries use tobacco packages to educate the public, primarily by requiring manufacturers to place a prominent warning label on each package. The acknowledged best practice in this area is the approach that has been implemented by Brazil and Canada, where half of the main display panels of cigarette packages must be devoted to a rotating series of bold, full-colour warning labels, using photos and other visual images, and conveying a strong health message [4]. The WHO FCTC makes this approach the global standard, requiring each Party to adopt and implement, within 3 years of the entry into force of the Convention for that Party, effective measures requiring large, clear health warnings, using rotating messages approved by a designated national authority *(28)*. The WHO FCTC provides that these warnings should cover 50% or more of the principal display areas, as is already done in Brazil and Canada; the warnings must occupy at least 30% *(29)*.

A second important role of packaging and labelling legislation is to prevent manufacturers from using packages to mislead consumers. The WHO FCTC requires that, within 3 years of the entry into force of the Convention for a State, each Party adopt and implement, in accordance with their national law, effective measures to ensure that: "(a) tobacco product packaging and labelling do not promote a tobacco product by any means that are false, misleading, deceptive or likely to create an erroneous impression about its characteristics, health effects, hazards or emissions, including any term, descriptor, trademark, figurative or any other sign that directly or indirectly creates the false impression that a particular tobacco product is less harmful than other tobacco products. These may include terms such as 'low tar', 'light', 'ultra-light', or 'mild'…" *(30)*. Given the importance of such measures, it would be highly desirable to include them in any comprehensive legislation on tobacco control, even in countries that are not Parties to the WHO FCTC.

- **Education, communication, training and public awareness (Article 12).** Large, sustained public information campaigns are an important way of changing the attitudes, beliefs and norms of society. The WHO FCTC requires Parties to adopt legislative, executive, administrative or other measures that promote public awareness and access to information on the addictiveness of tobacco, the health risks of tobacco use and exposure to smoke, the benefits of cessation and the actions of the tobacco industry.

- **Tobacco advertising, promotion and sponsorship (Article 13).** The WHO FCTC requires each Party, "in accordance with its constitution or constitutional principles, [to] undertake a comprehensive ban of all tobacco advertising, promotion and sponsorship. [...] within the period of 5 years after entry into force of this Convention for that Party …". [5] This is a centrepiece of an evidence-based programme.

---

[4] Examples of the warning labels required in Brazil and Canada may be found at http://www.anvisa.gov.br/divulga/ noticias/040601_1.htm (Brazil) and http://www.hc-sc.gc.ca/english/media/photos/tobacco_labelling/(Canada).

[5] WHO Framework Convention on Tobacco Control, Article 13. The treaty defines "tobacco advertising and promotion" as "any form of commercial communication, recommendation or action with the aim, effect or likely effect of promoting a tobacco product or tobacco use either directly or indirectly". "Tobacco sponsorship" is defined as "any form of contribution to any event, activity or individual with the aim, effect or likely effect of promoting a tobacco product or tobacco use either directly or indirectly". Article 1.

Parties whose constitution or constitutional principles do not allow them to undertake a comprehensive ban must apply a series of restrictions on all advertising, promotion and sponsorship of tobacco products *(31)*.

- **Demand reduction measures concerning tobacco dependence and cessation (Article 14).** Measures to encourage tobacco users to quit are an integral part of a comprehensive approach; they complement strategies focused on education and prevention. The WHO FCTC requires Parties to discharge this duty by endeavouring to:
  - create cessation programmes, not only in health care facilities, but also in workplaces, educational institutions and other settings;
  - include diagnosis and treatment of nicotine dependence in national health programmes;
  - establish programmes for diagnosis, counselling and treatment in health care facilities and rehabilitation centres;
  - collaborate with other countries to increase the accessibility of cessation therapies, including pharmaceutical products *(32)*.

Regarding the supply side of tobacco control, the WHO FCTC calls upon the Parties to enact, update and implement effective legislative, executive, administrative or other measures in the following areas:

- **Illicit trade in tobacco products (Article 15).** The WHO FCTC recognizes that eliminating smuggling and other forms of illicit trade in tobacco products is an essential component of tobacco control *(33)*. The WHO FCTC requires Parties to take a number of steps such as:
  - strengthening anti-smuggling laws;
  - ensuring that all tobacco packages are marked to assist tracing;
  - requiring that packages be marked to indicate their country of destination;
  - cooperating with other countries to monitor and control the movement of products and investigate their diversion;
  - developing a tracking and tracing regime;
  - gathering and exchanging data on cross-border tobacco trade in illicit products; and
  - seizing and destroying contraband products and confiscating the proceeds of illicit trade *(34)*.

Parties should also try to adopt additional measures, including, where appropriate:
  - licensing, which can be used to identify, monitor and control the actors in the chain of distribution. Beyond these steps, the WHO FCTC calls for regional, subregional and international cooperation in combating illicit trade, including investigating and prosecuting violations. These treaty obligations provide a checklist of possible legislative elements.

- **Sales to and by minors (Article 16).** This article contains provisions on sales methods that include:
  - restrictions on the quantity in which tobacco products can be sold. In accordance with the WHO FCTC, Parties must try to prohibit the sale of cigarettes individually or in small packets that are more affordable for minors *(35)*;

– requirements that signs be posted at retail locations. Depending on the approach taken, signs may further the government's health goals or detract from them. Some signs, particularly those created in tobacco industry "youth smoking prevention" programmes, may actually send subtle messages that encourage youth smoking, while strong visual images combined with informational messages may reinforce the law and educate the public;

– prohibition of any visible display of tobacco products, to prevent the product packages themselves from being used as a promotional vehicle. Subnational governments in Australia and Canada have restricted or banned displays *(36);*

– a ban on the sale of tobacco by minors. The WHO FCTC provides that countries should take measures to prohibit the sale of tobacco by minors *(37).*

- **Support for economically viable alternative activities (Article 17)**. In this and other articles of the Convention, the WHO FCTC recognizes the need to assist tobacco growers and workers whose livelihoods are seriously affected by tobacco control programmes *(38),* and encourages countries to support crop diversification and other economically viable alternatives as part of sustainable development strategies *(39).*

Another novel feature of the WHO FCTC is the inclusion of the issue of liability as a core provision of the treaty *(40).* Liability issues have not typically been included in other framework conventions, mainly because such issues are often controversial and risk stalling the negotiations on other core provisions. Despite this, the negotiators of the WHO FCTC forged ahead to draft a provision on liability. The WHO FCTC notes that issues related to liability represent another important part of comprehensive tobacco control *(41).* Moreover, the WHO FCTC specifically directs countries to consider using legislation to deal with civil and criminal liability *(42).*

One of the core functions of many treaties is to facilitate scientific cooperation and exchange of information. Provisions concerning such important issues are contained in the following articles of the WHO FCTC:

- Article 20 – Research, surveillance and exchange of information;
- Article 21 – Reporting and exchange of information;
- Article 22 – Cooperation in the scientific, technical and legal fields and provision of related expertise.

Not all treaties provide for funding and technical assistance for the implementation of the instrument. The WHO FCTC, however, belongs to the unique family of international agreements that undertakes to provide for such resources. These provisions are enshrined in Article 26 of the treaty. The treaty commits Parties to provide resources for their national tobacco control measures, and also encourages the use of innovative funding mechanisms and financial resources, including transfer of technology to enable developing country Parties and Parties with economies in transition to meet their obligations under the Convention.

Finally, it should be noted that the WHO FCTC represents a global minimum standard. This is acknowledged in Article 2 of the Convention where "Parties are encouraged to implement measures beyond those required by this Convention and its protocols…" *(43).*

Following the adoption by the World Health Assembly, the text was deposited with the Secretary-General of the United Nations and opened for signature.

POST-ADOPTION PHASE OF THE WHO FCTC PROCESS

A crucial phase of the work on the WHO FCTC commenced after its adoption in May 2003. After adoption, much of the work surrounding the treaty shifted from the international to the national and subregional levels. Article 36 of the final draft of the Convention stipulates that 40 ratifications or its equivalent will be required before the treaty enters into force, in other words before it has legal effect or becomes legally binding for those countries that ratify the treaty. The WHO FCTC was formally opened for signature from 16 to 22 June 2003 in Geneva, and thereafter at the United Nations headquarters, the depositary of the treaty, from 30 June 2003 to 29 June 2004. Under international law, the only three authorities that may sign treaties without further formalities are heads of state, heads of government and ministers of foreign affairs. Any other authority, including ministers other than the minister for foreign affairs, needs to submit full powers in order to sign the Convention. The power of the political support behind the WHO FCTC is evidenced by the impressive number of signatories of the Convention: in the first 6 months after the treaty opened for signature, almost one half of WHO Member States signed the WHO FCTC. Additionally, several countries proceeded to become Parties to the Convention shortly after 16 June 2003.

The signing of the WHO FCTC by a State indicates its intention to become a Party to the Convention but does not yet carry substantial obligations. The signature of a treaty, however, also produces some limited rights and obligations even before its entry into force. For example, a signatory has the right to receive notifications by the depositary concerning the treaty. Conversely, a signatory is under an obligation to refrain from acts that would defeat the object and purpose of the treaty, until it shall have made clear that it does not intend to become a Party to the treaty (Article 18 of the Vienna Convention).

Becoming a Party to the WHO FCTC commits a State to implementing the provisions of the treaty. The WHO FCTC will come into force 90 days after the date of deposit of the fortieth instrument of ratification or its equivalent with the United Nations Depositary. At that time, those States that have become Parties to the WHO FCTC will be legally bound by its provisions. For any State that becomes a Party to the treaty following the 40th ratification or its equivalent, the treaty will come into force 90 days after that Party's deposit of its instrument of ratification or its equivalent. States or regional economic integration organizations, for example the European Community, that do not become Parties to the treaty are not bound by its provisions.

The phase of becoming a Party to the convention is clearly a critical one for the WHO FCTC. Aside from the goal of achieving 40 ratifications or its equivalent to ensure its entry into force, this phase can be used by countries to examine their national tobacco control capacity (in terms of the necessary human resources, technical expertise, financial resources and political will) and ability to become a Party to and implement the treaty *(44)*. The domestic requirements for entry into force are governed by national law, frequently the national constitution. Domestic requirements "specify which treaties may be entered into on the sole authority of the executive, and which require some sort of legislative concurrence and, if so, by what house(s) and what majorities... They may also specify certain matters that a state may not do, and therefore which it cannot commit itself to by treaty" *(45)*. At the domestic level, approval of ratification of the WHO FCTC, or its equivalent, requires a series of steps that may include:

> translation of the WHO FCTC and ancillary documents into the national language; a survey of the State's existing international legal obligations to assess whether conflicts exist between those treaties and the WHO FCTC; a similar survey of the State's constitutional and statutory prescripts; and an assessment of whether the legal regime established by the Convention is beneficial to the State *(46)*.

What authorities are responsible for these steps will vary widely from one state to another depending on the structure of government and the distribution of authority.

CONCLUSION

The WHO FCTC provisions are laying the foundation of the national capacity-building process. General obligations are defined as follows:

- establishment or strengthening and financing of national coordinating mechanisms or focal points for tobacco control;
- adoption and implementation of effective legislative, executive, administrative and/or other measures and cooperation as appropriate, with other Parties in developing appropriate policies for preventing and reducing tobacco consumption, nicotine addiction and exposure to tobacco smoke.

The post-adoption phase highlights the need for country-level actions and for the political and logistic infrastructure to address core issues for a successful tobacco control programme. Success in controlling the tobacco epidemic is a question of resources and political will. The problems and solutions are clear, and political will has increased as a result of the WHO FCTC process. In order to sustain progress, it is essential that country capacity for tobacco control be strengthened and sustained, particularly in developing countries and countries in transition, to enable them to meet key obligations in the WHO FCTC and to implement related policies and programmes. The global community now has the opportunity to sustain both country-based and international efforts. Thanks to the momentum generated by an international treaty it can make significant global progress against the gains of the tobacco industry.

With the advent of the WHO FCTC, comprehensive tobacco control has effectively been redefined. In the past, the implementation of comprehensive tobacco control strategies focused predominantly on national and local actions. With the realization that even the best national tobacco control regimes can be undermined by cross-border factors, the need to implement global measures, as contained in the WHO FCTC, has become imperative. Countries aiming to implement comprehensive tobacco control strategies in the future will need to enact the WHO FCTC provisions as a complement to their national and local measures.

Therefore, in order to maximize use of the WHO FCTC as a tool for public health, we need to make it a reality at country level by utilizing it as a complement to, rather than a substitute for, the work that needs to be done there. The web of partnerships developed during the negotiations of the WHO FCTC will help to prepare the implementation of the WHO FCTC at country level. In the words of WHO's Director-General, Dr Jong-Wook Lee:

> The WHO FCTC negotiations have already unleashed a process that has resulted in visible differences at country level. The success of the WHO FCTC as a tool for public health will depend on the energy and political commitment that we devote to implementing it, in countries in the coming years. A successful result will be global public health gains for all.

In order to obtain this result, the drive and commitment, which characterized the negotiations, will need to spread to the national and local levels so that the idea of the WHO FCTC becomes a reality.

References

1. Daulaire N. *Globalization and health.* Paper presented at the International Round Table on Responses to globalization: rethinking equity and health. Geneva, July 1999.

2. Taylor A, Bettcher DW. WHO Framework Convention on Tobacco Control: a global "good" for public health. *Bulletin of the World Health Organization*, 2000, 78(7):920.

3. Taylor A, Bettcher DW, Peck R. International law and the international legislative process: The WHO Framework Convention on Tobacco Control. In: Smith et al., eds. *Global public goods for health.* Oxford, Oxford University Press, 2003:Chapter 11.

4. Yach D, Bettcher DW. The globalization of public health: threats and opportunities. *American Journal of Public Health,* 1998, 88(5):735–38.

5. Resolution WHA 51.7. Health for all in the twenty-first century. In: *Fifty-first World Health Assembly, Geneva, 11–16 May, 1998. Volume I. Resolutions and decisions, and list of participants.* Geneva, World Health Organization, 1998 (WHA51/1998/REC/1).

6. Chen LC, Evans TG, Cash RA. Health as a global public good. In: Kaul I, Grundberg I, Stern MA, eds. *Global Public Goods.* New York, Oxford University Press, 1999:284–304.

7. Kaul I, Grundberg I, Stern MA. Defining global public goods. In: Kaul I, Grundberg I, Stern MA, eds. *Global Public Goods.* New York, Oxford University Press, 1999:xix-xxxviii.

8. Taylor A, Bettcher DW. WHO Framework Convention on Tobacco Control: a global "good" for public health. *Bulletin of the World Health Organization*, 2000, 78 (7):922.

9. Taylor A, Bettcher DW, Peck R. International law and the international legislative process: The WHO Framework Convention on Tobacco Control. In: Smith R et al., eds. *Global public goods for health.* Oxford, Oxford University Press, 2003: Chapter 11.

10. *The world health report 2002: reducing risks, promoting healthy life.* Geneva, World Health Organization, 2002:225.

11. *Basic Documents, 42nd ed.* Geneva, World Health Organization, 2002:7.

12. Doll R. Uncovering the effects of smoking: historical perspective. *Statistical Methods in Medical Research*, 1998, 7: 87–117.

13. Jha P, Chaloupka FJ, eds. *Curbing the Epidemic: Governments and the Economics of Tobacco Control.* Washington, DC, The World Bank, 1999.

14. Yach D, Bettcher DW. Globalisation of tobacco industry influence and new global responses. *Tobacco Control,* 2000, 9(2):206–216.

15. Da Costa e Silva VL, Nikogosian H. Convenio marco de la OMS para el control del tabaco: la globalizacion de la salud publica.[WHO Framework Convention on Tobacco Control: the globalization of public health.] *Prevencion del Tabaquismo* [Prevention of tobacco addiction], 2003, 5(2):71–75.

16. Bettcher DW. International law and health – Two approaches: the World Health Organization's Tobacco Initiative and international drug controls. In: *Proceedings of the 94th annual meeting of the American Society of International Law.* Washington, DC, American Society of International Law, 2000:196.

17. Bodansky D. *The Framework Convention Protocol Approach.* Geneva, World Health Organization, 1999 (WHO/NCD/TFI99.1).

18. Taylor AL, Roemer R. *An international strategy for tobacco control.* Geneva, World Health Organization, 1996 (WHO/PSA/96.6).

19. WHO Framework Convention on Tobacco Control. Geneva, World Health Organization, 2003. Article 3.

20. WHO Framework Convention on Tobacco Control. Geneva, World Health Organization, 2003. Article 5, paragraph 2.

21. Personal communication, Hatai Chitanondh, President of Thailand Health Promotion Institute, 2003.

22. *Curbing the epidemic: Governments and the economics of tobacco control.* Washington, DC, The World Bank, Development in Practice series:39–43, 1999 (http://www1.worldbank.org/tobacco/reports.htm)

23. WHO Framework Convention on Tobacco Control. Geneva, World Health Organization, 2003. Article 6, paragraph 1.

24. WHO Framework Convention on Tobacco Control. Geneva, World Health Organization, 2003. Article 8, paragraph 2.

25. Wakefield M et al. The cigarette pack as image: new evidence from tobacco industry documents. *Tobacco Control*, 2002, 11:73i–80.

26. Feighery EC et al. Cigarette advertising and promotional strategies in retail outlets: results of a statewide survey in California. *Tobacco Control,* 2001, 10:184–188.

27. Mahood G. Warnings that tell the truth: breaking new ground in Canada. *Tobacco Control,* 1999, 8:356–362.

28. WHO Framework Convention on Tobacco Control. Geneva, World Health Organization, 2003. Article 11, paragraph 1.

29. WHO Framework Convention on Tobacco Control. Geneva, World Health Organization, 2003. Article 11, paragraph 1(b).

30. WHO Framework Convention on Tobacco Control. Geneva, World Health Organization, 2003. Article 11, paragraph 1(a).

31. WHO Framework Convention on Tobacco Control. Geneva, World Health Organization, 2003. Article 13, paragraphs 3–8.

32. WHO Framework Convention on Tobacco Control. Geneva, World Health Organization, 2003. Article 14, paragraph 2.

33. WHO Framework Convention on Tobacco Control. Geneva, World Health Organization, 2003. Article 15, paragraph 1.

34. WHO Framework Convention on Tobacco Control. Geneva, World Health Organization, 2003. Article 15, paragraph 4.

35. WHO Framework Convention on Tobacco Control. Geneva, World Health Organization, 2003. Article 16, paragraph 3.

36. WHO Framework Convention on Tobacco Control. Geneva, World Health Organization, 2003. Article 16, paragraph 1.

37. WHO Framework Convention on Tobacco Control. Geneva, World Health Organization, 2003. Article 16, paragraph 7.

38. WHO Framework Convention on Tobacco Control. Geneva, World Health Organization, 2003. Article 4, paragraph 6, and Article 17.

39. WHO Framework Convention on Tobacco Control. Geneva, World Health Organization, 2003. Article 26, paragraph 3.

40. WHO Framework Convention on Tobacco Control. Geneva, World Health Organization, 2003. Article 19.

41. WHO Framework Convention on Tobacco Control. Geneva, World Health Organization, Article 4, paragraph 5; Blanke D. *Towards health with justice: litigation and public inquiries as tools for tobacco control*. Geneva, World Health Organization, 2002 (http://repositories.cdlib.org/tc/reports/WHO1).

42. WHO Framework Convention on Tobacco Control. Geneva, World Health Organization, 2003. Article 19, paragraph 1.

43. WHO Framework Convention on Tobacco Control. Geneva, World Health Organization, 2003. Article 2, paragraph 1.

44. Blanke D. *Tobacco control legislation: an introductory guide*. Geneva, World Health Organization, 2003: Chapter IV.

45. Szasz P. General law-making processes. In: Joyner C, ed. *The United Nations and international law* . Cambridge, Cambridge University Press, 1995:87.

46. Blanke D. *Tobacco control legislation: an introductory guide*. Geneva, World Health Organization, 2003: Chapter XII.

Part II

Putting theory into practice

Part II
Putting theory into practice

5

Developing a national plan of action

*In nothing do men more nearly approach
the gods than in giving health to men.*

—*Cicero*

Nearly all countries proclaim their commitment to providing health for the people *(1)* in national policy, seeking to live up to the noble expectations of Cicero's statement.

Yet, if governments are sincere about their proclaimed commitment to provide health comprehensively and equitably for their people, they must deal with tobacco use, which is one of the major preventable causes of death worldwide *(2)*. Tobacco-related diseases are perhaps the world's most easily preventable ones because the 'causative agent' – tobacco – is not necessary for life or good health. Indeed, cessation of tobacco use is associated with improved health and quantifiable socioeconomic benefits to the users, their family, their friends, the community and the nation at large.

While tobacco control activities can be carried out at various levels in society, experience demonstrates that meaningful changes in tobacco consumption result from coordinated and strategic national efforts. Building a national plan of action for tobacco control and establishing the infrastructure and capacity to implement the plan of action are key steps in the successful mitigation of the tobacco epidemic.

The national plan of action for tobacco control is a document that explicitly describes the goals and objectives of a country in relation to its health priorities, the strategies and activities that are needed to achieve these goals and objectives, the resources that the government is willing to commit, the parties responsible for each activity, and the mechanism for tracking progress. It is essentially a roadmap outlining how a country intends to deal with the tobacco epidemic and setting a time line and target date for completion. This chapter provides an overview of the process of developing a national plan of action.

FINDING THE ARCHITECTS OF THE PLAN: ESTABLISHING A NATIONAL COORDINATING MECHANISM

Building institutional capacity is essential for the long-term sustainability of tobacco control efforts. It is also critical to the development of a comprehensive and relevant national plan of action for tobacco control, and to the plan's successful implementation.

Designating a national focal point for tobacco control

The Ministry of Health is the logical government agency to spearhead the process of developing capacity for tobacco control. In practice, the first step to attaining institutional capacity is the official designation of a national focal point for tobacco control within the government. Often, the focal point is an individual within a unit of the Ministry of Health or related administrative agency. The focal point's main responsibility is to coordinate the country's response to the tobacco epidemic. This requires mobilizing other ministries and agencies, building alliances with civil society, enhancing public information and advocacy, training a core group of advocates and champions, and setting up a mechanism to coordinate the implementation of a national plan of action. Ideally, the focal point does not work alone, but leads a team within the Ministry of Health: the National Tobacco Control Programme (NTCP). The NTCP is directly responsible for the implementation of the action plan, and is usually independent of the National Steering Committee for Tobacco Control (see below), although it often serves as the Steering Committee's technical support group or secretariat. Establishing the NTCP is discussed in Chapter 6.

Creating a national steering committee for tobacco control

A successful national plan of action to control the tobacco epidemic requires broad popular support, so various key stakeholders must be involved in the development of the plan. The experience of many countries with progressive tobacco control programmes indicates that this is best achieved through the creation of a multisectoral national committee, task force, working group or steering committee for tobacco control. In larger countries it may be necessary to establish multisectoral committees for tobacco control at the state, district and provincial levels in order to set up an appropriate plan of action at those administrative levels.

The purpose of those committees is to develop a national plan of action for tobacco control, to select and coordinate the appropriate components and activities involving policy and legislation, smoking cessation, education and advocacy, and to integrate other elements embodied in the WHO FCTC. Ideally, the committees should have a regular reporting mechanism to ensure accountability and allow public involvement and participation. While national tobacco control committees can initially be created on an ad hoc basis, over time, they should be made official, permanent, established in law and provided with national funding.

The composition of these committees should be carefully studied. As a general rule: aim for the broadest possible representation but take care not to include those who would impede or counter the committee's efforts at controlling the tobacco epidemic. The following groups or institutions should be carefully evaluated for their potential to advance the development of the national plan of action for tobacco control, based on the particular situation in each country. Select only the essential members to keep the size of the committee manageable.

Government ministries

- Health ministry – It usually has the lead role in tobacco control. The health ministry often has data on the impact of tobacco use on the nation's health indicators, and technical expertise in training, health education and smoking cessation. Many countries have national health policy and sector strategy papers that set the frame for the scope of state-supported health services. When there is a possibility for stakeholder dialogue during development or review of such documents, the importance of including a reference to the national plan for tobacco control should be emphasized. The national infrastructure for public health is a critical component of the implementing network once the plan is ready to be set into motion, and should be taken into account already during the development of the plan.

- Finance and treasury ministries – The ministry of finance and the treasury establish tax policy and tax collection procedures, which are key elements in tobacco control.
- Customs and excise ministries – These ministries can:
  - provide information on tobacco smuggling, and advise on developing and enforcing anti-smuggling measures;
  - provide information on current and past tobacco taxation levels, tobacco sales and tobacco tax revenues;
  - alert the national committee to tobacco industry tactics to circumvent the intent of tobacco tax laws, or to exploit favourable tax treatment of particular tobacco products.
- Trade and commerce ministries – These ministries can provide economic alternatives to tobacco growing and manufacturing. Licensing authorities can also be used to prohibit the sales of tobacco products to minors.
- Consumer affairs ministry – This ministry implements regulatory requirements on tobacco marketing, advertising, packaging and labelling, tobacco testing and disclosure of information on tobacco additives and toxic ingredients.
- Agriculture ministry – This ministry can facilitate the realignment of national agricultural policies away from tobacco agriculture.
- Ministries of international trade and foreign affairs – Coordinated international policy for tobacco control is envisioned in the WHO FCTC. In addition, these ministries can:
  - analyse the balance of payments for tobacco;
  - advise on international law implications of tobacco control policy proposals;
  - assist in developing complementary tobacco control strategies in neighbouring countries;
  - respond to challenges by foreign tobacco companies that might attack domestic tobacco policies.
- Law and justice ministries – Their collaboration is vital when developing, implementing and enforcing legislative measures to control tobacco use. In addition, the justice ministry can also:
  - defend against legal challenges to tobacco control legislation;
  - advise on constitutional matters and international treaty obligations;
  - assist in developing and drafting tobacco control laws and legislation.
- Ministries of labour, transport and public service personnel – The participation of these ministries is essential when developing and implementing interventions to protect the public from second-hand smoke exposure in workplaces, public transportation and other public places.
- Education ministry – A comprehensive national plan of action for tobacco control requires the involvement of the education ministry.
- Defence ministry – The armed forces can contribute to a national plan of action by promoting a fit and tobacco-free lifestyle among their personnel, assisting in the enforcement of tobacco control laws and requiring that all tobacco products sold

in military establishments (e.g. army shops and PX stores) be sold at a price that is at least as high as in non-military stores.

- Culture and sports ministries – Involvement of culture and sports ministries in the development of national plans of action can facilitate the elimination of tobacco sponsorships from cultural and sports events.

- Ministry of the environment – This ministry should participate in the development of interventions to reduce the adverse impact of tobacco use on both outdoor and indoor environments.

- Religious ministries – Where present, religious ministries can support the creation of a feasible national plan of action by marshalling support for tobacco control within religious communities, ensuring that places of worship are smoke-free and encouraging religious leaders to serve as role models for a tobacco-free life.

The private sector: legitimate stakeholders

A truly multisectoral tobacco control programme should involve the private sector. In most countries, the national steering committee includes several representatives of this sector. The WHO FCTC recognizes the importance of participation of civil society to achieve the goal of reducing tobacco-related mortality and morbidity. In some instances, the impetus for developing a national tobacco control programme comes from the private sector, and in a number of countries it is this sector that leads the national tobacco control committee.

Stakeholders in tobacco control within the private sector include:

- The media – The media can help develop a communications strategy to support the national plan of action for tobacco control.

- NGOs involved in tobacco control – In a number of countries, dynamic tobacco control NGOs have become the driving force behind government action, directly addressing issues that government agencies may not be in a position to tackle. When political constraints require moderation in the official government stance on particular tobacco control issues, NGOs can be outspoken, insisting that policies adhere to scientific evidence for efficacy. Competing interests can distract the government's attention from tobacco control, but NGOs can maintain a single-minded focus on reducing tobacco consumption. Governments come in and out of power, but NGOs can provide the continuity needed for a national plan of action to come to fruition. Finally, when tobacco companies try to influence government policy, NGOs can bring this to public attention and support government officials to refuse the industry's overtures.

- Health professionals – Health professional organizations can incorporate tobacco control in their agenda to support the national plan of action for tobacco control.[1]

- Lawyers – Lawyers are needed to bring about effective legislative changes, to draft and amend laws, to respond to the tobacco industry's attempts to delay legislative progress, to monitor the enforcement of existing laws, to explore ways of applying general laws (e.g. consumer protection laws, children's rights, environmental laws)

---

[1] WHO Informal meeting of health professional organizations and tobacco control. http://www.who.int/tobacco/events/30jan_2004/en/

to tobacco control and to investigate the possibility of litigation against the tobacco industry.

- Economists – They can provide the economic analyses that demonstrate the cost effectiveness of tobacco control and the adverse long-term economic impact of continued tobacco use.
- Business, industry and labour unions.
- Other stakeholders – Other potential partners for tobacco control include women's and children's rights groups, environmental groups, religious groups, consumer organizations, teachers and youth groups, and parents' organizations.

Who are not legitimate stakeholders in the control of the tobacco epidemic?

The tobacco industry and its affiliates often present themselves as stakeholders in tobacco control, and usually attempt to gain entrance into national planning committees or bodies for tobacco control. Ultimately, sales of tobacco products – which is the business the tobacco industry is in – implicitly promote tobacco use. This is directly in opposition to the goal of tobacco control. At present it is highly unlikely that the tobacco industry and its representatives will earnestly work for effective strategies to reduce tobacco promotion and sales. National focal points and other legitimate members of the national steering committee need to carefully consider the consequences of allowing the tobacco industry into the planning process for tobacco control. WHO strongly urges its Member States not to engage the tobacco industry when designing, implementing and evaluating plans of action for tobacco control.

DETERMINING NEEDS AND RESOURCES: CONDUCTING A SITUATION ANALYSIS (3)

In policy-making, evidence is power. In no other public health area is this truer than in tobacco control. Once the national tobacco control committee is in place, the next step in developing a relevant plan of action for tobacco control is to conduct an analysis of the current situation in the country. Deciding on the policy mix for the national plan will depend on the specific needs of the country, and the resources available to meet those needs.

Developing the capacity to collect and generate reliable data is an indispensable step because the right information can:

- facilitate public understanding and support for measures to reduce tobacco consumption;
- determine the specific policies and interventions in the national plan of action;
- persuade political decision-makers to adopt tobacco control policy and legislative recommendations;
- provide the baseline for measuring progress in tobacco control efforts;
- ensure regular feedback to improve existing policies and interventions.

In general, four types of information are needed at the outset. The first involves mapping out the political environment in relation to tobacco control. The successful national plan of action for tobacco control requires political will. Essential aspects of the political environment include:

- the state of tobacco control in the country, including existing policies, practices, visions, debates and the stakeholders involved;
- the role of the tobacco industry in the country, including its resources, programmes and activities, its allies and affiliates, its links – both informal and formal – to government officials and agencies, the extent of its influence on government policy and the ability of the government to influence tobacco industry strategies (for example, in the case of state-owned industries);
- the role of tobacco control advocates in the country, including concerned professional associations (health, legal professions), consumer groups and other NGOs, academia, government bodies;
- the current attitude of key institutions such as the media and the business community, their likely reactions to the advancement of tobacco control.

The second category of information revolves around the health and economic impact of tobacco use, and the effectiveness of various tobacco control interventions. Drawing on the experience of many countries, WHO has identified a list of indicators which should be monitored by each country to support the health policy process. These include:

- sociodemographic characteristics;
- tobacco production, trade and industry;
- tobacco consumption patterns;
- estimates of the health and economic impact of tobacco use;
- population coverage regarding access to information and support for cessation of tobacco use, prevention of uptake and tobacco control policies.

The third set of information encompasses public knowledge, opinions, beliefs and attitudes. Opinion surveys can identify critical gaps in knowledge. More importantly, these surveys indicate areas where public support for tobacco control needs to be reinforced through advocacy and education. On the other hand, proof of strong public support for specific tobacco control interventions can sway policy leaders to back these interventions through the enactment of laws and/or the adoption of policies.

Finally, and importantly, effective capacity for tobacco control includes the ability to monitor and expose the tobacco industry's activities. In many countries, the main sources of this type of information are the internal documents of the tobacco industry, which are now publicly available as a result of litigation in the United States. Every country should attempt to search these documents for country-specific information that could shed light on attempts to undermine local tobacco control efforts in the past. Relationships with political and health leaders can be identified, and strategies to obstruct progress in tobacco control can be exposed. Studying the internal documents of the tobacco industry can provide valuable insight when planning for future tobacco control interventions.

Collecting all these types of information may seem a daunting task, particularly in countries where resources are scarce and research capacity is not fully developed. However, there are several sources of data in government agencies and academia, and having representatives of these bodies on the national steering committee can facilitate data collection. If national data are unavailable, it may be possible to derive estimates using existing local, regional or global information. Academic institutions, foundation-funded programmes and external groups can be tapped for technical assistance in designing formal data collection mechanisms.

SETTING THE STRATEGIC DIRECTION (4)

Definitions

A vision describes an ultimate state or condition where all outcomes are achieved under ideal conditions. In general, vision statements should be:
- understood and shared by members of the community;
- broad enough to allow a diverse variety of local perspectives to be encompassed within them;
- inspiring and uplifting to everyone involved;
- easy to communicate (short enough to fit on a T-shirt).

A mission statement describes the overall purpose of an organization; in this case, the NTCP. It should describe what the NTCP is going to do, and why it is going to do it. The mission statement should be:
- Concise – although not as short a phrase as a vision statement, a mission statement should still get its point across in one sentence;
- Outcome-oriented – mission statements explain the overall outcomes the NTCP is working to achieve;
- Inclusive – while mission statements highlight the programme's overarching goals, it is very important that they do so very broadly; good mission statements do not restrict the strategies or sectors of the community that may become involved in the project.

A goal is a desired general end point that an organization or programme wants and expects to accomplish in the future.

An objective is a specific measurable result expected within a particular period of time, consistent with a goal. It is a means by which the success of a goal is attained, the end result of a set of actions or activities.

The vision of all tobacco control programmes is to create a tobacco-free society. The mission of a national tobacco control programme is to foster individual, community and government responsibility to prevent and reduce tobacco use by enabling multisectoral participation in tobacco control.

The goal of a national plan of action for tobacco control should be to reduce the mortality and morbidity caused by the use of tobacco products. The objectives that will guide the achievement of this goal should include:

- helping those who do not use tobacco to stay tobacco-free;
- promoting cessation of tobacco use by assisting and encouraging current tobacco users to quit;
- protecting the health and rights of non-smokers by eliminating exposure to tobacco smoke.

A national plan of action for tobacco control should be developed with the vision, mission, goal and objectives in mind. While the specific elements of the plan may vary from country to country, depending on national capacity, availability of resources, political will and unique sociocultural features, the overall plan should be designed to attain the goal of reducing the health burden from tobacco use.

DEVELOPING THE BLUEPRINT FOR ACTION: DRAFTING THE NATIONAL PLAN

Once the national steering committee is in place and a current assessment of the tobacco control situation, needs and resources of a country has been carried out, drafting of the national plan of action can begin. International experience attests to the importance of including a comprehensive mix of policies, legislation and interventions for successful tobacco control *(5, 6)*. The various elements that should be considered for inclusion in the national plan are outlined in the WHO FCTC, and every effort should be made to incorporate strategies for the ratification of the WHO FCTC in the plan of action. In addition, country planners should heed the lessons learned by other countries that have already gone through the process of tobacco control planning and implementation. The experiences of those countries can highlight pitfalls to avoid and successful strategies to incorporate in the national plan.

Some of the legislative, economic and programme elements of the national plan of action are discussed in detail in the succeeding chapters of this handbook. The situation analysis will determine the selection of particular elements for each country, and the order of their implementation. The plan should be practical and viable in the country for which it has been designed, while adhering to the evidence for effectiveness. This means it must be carefully adapted to the country's unique sociocultural and politicoeconomic qualities without sacrificing the principles that render interventions effective.

The plan of action should clearly identify general and specific objectives, and the corresponding strategies and activities required to achieve these objectives. Strategies explain how the initiative will reach its objectives. Five specific strategies can help guide most interventions:

- providing information and enhancing skills (e.g. offering skills in cessation counselling);
- enhancing services and support (e.g. starting a quit line for smokers);
- modifying access, barriers, and opportunities (e.g. expanding prevention programmes to cover young people who are not attending school);
- rewarding efforts (e.g. providing incentives for restaurants to become smoke-free);
- modifying policies (e.g. changing consumer laws to ban all tobacco advertising);
- anchoring tobacco control strategies and activities in relevant planning documents at national and other levels (e.g. ensuring a reference to the national plan of action for tobacco control in the formulation of a national health policy).

Expected outputs should be listed for each objective, and responsible people/agencies assigned to each activity. Resources needed to carry out the activities must be ascertained and potential sources of funding pinpointed. A timeline should be set up, with target dates for completion. Finally, indicators of progress and an evaluation mechanism should be specified. Good planning provides for careful evaluation of progress, successes and failures as policy and programme implementation proceed. The results of such evaluation should then be used to revise, improve and update successive planning and programming, in a continuing effort to reduce tobacco consumption. Annex 1 provides a sample template for a national plan of action.

While countries share the same goal for tobacco control, no two national action plans will be identical. However, there have been sufficient similarities among countries within the same WHO region to allow the development of regional plans of

---

Overview of the elements of an action plan

1. State the vision. The vision should communicate what the NTCP believes is the ideal condition for the nation.

2. Develop the mission statement. The mission statement should clearly describe what the NTCP is trying to accomplish.

3. Draft a brief background that summarizes key findings of the situation analysis, and outlines the rationale for taking action.

4. Set the goal and objectives.

5. For each objective, select the strategies and expected results needed to achieve the objective.

6. Identify specific activities within each strategy.

5. Indicate who is responsible for each activity.

6. Note down the target date for completion of each activity.

7. Determine the resources needed to complete each activity.

8. Note down the progress indicator to measure the effectiveness of implementation.

action for tobacco control. Countries may use these regional action plans as a basis for the development of their own national plans, adapting certain sections to address their specific needs. More importantly, countries should strive for consistency with the recommendations of the WHO FCTC.

ENSURING LEGITIMACY: OFFICIAL ADOPTION OF THE NATIONAL PLAN OF ACTION

A national plan of action is only a piece of paper until it is ready to be implemented. Successful implementation requires at least two additional steps:
- broad consultation to establish ownership of the plan among the implementing and enforcing parties;
- rormal recognition of the national plan, granting it official status.

The careful selection of members of the national steering committee, and the provision of opportunities for other stakeholders to provide feedback and input into the national plan, help it gain acceptability among key stakeholders. Once the plan has been revised in consultations with those stakeholders, the committee needs to go one step further and secure legitimacy for the plan by ensuring its official adoption by the government. Only at that point can implementation begin.

LAUNCHING THE NATIONAL PLAN OF ACTION

The creation and official adoption of the national plan of action should be widely publicized so that the nation is informed of the country's intention to reduce tobacco consumption. This can be done in various ways, such as through a press conference or other media events (see Chapter 9). A number of countries have launched their national plans of action to coincide with the celebration of World No Tobacco Day. This is an effective way of capturing the public's attention and ensuring broad media coverage.

CONSIDERATIONS

In smaller countries, the adoption of a national plan of action is sufficient to initiate a sustainable process for controlling tobacco use. However, in large or heavily populated countries, the administration of tobacco control policies is often delegated to local governments. In some cases, local governments are ahead of national action on tobacco control. Where local government plays a role in tobacco control, the establishment of a complementary infrastructure and plan of action at the local level can be extremely helpful in ensuring the success of efforts to reduce tobacco consumption. National authorities and bodies, such as the national steering committee, should provide support and encouragement to their local counterparts, and maintain open lines of communication to foster coordination. The process for developing a plan of action at the local government level is similar to the one described in the preceding sections, although the scope and activities may have to be adapted to correspond to the local situation. Establishing the infrastructure to ensure coordination among the various levels is discussed in the next chapter.

CRITICAL ISSUES TO CONSIDER WHEN DEVELOPING A PLAN OF ACTION

It is useful to identify common problems and obstacles that hinder tobacco control in many countries. These must be addressed in any meaningful plan of action for tobacco control.

Low political will

In many countries, particularly among the developing nations where infectious diseases still pose a major challenge to health and survival, the tobacco epidemic is generally not viewed as a priority health problem. In countries where the state owns or subsidizes the tobacco industry, government may be reluctant to enact policies meant to reduce consumption, as these may be viewed as being in direct conflict with the economic interests of the state. in addition, political leaders who receive support from the tobacco industry may withhold support or, worse, directly oppose tobacco control efforts. An effective control plan must build political will, identifying those factors that oppose the successful establishment of a tobacco control programme, and choosing interventions to persuade political decision-makers to support efforts to curtail tobacco use. This may require strategic political mapping and targeted advocacy to educate policy-makers about the magnitude of the tobacco problem and the effective interventions needed to address this problem. Beyond education, political decision-makers need to be convinced and persuaded that tobacco control is in the best interest of their careers, their political parties and their constituencies.

Lack of data on tobacco control policy

Data that are inadequate or ineffectively communicated reinforce the lack of political will for action on tobacco control. An effective plan of action must tackle this problem by:
- making provisions for local studies and surveillance of the health and economic impact of tobacco use, the effectiveness of interventions for tobacco control and the factors that hinder efforts to control the tobacco epidemic (including the activities of the tobacco industry), using standardized and innovative approaches for data analysis and information dissemination so that effective messages are communicated to policy leaders;
- ensuring optimal use of existing data, which may be achieved by pooling and reanalysis.

Inadequate resources for tobacco control

Closely linked to 'low political will' is the issue of 'inadequate resources' for tobacco control, largely due to allocation of resources to other perceived priority health problems. This is especially critical in developing countries where health resources are extremely limited to start with. Resource mobilization must thus feature prominently in a tobacco control plan of action (POA), recognizing that there can be innovative ways of identifying funds within government for tobacco control (e.g. through earmarked taxes). In addition, external funds exist (e.g. from bilateral and multilateral grants or from philanthropic institutions); these should be sought, identified and utilized. Substantial efficiency gains can be achieved by designing tobacco control activities as part and parcel of national health services.

Ineffective tobacco control policies

Some governments adopt weak tobacco control policies as a compromise position, erroneously believing that stronger policies might have harmful economic consequences (7). This is especially true for the few countries that derive a substantial portion of their national revenue from tobacco agriculture, manufacturing or trade. A meaningful plan of action for tobacco control must take this into account and ensure that policy-makers accept the truth about tobacco's adverse impact on national economies and the substantial economic benefits of tobacco control.

In addition, enforcement strategies of national tobacco control policies are too often not devolved to subnational or local levels, resulting in inconsistent and ineffective implementation. A plan of action for tobacco control needs to be designed so that implementation and monitoring can be readily decentralized.

The influence of the tobacco industry

The tobacco industry continues to counteract effective tobacco control *(5)* through its various activities, both overt and covert, particularly in developing countries where tobacco control legislation is either non-existent, weak or poorly enforced. An effective tobacco control plan must tackle the tobacco industry's influence on the development of national tobacco control policy through effective counter-mechanisms (see Chapter 13). It must also emphasize the need for strong legislation and public dissemination of information about the industry's real motives.

Tobacco control relegated to the health sector

Tobacco control activities are often relegated to the health sector even though the problem transcends this domain. It is a multisectoral concern involving agriculture, environment, finance, education, information, sports, arts and culture ministries. Furthermore, the private sector, NGOs, international agencies and various community groups have crucial roles to play in tobacco control. An effective control plan should therefore involve as many relevant sectors and stakeholders as possible in the development, implementation and dissemination of tobacco control interventions. It should not only provide the required direction and focus, but also ensure that all relevant sectors have the opportunity to build a strong alliance for the effective control of the tobacco epidemic.

References

1. Dhillon HS, Phillip L, eds. *Health Promotion and Community Action for Health in Developing Countries*. Geneva, World Health Organization, 1994.

2. Warren CW et al. Tobacco use by youths: a surveillance report from the Global Youth Tobacco Project. *Bulletin of the World Health Organization*, 2000, 78(7):868–876.

3. Blanke D, ed. *Tobacco control legislation: an introductory guide*. Geneva, World Health Organization, 2003.

4. Work Group on Health Promotion and Community Development. Community tool box: Strategic planning tool kit. University of Kansas, Kansas, USA (http://ctb.ku.edu/).

5. Wakefield M, Chaloupka FJ. Effectiveness of comprehensive tobacco control programs in reducing teenage smoking in the USA. *Tobacco Control*, 2000, 9(2):177–186.

6. Stephens T et al. Comprehensive tobacco control policies and the smoking behaviour of Canadian adults. *Tobacco Control*, 2001,10:317–322.

7. Economic, social and health issues. Report of the WHO International Meeting, Kobe, Japan, 3–4 December 2001. Geneva, World Health Organization, 2003.

Bibliography

Eriksen MP. Best practices for comprehensive tobacco control programs: opportunities for managed care organisations. *Tobacco Control*, 2000, 9(Suppl 1): i11-i14.

Laugesen M, Swinburn B. New Zealand's tobacco control programme 1985–1998. *Tobacco Control*, 2000, 9:155–162.

Robbins H, Krakow M. Evolution of a comprehensive tobacco control programme: building system capacity and strategic partnerships – Lessons from Massachusetts. *Tobacco Control*, 2000, 9:423–430.

Annex 1. Sample template of a national plan of action for tobacco control

■ **VISION:** A world free from tobacco. ■ **MISSION:** The mission of the National Tobacco Control Programme is to foster individual, community and government responsibility to prevent and reduce tobacco use by enabling multisectoral participation in tobacco control. ■ **GOAL:** To reduce the mortality and morbidity caused by the use of tobacco products.
■ **BACKGROUND:** Please insert background information and rationale for action in your country here.

	Strategy	Expected result	Activities	Responsible agencies	Resources needed	Target date of completion	Potential barriers	Progress indicators
Objective 1: preventing tobacco use								
Objective 2: Reducing tobacco consumption among current users of tobacco products								
Objective 1: Protecting non-smokers from exposure to second-hand smoke								

6

Establishing an effective infrastructure for national tobacco control programmes

Careful planning will lead to success.
—*Sun Tzu*, The Art of War, *500 BC*

A S THE DEVELOPMENT of a national plan of action unfolds, the national focal point or the equivalent official must begin to establish the infrastructure to implement it. The specific requirements for this will vary from one country to another. Ministries of health usually take the initiative by creating an instrument of implementation, most often a NTCP, whose responsibility is to ensure the successful implementation of tobacco control interventions, with the national focal point as the lead programme officer. Usually, the NTCP functions independently of the national steering committee or task force for tobacco control, although it often serves as the technical support group for either of them. This chapter outlines a model for setting up a national network and infrastructure for tobacco control that is driven by the NTCP.

OVERVIEW

A successful NTCP must, by definition, cover the entire population. Strategic planning for the NTCP usually occurs at the central level, within the Ministry of Health. In larger countries, however, the programme must be designed for flexible implementation, through decentralization of authority to the municipal and county/village levels so that interventions can target and reach each and every citizen.

This requires resources and skills at all levels of the programme management infrastructure. In addition to human resources, the NTCP needs material and financial resources. No national programme can become operational without logistic support. The capacity and resources to manage a programme of such magnitude are usually available at the central level, but in many developing countries, few resources are allocated to local authorities. Since the programme is carried out at the local level, therefore, success depends on ensuring the availability of adequate resources and building the capacity of local public health professionals and government leaders.

Where central and local levels possess adequate capabilities and resources, and work in synergy, an integrated organizational framework can be used to disseminate and implement the proven effective interventions for tobacco control contained in the WHO FCTC.

Tapping existing resources and networks is a pragmatic way of keeping down the implementation costs of the NTCP. In most cases, the physical and human resources needed for the NTCP are already in place within ministries of health, under related programmes such as prevention of noncommunicable diseases (NCDs), health promotion, and control of substance abuse. Using the existing resources and infrastructure also allows the NTCP to take advantage of lessons learned from successful disease prevention and health promotion activities.

The WHO FCTC defines the proven tobacco control interventions for all countries. However, because countries are so different from one another, each NTCP, guided by the national plan of action, will need to decide which implementation strategies are appropriate and most likely to succeed with its own health system in the political, sociocultural and economic circumstances.

Countries with a central unit for planning and policy development in the Ministry of Health and local units for implementation and enforcement, are well placed to carry out tobacco control activities. In countries where central and local levels of health governance function independently of each other, the central level can still play an important role in the development of national policy guidelines and standards, national surveillance and monitoring, and information dissemination. In all cases, it is of the utmost importance for the central level to respect local priorities.

The size and complexity of the NTCP infrastructure depends also on variables such as the country's area, population, and geopolitical divisions. Given that some 72% of countries have populations of under 10 million, the framework suggested above, with a decentralized system that links central and local levels within the public health network, appears feasible. This framework will be used as the reference for the rest of this chapter.

Other important variables that can affect the successful establishment of the NTCP include the political environment, socioeconomic conditions and the cultural peculiarities of individual countries. These can work for or against tobacco control. Ministry of Health officials and staff running NTCPs, and their partners in civil society, face the unique challenge of determining the most effective way to take advantage of their countries' particular circumstances to bolster their efforts to control tobacco consumption and garner support for the NTCP.

Coordination of the NTCP, at the central and local levels, will be essential to ensure that the tobacco control interventions reach the target population. In addition, a system for monitoring the implementation process and its outcomes, including a periodic assessment of the NTCP's impact on health indicators, is necessary. The following sections address these issues in greater detail.

NATIONAL COORDINATION OF THE NTCP

Where to place the national coordination of the NTCP

Ideally, before the NTCP is established, there must be an official government mandate for tobacco control. As part of this mandate, the role of coordinator of the NTCP should be clearly defined and officially designated within the Ministry of Health. Careful analysis of the organizational set-up of the Ministry and its affiliated institutes is important to determine the most suitable position of the coordinator within the overall structure.

Depending on the level of political commitment to tobacco control, three scenarios are possible.

1. The Member State is not considering signing, ratifying or acceding to the WHO FCTC.

In this case, one must seek other avenues to support tobacco control activities and sensitize decision-makers into recognizing the urgency of establishing tobacco control as a national public health priority. In some countries, actions to institute and coordinate national and subnational tobacco control activities were initiated by NGOs, nationwide institutions such as National Cancer Centres and National Health Promotion Centres, and at the subnational level, by academic or even government institutions such as municipal health bureaus. The experience of Brazil, Mexico, Peru and Thailand demonstrates how NGOs, universities and other groups can assume leading roles in tobacco control activities. The rationale of the involvement of multiple sectors of society in tobacco control programmes is that when governments fail to take the lead in tobacco control, an alternative grass-roots approach can be explored and vice versa.

In some countries, potential tobacco control leaders sought and received technical support from WHO through its representatives and country offices – WHO representatives (WRs) and country liaison officers (CLOs). Responding to requests from countries, WHO provided technical and logistical support for capacity-building, helping countries to acquire the necessary skills and tools for effective tobacco control.

One potential media event is WHO's World No Tobacco Day, which is celebrated by virtually all of its Member States. By strategically developing an advocacy campaign around this day, several countries have successfully raised the profile of tobacco control, winning greater political commitment for a national campaign to prevent and reduce tobacco use.

2. The Member State has signed and ratified, or is preparing to ratify the WHO FCTC, but it does not have an official NTCP and has not yet designated an official coordinator or coordinating body for tobacco control.

Once a country has officially signed and ratified the WHO FCTC, the Ministry of Health is in a particularly strong position to establish a NTCP. Following the official signing, it must be ensured that the government ratifies the WHO FCTC, because the sooner the WHO FCTC comes into force, the sooner signatories become bound to honour their commitment to the treaty. Allies outside the Ministry of Health can help persuade the government to formally mandate the establishment of an NTCP under the Health Ministry, in anticipation of the treaty's entry into force. These allies include prominent members of the legislature who support tobacco control, allies in civil society and representatives of bilateral, multilateral and international partners who recognize the benefits of tobacco control for the country.

3. The Member State has signed and ratified, or is moving towards ratification of the WHO FCTC, and an NTCP is in place.

The best possible scenario is when a country has endorsed the treaty and the Health Minister has officially designated a coordinator or coordinating body and a central structure for the NTCP. In most cases, national coordination of the NTCP should be directly under the Health Ministry. It is the most appropriate governmental institution to oversee tobacco control, given its mandate to preserve and protect public health. An additional advantage is its ability to tap into an extensive, official governmental network and to access other government ministries and agencies that need to play a role in tobacco control.

Alternatively, it is possible to entrust national coordination of the NTCP to an independent institution outside the Health Ministry. This is occurring with varying degrees of success in a number of countries. However, even in those countries with highly successful tobacco control activities, such as Canada, tobacco control experts admit that bridging the gap between the private and public sectors can be a challenge. Moreover, when national tobacco control efforts emanate from outside the government, synchronization between the interventions proposed by the NTCP and the required governmental actions to support them can be difficult *(1)*.

Basic requirements for national coordination of the NTCP at the central level (Health Ministry)

The basic requirements for successful establishment and coordination of the NTCP at the central level include human, material and financial resources.

Human resources at the central level

Nominating the coordinator

Ideally, the Minister of Health should nominate the coordinator of the NTCP. Selecting this person, if possible from existing public health staff, saves time otherwise spent in the selection process and obviates the need to increase staff costs. Usually the coordinator is also the designated national focal point for tobacco control.

The person selected should possess the skills and knowledge of a public health professional. While familiarity with tobacco control interventions is an advantage, what is more critical is the individual's commitment to and interest in tobacco control. It is possible to rapidly acquire the knowledge about the tobacco epidemic and effective interventions to control it, but tobacco control cannot be successfully overseen by someone who lacks the passion for and dedication to the field. Most importantly, the person selected should have neither personal nor professional relations or pecuniary interests in the tobacco industry. The integrity of the individual selected to oversee the country's NTCP is extremely important, and the person should be willing to make an affidavit stating that he or she has no conflict of interest in this regard.

Other desirable qualities for this position include:
- the ability to think and plan strategically and creatively;
- the ability to inspire confidence, to act as team leader and to successfully manage other staff members and implementing partners at the local level;
- the ability to communicate effectively, both verbally and in writing;
- the ability to administer day-to-day tasks required to keep a national programme running in an organized and result-oriented manner;

- the ability to interact effectively with others, and to build partnerships and alliances to expand the tobacco control network within the country;
- the ability to work well under pressure, particularly in the face of overt or covert pressure from the industry and its supporters;
- the ability to identify opportunities for maximizing resources, given the meagre budgets that most health ministries are allocated;
- the ability to fully understand the political context of tobacco control and to interact with political decision-makers in a compelling and persuasive manner.

Other qualifications depend on the particular situation of a given country. Technical expertise in the field of tobacco control is desirable, but it should not be the sole or major criterion. Experts are not always the best managers. Instead, the ability to successfully manage the intricacies of running a national programme and an unswerving commitment to tobacco control should be at the top of the list.

Staffing the tobacco control team

Depending on the size of the country and population, the NTCP coordinator may need to look for other staff members. The ideal NTCP team would include:

- other public health professionals with skills and experience in programme management, health policy development, epidemiology and surveillance, advocacy, health promotion and prevention of NCDs, management of substance abuse, environmental health, health education and training;
- a health economist;
- a legal counsellor who is familiar with the WHO FCTC and legal issues pertaining to tobacco control;
- a media and communications person;
- support/secretarial staff with good computer skills, particularly in word processing, spreadsheets, database management, Internet searches, and the like.

In all cases, it would be best to choose the necessary personnel from existing Ministry staff. This minimizes the need for establishing new posts and securing the budget lines to fund them. In some cases, however, the Health Ministry may need to hire new staff. If so, a thorough search to identify the best qualified and committed individuals to fill these posts is required, keeping in mind the essential qualities discussed in the preceding section. It is extremely important to ensure that those being considered for posts within the NTCP have no links whatsoever with the tobacco industry.

Realistically, in many developing countries, and in developed countries where tobacco control is not among the top priorities of the Ministry of Health, staffing will be a challenge: in a number of those countries, NTCP staff may be limited to one or two people. However, establishing a successful NTCP takes time, and progress is often gradual. When the Ministry of Health assigns dedicated staff to tobacco control, even if the number of people is limited, it should be considered the first in a series of successes.

Some countries, such as Brazil, South Africa and Thailand, started with a limited programme, but eventually developed successful NTCPs *(2)*.

Preparing the tobacco control team

The NTCP coordinator and the tobacco control team need to prepare for the challenging and often gruelling work ahead. They must be knowledgeable about:

- the evidence of the adverse health effects of tobacco and second-hand tobacco smoke;
- the proven as well as the less effective interventions to reduce and prevent tobacco use, and the provisions of the WHO FCTC;
- the strategies of the tobacco industry and how best to counter them;
- the state of the tobacco epidemic in a particular country, using all available local data and a thorough assessment of the political and economic environment that may affect the work of the NTCP.

A number of countries began by asking WHO to help with training courses on capacity-building and technical advice from tobacco control consultants. WHO regional offices can assist Member States in this process if requested by governments. Furthermore, all the WHO regions have regional action plans for tobacco control, which are developed by Member States on the basis of the specific needs and resources available within each region. The action plan for your region can be a helpful starting point when the tobacco control team draws up its strategies and workplan. If a national plan of action for tobacco control is already in place, this should be used as well.

The duties and responsibilities of the NTCP team

They are as follows:

- Collection of local data and the building of a national tobacco control database to support the development and implementation of a strategic national plan of action, and the preparation of related technical and advocacy material.
- Regular conduct of awareness-raising activities for both the general public and selected target audiences on the magnitude of the tobacco epidemic and the urgent need for action to control tobacco. Target audiences include political decision-makers, community opinion leaders, special interest groups such as environmental groups and children's rights groups, and the media. Remember to adapt your message to the specific concerns of each of your target audiences. For example, political decision-makers need to hear about the economic benefits of raising tobacco taxes, while environmental and children's rights groups would be interested in the issue of second-hand tobacco smoke as an environmental pollutant that impairs the health of children.
- Compilation of a directory of all potential stakeholders of tobacco control in the country and creation of relevant mailing lists using this directory. This is best achieved using electronic mail, and several types of software exist for this purpose. However, in countries where the Internet is not readily available, the use of fax, telephone and regular mail will achieve the same purpose. The key is a system for readily reaching those whose support for the NTCP is vital. This type of readily accessible directory can facilitate day-to-day communication, provision of regular updates to relevant stakeholders on issues related to tobacco control, distribution of educational and advocacy materials, mobilization of supporters for specific activ-

ities such as World No Tobacco Day, and lobbying of legislative decision-makers for particular tobacco control policies or legislation. Where possible, the database should contain the complete contact details of each individual, including institutional, professional and personal postal addresses, phone numbers and e-mail addresses.

- Forging of partnerships with other public health programmes within the Ministry of Health, such as health promotion, NCD control, prevention of substance abuse, and environmental health.

- Development and maintenance of good relationships with the media, providing them with regularly updated information on tobacco-related issues and responding in a timely manner to their requests for information and interviews.

- Facing the tobacco industry whenever required, ensuring that the official spokesperson is fully prepared to counter the industry's allegations with facts and compelling arguments to support measures that lead to a reduction in tobacco use.

- Preparation of studies, in partnership with different institutions and groups, to collect and assess local epidemiological data, to develop and test intervention and evaluation strategies, including methodology and instruments, to create and test educational and advocacy materials; the results of these studies must be disseminated to the relevant audiences and the general public in a timely and informative manner.

- Establishment, in partnership with different stakeholders, of a network to decentralize the coordination and implementation of the NTCP; linking states, municipalities and other levels of local governance with the relevant government agencies, partners in the private sector, academia and the NGO community.

- Coordination of regular national campaigns, such as World No Tobacco Day, providing technical support to participating partners.

- Dissemination of information on the country's progress in tobacco control and recent actions and controversies through various media, including print (newspaper articles, fact sheets and newsletters), radio and television, and the electronic media (Internet bulletins and web pages).

- Organization of technical seminars, meetings and congresses to stimulate discussion and information exchange on tobacco issues among various groups within the country.

- Provision of technical support to other ministries on pertinent tobacco-related issues.

- Provision of technical support and information on tobacco-related issues to legislators.

- Promotion and provision of technical assistance for the establishment of comprehensive national tobacco control policies and legislation.

- Coordination of advocacy activities to persuade legislators to support effective tobacco control legislation.

- Promotion and support for the establishment of an interministerial committee for tobacco control to support the NTCP and to facilitate the ratification of the WHO FCTC.

- Encouragement and technical support for local governments, individuals and institutions, nongovernmental and governmental organizations interested in tobacco control.
- Encouragement of open communication between governmental and nongovernmental organizations, in order to maintain and reinforce good working relationships between these two sectors.
- Coordination of tobacco control monitoring with relevant partner agencies, and local government counterparts, ensuring continuity over time.
- Encouragement and support for universities and research institutions in the development and conduct of research related to tobacco issues.
- Representation of the Ministry of Health on tobacco-related topics, whenever needed, particularly when dealing with WHO and other national and international organizations concerned with tobacco control.
- Convening of an annual meeting on tobacco control evaluation and planning for national and subnational counterparts of the NTCP, to monitor national progress and to decide about future priorities and activities.

Basic material infrastructure

Office space

It is important to have an officially designated location for the NTCP: it provides a point of reference for individuals and groups interested in tobacco issues around the country, an address from which information, educational, advocacy and training materials can be obtained, and where the NTCP staff can be reached.

The availability of resources will determine the location, size and set up of the NTCP office, but even when resources are meagre, it is often possible to find a suitable space. The NTCP office should be large enough to allow the coordinating team to perform its activities, hold meetings, interviews, research, studies and workshops, and accommodate basic equipment, furniture, document files and a supply of technical and advocacy materials.

Furniture

Internal documents, reports, publications and files are vital for the development and management of the NTCP. The proper organization and storage of these files and documents calls for shelves, filing systems and cupboards. Confidential documents may require security systems such as locked storage cabinets and paper shredders. Other basic furniture requirements include computer desks, a meeting table, work tables, chairs, a blackboard, message boards, flipcharts, and a projection screen.

Equipment

The basic equipment should include the following:

- computers with CD-ROM drive, text editor software, slide editor software, direct mail programme and an epidemiological statistics programme (ideally Epi-Info), at a ratio of one computer for every two members of staff; at least one laptop for training and presentation purposes
- printer

- typewriter
- fax machine
- telephone lines with extensions
- audio and video recorders
- Internet access with e-mail address
- TV and VCR
- overhead and slide projectors, multi-media projector
- camera
- photocopier with a supply of paper.

Support material

Office supplies: these should include a defined mailing budget. General office supplies will also be needed, such as writing paper, pens, clips, pencils, fax paper, address labels, files, rubber bands, staples, briefcases, markers, stickers, diaries and organizers.

Technical, educational and advocacy materials: these include reference materials, practical guides, manuals, bulletins and posters, folders and stickers. Estimate the amount needed for planned activities, with sufficient copies for states/regions/provinces/municipalities/counties and interested parties.

Transportation

Transport is essential to enable the coordinating team to perform its duties. The team will often be on the move for various reasons: training, advocacy, technical support, meetings and conferences, research, surveillance and monitoring. The type of transport will be dictated by available resources and by topography. For example, in mountainous areas without paved roads, mountain bikes and animal transport may be needed. In countries where communities are separated by large bodies of water, such as in the Amazon and the Pacific, boats are essential.

Financial resources

The NTCP needs to have a working budget. This is often the biggest challenge faced by tobacco control advocates within the Ministry of Health, as health budgets are notoriously small, and a new national programme for tobacco control will have to compete with other programmes for its share of the funds. Nevertheless, the NTCP team must use all of its persuasiveness to convince decision-makers that tobacco control is an urgent national priority, so that specific resources are allocated to the NTCP.

Every country has regular meetings attended by the minister of health and secretaries of state. They should be presented with compelling evidence of the seriousness of the tobacco epidemic, and the specific actions they need to take, including allocation of a budget for the NTCP. This strategy was successfully adopted in Brazil: it won official commitment and a specific budget for NTCP approved by the Health Ministry.

In addition to government resources, the NTCP national coordinator should always look for opportunities to secure funding from other legitimate sources. Sometimes donations or grants from national NGOs or international funding agencies are available to provide start-up funds for the programme. In Thailand, for example, the Rotary Club helped to support the first set of activities of the country's NTCP.

Another innovative option is the realignment of funds allocated to related programmes, such as cardiovascular disease control, for tobacco control. By linking tobacco control to other programmes within the Ministry of Health, it may be possible to access additional funding for the NTCP.

Support from international multilateral organizations is another potential source of funding for the NTCP. The WHO FCTC includes provisions that discuss the various options for funding tobacco control activities, particularly in less developed countries. Recently, the European Union expressed interest in reviewing proposals for grant funding wherein tobacco control is integrated with the development process.

One source of funding that should not be sought by the NTCP is the tobacco industry, its partners and representatives. In the past, the industry has offered support to governments, but given the nature of the NTCP, this would give rise to a direct conflict of interests and should not be pursued.

Financial resources must be sufficient to cover costs for staffing, office space and equipment, transportation and supplies, as well as the costs for the implementation of NTCP activities.

Decentralizing the coordination of the NTCP to establish an implementation network

Once a country has established its centrally coordinated NTCP, a strategy to ensure that the programme interventions are widely and properly implemented needs to be developed. In most cases, this involves decentralization of authority to partners at the various local levels of governance who have the autonomy to implement and enforce the interventions recommended by the NTCP. Integration of these various levels of local governance with the NTCP is essential.

Within most national health systems, it is possible to designate tobacco control focal points at each level of local governance. These focal points must have the capacity to deal with tobacco control issues and to manage the required infrastructure at the local level. Identifying the focal points, securing their commitment to the NTCP and integrating them into a national network for tobacco control is the first step to ensuring effective implementation of NTCP interventions.

Building and maintaining the decentralized network

Actions needed at the central level:
The NTCP coordinator and programme staff need to take the following steps:
- Secure the support of the Health Minister to request that health officials at the state, regional and provincial levels designate local coordinators or focal points for the NTCP, and to meet the basic requirements for a corresponding local tobacco control programme.

- Define the terms of reference for the local coordinator or focal point for tobacco control and outline the basic parameters of a local tobacco control programme.
- Oversee training workshops on capacity-building at each level of local governance where a tobacco control programme is to be established. These workshops should bring together in each region, the official state, regional and provincial coordinators (or the equivalent in the administrative structure of the country) and selected staff members.

Local health officials might not be eager to establish a local tobacco control programme. If this is not a priority for a particular local government unit, the NTCP should explore alternatives. Academic institutions or NGOs may be interested in the role of local coordinator for that particular area. If so, the NTCP should support and enable them to do so.

The process of securing the commitment of each successive level of local governance should be repeated until the smallest local government unit is reached, a local coordinator for tobacco control is selected and trained, and a local version of the tobacco control programme is established at each level. Each local tobacco control coordinator or focal point is responsible for initiating the process at the next level down. This creates a 'cascade' system, very much like the 'ripple effect', which multiplies the number of designated tobacco control workers within the country. The cascade system should also be used for training: NTCP staff train state-level health workers, who, in turn, train regional health professionals; these will train provincial health workers, and so on, until health workers in the smallest government unit are trained.

Actions required of all local government tobacco control coordinators and their staff

Once designated and trained, the coordinators or focal points and staff of the local tobacco control programme should take the following steps:

- build a database of important contacts at their level of governance, with the names of local official representatives and other stakeholders;
- convene an annual evaluation and planning meeting, prior to the national evaluation and planning meeting, to assess the state of implementation at local level of the national plan of action for tobacco control and to map out the next year's priorities and activities;
- provide technical support and materials to the next level down in governance, to enable it to conduct local tobacco control activities effectively;
- conduct local surveillance, monitoring and research in accordance with the NTCP plan of action, and report the results of those activities to the NTCP;
- maintain an open channel of communication for all levels of management in the NTCP.

Duties and responsibilities, required resources and operational processes for local counterparts of the NTCP will closely parallel those of the national programme, although they will need to be scaled down and adapted to each particular location. Staff of the local tobacco control programme will be working more closely with communities and the population in general, addressing tobacco control issues at the micro level.

The cascade system, by generating capacity for tobacco control at each level of governance, promotes the establishment of an effective network for the successful implementation of tobacco control interventions throughout the country. This process must complement and support the development of a national action plan. Together, they comprise the basic infrastructure that will enable countries to effectively tackle the tobacco epidemic.

References

1. Da Costa e Silva Goldfarb LM. Government leadership in tobacco control: Brazil's experience. In: De Beyer J, Waverley Brigden L, eds. *Tobacco control policy: strategies, successes & setbacks*. Washington, DC, The World Bank, 2003:38–70.

2. De Beyer J, Waverley Brigden L, eds. *Tobacco control policy: strategies, successes & setbacks*. Washington, DC, The World Bank, 2003.

Bibliography

Da Costa e Silva VL et al. *Practical guidelines to implement a tobacco control programme*, 1st ed., Rio de Janeiro, National Cancer Institute/Ministry of Health, 1998 (in Portuguese).

Goldfarb LM et al. *Basis for the implementation of a tobacco control programme*, 1st ed., Rio de Janeiro, National Cancer Institute/Ministry of Health, 1996 (in Portuguese).

7
Training and education

The end of all education should surely
be service to others. We cannot seek
achievement for ourselves and forget about
progress and prosperity for our community.
—Cesar Chavez

INTRODUCTION

Successful tobacco control depends largely upon the availability of human resources to develop and implement a range of activities at different levels. The activities described in this handbook call for specific knowledge and skills, some of which may not exist in a particular country. Hence, training and education needs should be identified and integrated into the country programme from the outset.

Education is the method of transferring information and understanding about tobacco control and tobacco use. Different target groups require different types of information in order to resist tobacco, cease using it, support cessation efforts or plan and implement a range of tobacco control measures.

Capacity-building is essential for effective tobacco control, and is a wise investment for every country. Appropriate policies cannot be developed if those making decisions do not know how to apply their knowledge to bring about change. New measures may fail if people lack confidence or skills in carrying out new duties, including the capacity to form partnerships. Successful programmes and interventions require skills in investigating the problem and in planning, monitoring and evaluating the necessary actions.

Education about how tobacco threatens health is rarely enough to make people quit smoking. People need to understand the process of behavioural change; they may need interventions that tackle obstacles to quitting within their society. Health professionals also need to understand how change happens and how they can support it. Those working in cessation clinics or telephone help lines require skills to meet the varied needs of clients.

People working to prevent tobacco use in the community need to know how to reach their target audiences. Young people, for instance, may need general life-skills training in order to avoid risk, while non-tobacco users may need support in saying no to cigarettes in the long term.

This chapter is a brief overview of a complex area, and is not intended to be comprehensive. Wherever possible, additional resources to support training and educational activities will be identified.

This chapter focuses on the following questions:
1. Who needs what type of education?
2. What materials are suitable for different targets?
3. How can these materials be located, adapted or developed?
4. Who needs to be trained?
5. What skills and training materials are needed for tobacco control?
6. Who can and should conduct training?
7. What training methods are likely to be effective?
8. How can you plan an effective training workshop?

Terminology and organization of the chapter

Training refers to the transfer of skills to build capacity in order to undertake effective tobacco control. Education means imparting knowledge and understanding about (a) methods of effective tobacco control; and (b) the dangers of tobacco and methods of cessation. There is not always a meaningful distinction between transfer of information and transfer of skills (e.g. theories versus techniques for quitting). However, information alone may be suitable and sufficient for some target groups (e.g. community awareness campaigns to increase support for smoking bans). The discussion about the content of education appears in the sections dealing with education and training.

Decision points, tips and examples

Throughout the chapter, the most important decisions, as well as helpful tips, guiding principles and examples of previously used or recommended training activities are highlighted in text boxes. The final section contains generic training guides, one for countries just beginning tobacco control activities, and another for countries with more established policies and programmes.

KNOW THE COUNTRY: LINKS BETWEEN NEEDS ASSESSMENT AND DECISIONS ON TRAINING AND EDUCATION

Chapter 5 described the crucial role of a situation analysis or needs assessment for developing a national plan of action. This should include training and education for tobacco control.

Any decision concerning who needs what knowledge or skills should be based on a needs assessment, which should reveal:
- who uses tobacco (age, sex, ethnicity, location, social class);
- the form of tobacco used by each subgroup (e.g. cigarettes, *bidis*, smokeless or chewing tobacco, cigars, etc.);
- influences on starting tobacco use (e.g. gender norms, image, cultural beliefs, peer pressure, advertising);
- what, if any, forms of control exist and whether they are implemented fully (e.g. advertising bans, taxes and price rises, bans on the use of tobacco in public places, age restrictions on purchase);
- what, if any, prevention or cessation programmes exist (e.g. cessation clinics, help lines, media campaigns, educational programmes, NTRs).

Training Needs Assessments

A training needs assessment (TNA) is the process of identifying systematically what knowledge and skills are needed, and what exists within the pool of human resources. This chapter will assist in this process. A TNA also helps reduce duplication by building upon existing strengths and identifying capacities and gaps.

Question 1. Who needs what type of education?

If the needs assessment revealed few control measures or programmes and high tobacco-use prevalence among men, women and young people, the targets would be broader. Education should probably focus on raising community awareness, promoting advocacy for restrictions and introducing knowledge about the methods and benefits of cessation.

If the country has adopted strong control measures and has achieved large reductions, the targets will be narrower. Education should then focus on stronger restrictions, prevention information for young people and specialized quitting interventions for particular subgroups.

For most countries, there will be two main target groups (there will be some overlap).

Target Group I – Those planning or supporting tobacco control measures and programmes

Targets in Group I require education about tobacco control processes and strategies:

- government officials from relevant ministries such as health, finance, agriculture and education at central, state, provincial and district levels
- key decision-makers from teachers' groups, youth associations, employers, employees' associations, and community groups
- legal community
- health workers
- media representatives.

Target Group II – Those involved in individual or community tobacco prevention and cessation activities

Targets in Group II require education about the health risks of tobacco and methods of quitting:

- tobacco users
- general community
- media representatives
- young people and others at risk of initiating tobacco use
- staff at cessation clinics, help lines, etc.
- health workers.

> **Decision point:**
>
> Compile a list of these two target groups in the country.

Question 2. What materials are suitable for different targets?

Educational materials should suit the degree of literacy, age, background, position of targets and expected learning outcomes.

Target Group I – Those planning and supporting tobacco control measures, such as policies, legislation and programmes, need more complex materials to explain complicated arguments, including economic and legal aspects. Others need simpler frameworks for use at the community level. Box 1 outlines information needs for different actors.

Box 1. Information needs for Group I

	Government officials	Teachers, employers, community groups	Youth leaders, employee representatives	Legal community	Health workers	Media
Health risks of tobacco	✓	✓	✓		✓	✓
Health and economic burden of tobacco	✓	✓	✓	✓		✓
Steps to quitting		✓	✓		✓	
Models for developing smoke-free schools, workplaces		✓	✓		✓	
Models of successful tobacco control measures	✓			✓	✓	
Price elasticity issues	✓			✓		✓

Target Group II – Those needing information about the harm caused by tobacco and how to quit include people from all walks of life. While good materials exist, it may be worth producing country-specific ones to ensure cultural acceptability for each target group. Box 2 outlines information needs for members of Group II.

Box 2. Information needs for Group II

	Tobacco users	General community	Media representatives	Young people and others at risk	Cessation clinic staff	Health workers
Health risks of tobacco	✓	✓	✓	✓	✓	✓
Quitting strategies	✓	✓	✓		✓	✓

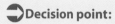

> **Decision point:**
> Using the lists under Question 1, make a table to identify the types of information needed by each subgroup.

Question 3. How can these materials be located, adapted or developed?

It is quite likely that the NTCP will want to use some existing resources and develop others, so this section covers both approaches.

Locating materials

The search will be influenced by the available time, budget, technology and links with national and international organizations.

- Convene an information-sharing meeting with people likely to have relevant materials (e.g. government departments, universities, research institutes, health promotion and health professional organizations and NGOs:
  - ask participants to bring along resources or reference details;
  - during the meeting, invite participants to suggest other sources;
  - during or after the meeting, invite selected participants to conduct a more systematic search;
  - conduct an electronic search (libraries and web browsers, such as *google.com)*, using key words, such as *tobacco, smoking prevention, health education, health promotion, health worker training, smokeless tobacco, bidi, smoking cessation.*
- Check the web site of the WHO Tobacco Free Initiative (TFI) (http://www.who.int/tobacco/en) regularly, or e-mail TFI at: tfi@who.int. The WHO regional offices may also have materials in the main languages of their respective regions. The web sites of the regional offices can be accessed from the TFI web site above.
- Visit relevant web sites on cancer control, health promotion, health education and youth health, such as
  - http://www.uicc.org/
  - http://www.tobaccopedia.org/
  - http://www.globalink.org/tobacco/news/
  - http://www.ash.org/
  - http://www.inwat.org/
  - http://tobaccofreekids.org/
- Contact the above organizations by telephone, letter or e-mail, asking for resources or suggestions. Many of these organizations provide copies of their materials free of charge.
- Select materials carefully, ensuring that the sources are reliable. The tobacco industry and its affiliated groups also put out materials allegedly in support of tobacco control strategies, particularly in the area of youth smoking prevention. However, research into these industry-generated materials indicates that the strategies they emphasize are either ineffective or minimally effective. To help you decide which materials are credible, ask for a copy of the TFI (WHO Regional Office for the Western Pacific) brochure *Seeing Beneath the Surface: The Truth Behind the Tobacco*

Industry's Youth Smoking Prevention Programmes by e-mailing: tfi@wpro.who.int. Also see the publication of WHO Eastern Mediterranean Regional Office, *The Tobacco Industry Documents: What they are, what they tell us and how to search them. A practical manual* (http://www.emro.who.int/tfi/TobaccoIndustry-English.pdf).

Adapting materials

Adapting is often cheaper than developing new materials.

- Compile existing materials and invite a team of health education and communications experts and representatives of the target population to review these materials and to provide feedback.
- Identify precisely what components are appropriate for the country in terms of content, style, length and language and what needs alteration, bearing in mind existing budgets and skills.
- When translating into another language, hire a professional to ensure the language is technically and culturally correct.

 Tip: Always pretest materials with target populations after initial modification.

Identifying the gaps

After searching for and adapting existing materials, identify the gaps in order to meet specific educational needs. Ask members of the teams described above to help make these strategic decisions (consider timing, budget and available human resources). List the types of material still needed, and for whom it is intended,[1] before deciding to prepare new documents.

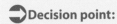 **Decision point:**

Identify what materials are needed and for whom; assess availability and decide whether to prepare new materials, modify existing ones, or both.

Developing materials

Materials developed by the NTCP are more likely to suit the country's needs. Even though existing material may initially be used, new materials may have to be developed if the existing ones are not effective. Key steps in developing materials are summarized below.

- Once gaps have been identified, determine the role and purpose of proposed materials. Some will be useful for both information and training, while others will be more appropriate for a specific task.

---

[1] For a clear, simple summary of why and how to assess what is needed for health education see: *(1)*.

Information materials should:
– be clear and easily understood by the target audience;
– counteract myths perpetrated by the tobacco industry;
– be appropriate in terms of length, language, and technical complexity for the intended target group;
– offer additional information, e.g. where to get help to quit.

Training materials (including manuals) should:
– have detailed explanations and step-by-step instructions;
– have many examples and exercises;
– be appropriate in terms of complexity, length and language;
– be realistic in terms of the time and resources of those expected to use it;
– list additional resources.

- Think about the best method of communication with the audience. Each of the following offers different advantages in different settings *(1, 2)*:
  – stories and plays
  – posters
  – flipcharts
  – photographs
  – audio and video tapes or CDs
  – newspaper or magazine articles
  – publications in journals or newsletters
  – manuals
  – electronic materials, through web sites or e-mail groups.

- A suggested sequence for preparing communication materials *(2)*:
  – decide the overall content and specific content
  – write a rough draft
  – review the draft with experienced people and target audience
  – pretest with target audience
  – modify where indicated
  – arrange for printing/production and distribution.

Question 4. Who needs to be trained?

Refer once again to the needs assessment. Countries with limited tobacco control and high rates of tobacco use will need to train more broadly. Where prevalence is lower and tobacco control more developed, targets will be narrower.

In determining who needs skills, use a framework similar to the one used to consider information needs.

Staff needing capacity-building might include:
- policy-makers and their advisers (government officials across sectors);
- programme/intervention designers (government and NGO);
- health professionals or counsellors who advise on smoking cessation;
- teachers, youth workers, others involved in prevention including life skills training;

- health promotion workers;
- tobacco users wanting to quit;
- public health advocates prepared to make a strong case for tobacco control;
- tobacco control NGOs.

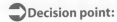**Decision point:**

List the types of people needing new skills.

Question 5. What skills and training materials are needed for tobacco control?

'Task analysis' *(2)* is used to identify precisely the capacities needed to do a job effectively. Tobacco control activities are varied, each with its own set of tasks. A task analysis will help select learning objectives, teaching materials and appropriate trainers. 'Tasks' typically involve learning attitudes and knowledge, as well as skills.

Activities and training needs

Table 1 below is a basic guide to identifying the skills needed for specific tasks, but the NTCP should develop its own list.

Table 1. Skills needed for tobacco control

Tobacco control activities	Required skills
Drafting and implementing policy measures (pricing, bans, sales restrictions) at all levels	• developing cross-sectoral partnerships • conducting health and economic analyses of impact of policy measures • drafting legislation and implementing appropriate rules and regulations that can be implemented
Advocacy at all levels	• conducting community surveys (including sampling, data gathering and analysis) on the acceptability of the measures • effective report-writing and presentation of data in a range of media to disseminate information and influence target groups • critically reviewing existing health data and countering tobacco industry arguments • identifying partners and building strategic alliances
Monitoring tobacco use patterns	• population-based survey techniques • data management and analysis • report-writing and dissemination of information
Planning and implementing interventions at national, provincial, district or organizational levels (eg. school-based education; media campaigns; smoke-free workplaces)	• accurate 'situation analysis' (qualitative, quantitative and rapid assessment investigation of influences on tobacco use) • data analysis and interpretation • strategic health programme planning, based upon situation analysis • designing appropriate curricula and educational materials • communicating persuasively with target groups • programme monitoring and evaluation
Smoking cessation programmes at provincial, district and community levels	• counselling for behavioural change and provision of support • managing and supporting counsellors
Avoiding or quitting smoking for individuals	• 'life skills' (ability to perceive risk and peer pressure, saying no, understanding decision-making) • techniques for quitting and staying off tobacco (with or without NRT and/or bupropion)

Capacities required by different personnel

Box 3 looks at the skills needed by the various categories of individuals targeted for training and education.

Building on existing human resources

People with the above skills probably exist in the country, even if they are not involved in tobacco control. It would be better simply to upgrade such people's skills to enable them, if they are keen, to work in tobacco control, rather than starting with complete beginners.

Box 3. Who needs what skills?

	Youth	Adults	Community groups	Teachers	Health workers	Cessation clinic staff	Programme planners	Policy-makers
Resisting pressure to use tobacco	✓	✓	✓	✓	✓	✓	✓	
Quitting & staying off tobacco	✓	✓	✓	✓	✓	✓	✓	
Counselling others to quit			✓	✓	✓	✓	✓	
Gathering data on tobacco use					✓		✓	✓
Analysing data					✓		✓	✓
Planning community interventions			✓		✓		✓	
Monitoring and evaluating interventions			✓		✓	✓	✓	
Disseminating information			✓		✓	✓	✓	✓
Conducting economic analysis for decisions on pricing								✓
Implementing media campaigns			✓		✓		✓	
Developing educational materials			✓	✓	✓		✓	
Building partnerships		✓	✓	✓	✓	✓	✓	✓
Developing policies			✓		✓		✓	✓

People with research and evaluation skills may be found in institutes and universities; economic modelling experts in government or universities; legal practitioners in universities and the legal profession; policy-makers in government departments; experts on advocacy and partnership building in NGOs; health planners in central and provincial health departments and university public health schools; writers, editors and communication experts in business, the media, publishing, universities and NGOs; behavioural change counsellors in adolescent health, drug abuse or violence prevention programmes; "life skills" experts in adolescent health and development organizations.

✱ **Tip:** Be sure that those invited to train or develop materials do not work for the tobacco industry or have other conflicts of interests.

⊃ **Decision point:**

Identify skills to be covered and where to find personnel.

Recommended educational and training materials

The list below, organized by topic, is a starting point for implementing tobacco control education and training. It is not comprehensive; references to other materials can be found in other chapters of this handbook.

✱ **Tip:** World Health Organization materials are often cheaper for developing countries.

1. Health consequences of tobacco use, cost–benefit analysis, decision-making on taxation and pricing, regulation, litigation, materials for advocacy.

Curbing the epidemic: governments and the economics of tobacco control. Washington, DC, The World Bank Development in Practice series, 1999 (http://www1.worldbank.org/tobacco/reports.asp).

Economic, social and health issues in tobacco control. Report of the WHO International Meeting, Kobe, Japan, 3–4 December 2001. Japan, World Health Organization, 2003.

Guindon GE, Boisclair D. *Past, current and future trends in tobacco use.* Washington, DC, The World Bank, 2003 (Health Nutrition and Population Discussion Paper, Economics of Tobacco Control, paper No. 6).

Mackay J, Eriksen M. *The tobacco atlas.* Geneva, World Health Organization, 2002.

Public support for international efforts to control tobacco: a survey in five countries. Toronto, Environics Research Group Limited, 2001.

The economics of tobacco use & tobacco control in the developing world. A background paper for the High-Level Round Table on Tobacco Control and Development Policy. Brussels European Commission in collaboration with WHO and the World Bank, 3–4 February 2003.

The European report on tobacco control policy – Review of implementation of the Third Action Plan for a Tobacco-free Europe 1997–2001. Copenhagen, WHO Regional Office for Europe, 2002.

Samet J, Soon-Young Yoon eds. *Women and the tobacco epidemic: Challenges for the 21st century.* Geneva, World Health Organization, 2001.

Tobacco control legislation: an introductory guide. Geneva, World Health Organization, 2003.

World Health Organization, Tobacco Free Initiative: http://www.who.int/tobacco/en

2. Smoking cessation methods, behaviour change, nicotine replacement therapies.

Addressing the worldwide tobacco epidemic through effective, evidence-based treatment. Expert meeting, Rochester, MN, USA, March 1999. Geneva, World Health Organization, 1999 (http://www.who.int/tobacco/health_impact/mayo/en/).

Helping smokers change: a resource pack for training health professionals. Copenhagen, WHO Regional Office for Europe, 2001.

Policy recommendations for smoking cessation and treatment of tobacco dependence. Geneva, World Health Organization, 2003

Regulation of nicotine replacement therapies: an expert consensus. Copenhagen, WHO Regional Office for Europe, 2001.

3. Training methods and materials design for effective learning.

Abbatt FR. *Teaching for better learning: a guide for teachers of primary health care staff, 2nd ed.* Geneva, World Health Organization, 1992.

Brookfield SD. *Understanding and facilitating adult learning.* San Francisco, Jossey-Bass Publishers, 1986.

Education for health: a manual on health education in primary health care. Geneva, World Health Organization, 1988.

The reading room: Training skills (http://www.reproline.jhu.edu/english/6read/6read.htm).

4. Planning and implementing smoke-free workplaces and communities.

Oakley P. *Community involvement in health development: an examination of the critical issues.* Geneva, World Health Organization, 1989.

Tobacco in the workplace: meeting the challenges. A handbook for employers. Copenhagen, WHO Regional Office for Europe, 2002.

5. Research methods, rapid assessment methods, health planning and evaluation, evaluation of tobacco control interventions, report writing.

Chollat-Traquet C. *Evaluating tobacco control activities: experiences and guiding principles.* Geneva, World Health Organization, 1996.

Giving adolescents a voice: conducting a rapid assessment of adolescent health needs. A manual for health planners and researchers. Manila, WHO Regional Office for the Western Pacific, 2001.

Guidelines for controlling and monitoring the tobacco epidemic. Geneva, World Health Organization, 1996.

Hawe P, Degeling D, Hall J. *Evaluating health promotion: A health worker's guide.* Sydney, Maclennan & Petty, 1990.

Health research methodology: a guide for training in research methods, 2nd ed. Manila, WHO Regional Office for the Western Pacific, 2001.

Minichiello V et al. *In-depth interviewing: researching people.* Melbourne, Longman Cheshire, 1990.

6. Prevention strategies among youth, building life skills, adolescent healthy development.

Programming for adolescent health and development. Geneva, World Health Organization, 1999.

Simantov E, Schoen C, Klein JD. Health-compromising behaviors: why do adolescents smoke or drink? Identifying underlying risk and protective factors. *Archives of Pediatrics & Adolescent Medicine,* 2000, 154(10):1025–1033.

The Global Youth Tobacco Survey Collaborative Group. Tobacco use among youth: a cross-country comparison. *Tobacco Control,* 2002, 11:252–270.

What in the world works? International Consultation on Tobacco and Youth. Singapore, 28–30 September 1999. Final Report. Manila, WHO Regional Office for the Western Pacific, 2000.

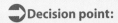**Decision point:**

Identify which materials are essential and which are desirable; assess availability, and decide whether or not to obtain them.

Question 6. Who can and should conduct training?

Tobacco control requires many skills and, therefore, many types of training. Do not worry if the country lacks designated 'tobacco control' trainers. Different sorts of individuals and groups can and should participate in training.

Using existing trainers

Trainers almost certainly already exist in the country, even if they work outside tobacco control. Contact government departments, NGOs, universities and institutes, social marketing organizations, and groups working in behaviour change, planning and evaluation, youth development and legislative change. Ask to speak to their training department or explain your needs. Trainers should have hands-on experience of the skills they will teach. Look for those willing to adapt their skills to a critical new area, but be sure they do not work for the tobacco industry.

Young people often learn more readily from another young person. If you reckon that age, sex, level of education, language and geographic and cultural background are relevant to the learning process, try and find trainers from the appropriate group.

> **Decision point:**
> Identify what trainers are needed, where they can be found, and whether they are suitable and available for training in tobacco control.

Training of Trainers (TOT)

TOT is a useful strategy for disseminating education and skills widely and quickly, particularly when used in a cascade system as described in Chapter 6. It is worth spending funds to develop master trainers in key areas. They will need to consolidate new information and skills, as well as training techniques. Be sure they have adequate resources, time and budget. Also, consider establishing a mentor programme, whereby one or two individuals offer support, feedback, additional materials or refresher training following TOT.

> **Tip:** Invite participants to evaluate training (anonymously) to ensure its quality, and find out whether trainers need further skills or have the interest and talent for this important role.

Question 7. What training methods are likely to be effective?

Most people learn best if they can practise the new skills they have learned. Adult learning techniques are relevant and useful. Most people adapt well to active learning, finding it enjoyable and effective even if they feel slightly embarrassed at first, but some societies consider it undignified for adults to role play or practise publicly, so always consider the cultural setting.

> **Tip:** Typical training methods are described in two training guides published by WHO *(1, 2)*. Select those most suitable to your audience and to the available skills, budget and materials.

The trainer's role

A good trainer makes learning meaningful and active, provides feedback, ensures assimilation of the lesson, is attentive to individual needs and shows commitment to the process. Abbatt *(2)* defines these qualities, and discusses methods of transfering knowledge, attitudes and skills.

Knowledge

A few key points for effective teaching:

- Do not try to teach everything: select key facts and use the appropriate pitch.
- Does the audience need information alone, or skills too?
- Offer several sources of information, providing resources and guidance so that trainees can acquire further information by themselves.
- Use 'real world' examples if possible.
- Plan the sequence (what should be learned first, second, etc.).
- Find out what they already know.
- Explain why the information is important.
- Begin with a brief summary.
- Use various methods (lectures, handouts, audiovisual aids, roleplays, exercises, group discussion, co-teaching, presentations by participants).
- Encourage questions and discussion.
- Adapt your language to the audience.
- At the end of each session summarize the main points and check that everybody has understood.

Teaching attitudes

The right attitudes are particularly important for smoking cessation counselling and advocacy.

- Provide information to shape attitudes (the harm caused by tobacco, obstacles to cessation in certain populations, cost–benefit analysis of tobacco use).
- Provide examples or models (e.g. increased sporting ability after quitting, a successful cessation clinic, advocacy leading to legislation, a video showing an effective counselling session).
- Provide group discussion and roleplays to explore attitudes and gain empathy (e.g. towards smokers, young people).

> **An example:**
>
> The resource pack *Helping Smokers Change,* published by the WHO Regional Office for Europe in 2001, includes a "pairs exercise" to gain empathy about behavioural change. In turn, participants identify a real habit they want to modify, discussing advantages and disadvantages of change versus non-change, while the other member fills in a grid.

Skills

- Do a "task analysis" *(2)* to identify what skills are needed and at what level, so that they can be analysed and taught in sequence.

- Describe and demonstrate tasks and enable every participant to practise, allowing time for repetition. Mastering skills may take 2–4 times longer than simply learning facts.
- Use roleplaying to build confidence (for interviews, counselling, public speaking). Ask others to provide feedback; however, never force anyone to do a roleplay.
- Use written case-studies (e.g. an effective partnership for tobacco control in another setting; a poorly-designed community intervention) for discussion or analysis.
- Job experience is the best way to consolidate skills, but it requires an understanding supervisor and opportunities for support, mentoring or further training.
- Helpful resources exist *(1, 3)* to support training for one-to-one counselling (e.g. skills for quitting).

> **An example:**
>
> WHO-sponsored workshops on Community Interventions for Tobacco Control in China in 2002 included daily small-group tasks leading to the completion of a draft intervention proposal submitted for competitive funding. This process consolidated skills in setting objectives, selecting strategies and activities and identifying indicators for monitoring and evaluation (see Box 7).

> **Decision point:**
>
> Undertake a task analysis and decide what types of training methods are most suitable for capacity-building.

Question 8: How can you plan an effective training workshop?

This section summarizes key components of planning and conducting training workshops and provides examples of actual workshops.

Workshops are generally short (2–10 days), highly focused and intensive. They are most suitable for training that can be practised within the classroom. Normally, workshops do not offer intensive training, so participants need materials to take home to refresh their learning, or opportunities for further training.

> **Tip:**
>
> When deciding who is to participate, consider that training workshops serve at least two purposes:
>
> 1. They offer time, space and the opportunity to gain new knowledge and skills (some applicable to other areas).
> 2. They help raise awareness and gain new allies and partners.

Workshop planning checklist
- Setting objectives:
  - be realistic about setting objectives, too many objectives may not be attainable;

- ensure that objectives are clearly explained and understood by participants;
- be aware of and acknowledge any hidden objectives (e.g. to gain allies).
- Thinking about the participants:
  - consider their role, capacity and willingness to attend the workshop and utilize new skills;
  - ensure balance of gender, ethnicity, geographical location and organizational background;
  - size: a group of 15–30 participants is large enough for exposure to different views and experience, and small enough to develop relationships and enable active participation;
  - avoid large power imbalances that inhibit open discussion;
  - select some 'aware' participants for an energetic start (dynamics are important);
  - invitation letters should explain the purpose, time commitment and expectations for the workshop;
  - invitations should be sent out in time for monitoring of responses.
- Timing
  - the chosen day/month/year should be appropriate for key participants;
  - the duration of training should be sufficient for the transfer of skills (additional workshops or other mechanisms may be needed to consolidate learning).
- Venue
  - choose a venue that is convenient and accessible for most participants;
  - ensure that the participants will not be disturbed by noise, traffic and other distractions;
  - the meeting room should be neither too small (too cramped) nor too large (too intimidating), and should provide a comfortable environment for the participants;
  - provide writing surfaces;
  - ascertain that refreshments and meals are provided or are conveniently available;
  - make sure that audiovisual requirements are met;
  - provide space and writing materials for group work.
- Workshop reading materials
  - moderate amount of reading materials is more likely to be read and used;
  - choose suitable materials for the type of education and focus;
  - provide a bound set to keep the materials secure, with provisions for add-ons;
  - offer tips to find additional materials and a list of references for future reading.

Limitations of workshops

Though popular and effective, workshops have some limitations:
- Learning styles and preferences: some people cannot focus during intensive sessions; some do not like group discussion.
- Intensity but no consolidation: many skills, such as research and counselling, require abundant practice and time for assimilation.
- Personality conflicts or strain due to inexperienced facilitators, or large power imbalances between participants, may impede learning.

Examples of tobacco control workshops

Box 4 outlines a generic workshop; Boxes 5, 6, and 7 summarize actual workshops held. A more detailed agenda of the workshops outlined in Boxes 5 and 7 can be found in Annex 1.

Box 4. Generic model of a 2-day awareness workshop on national tobacco control

Objectives

- Increasing knowledge of the health burden of tobacco and producing appropriate responses in key stakeholders.
- Building partnerships.
- Raising awareness of the WHO Framework Convention on Tobacco Control.

Target audience

- Mid- to high-level representatives from relevant ministries (health, finance, education, agriculture, etc.).
- Representatives of major health organizations (e.g. Cancer Council, Heart Council).
- Representatives of major community organizations.

If possible, ensure gender and age balance of target audience.

Presenter/facilitator

Someone at senior level, experienced in building participative exchange and partnerships, with no vested interests in tobacco.

Contents

- Health risks, the benefits of quitting, burden of disease internationally and nationally, trends.
- Economic and social costs.
- The WHO Framework Convention on Tobacco Control and why it is needed.
- The role of health professionals in smoking prevention and cessation.
- Successful models of tobacco control regulations, interventions, cessation and prevention programmes.
- Forming partnerships for tobacco control.
- Developing action plans.

Box 5. Workshop on building and strengthening national capacity for tobacco control [2]

Objectives

- Strengthening and supporting the capacity of countries to assess, plan, monitor and evaluate comprehensive tobacco control programmes that reflect national priorities and realities.
- Building on existing public health systems and strengthening their human and institutional capacity in managerial, technical and political areas.
- Developing a pilot project for similar training workshops on national capacity-building for tobacco control.

Target audience

Representatives of ministries of health.

Facilitators

Director, Tobacco Free Initiative, World Health Organization.

Contents

- Global and national issues in tobacco control.
- Making an impact on decision-makers in the area of tobacco control.
- The experience of Brazil.
- Use of communication tools to create a favourable environment for tobacco control.
- The role of civil society in tobacco control.
- National Tobacco Control Programmes: structural issues, coordination mechanisms and self-sustainability.
- Legislative and economic measures.
- How to search tobacco industry documents.

---

[2] Based on a 4-day workshop on strengthening national capacity for tobacco control, intended for Portuguese-speaking countries, held in Brazil in April 2003. The workshop was hosted by the National Cancer Institute (INCA), Brazil, and cosponsored by WHO/TFI and INCA, Brazil.

Box 6. Tobacco control and gender workshop[3]

Objectives

- Use of social models of health to explore gender dimensions of tobacco use among men and women.
- Understanding of the health impacts of tobacco and sex-related differentials.
- Assimilation of research tools in order to contribute to gender-sensitive programmes and policy design.
- Preparation of action plans to bring gender into tobacco control.

Target audience

Researchers, officials, programme planners familiar with health research and planning.

Facilitators

People with expertise in training, health policy, tobacco control and gender research.

Contents

- Recent epidemiological evidence about health impacts and patterns.
- What is tobacco control?
- Research evidence about sociocultural influences on tobacco use
- Exercises to identify gender issues in individual countries.
- Qualitative and quantitative methods to investigate tobacco use.
- Policy issues for gender and tobacco control.
- Developing effective interventions (planning, monitoring and evaluation).
- Action planning and peer review.

Box 7. Planning community interventions for tobacco control[4]

Objectives

- Becoming familiar with:
  - strategies for tobacco control in different settings
  - smoking cessation methods, process, impact and outcome evaluation
  - strategies to involve the community in the Chinese context.
- Preparing a proposal for a community intervention.

Target audience

- Researchers, policy and programme designers in health education.
- Members of community organizations.

Facilitators

Experts in programme planning and evaluation for tobacco control at the community level.

Contents

- Explaining tobacco control.
- The role of social factors in tobacco use.
- How to bring about behavioural change.
- Planning a community intervention.
- Conducting a situation analysis.
- Defining objectives and strategies.
- A practical model for smoking cessation.
- Possible activities in the context of China.
- Monitoring and evaluation of tobacco control.

---

[3] A 9-day workshop held by the University of Melbourne in December 2000, for 13 South-East Asian participants.

[4] WHO-sponsored workshops in Beijing and Chengdu, China, held in October 2002. Selected interventions developed during the workshop were funded and implemented in 2003.

Suggested framework for education and training in different settings

In the next two subsections we suggest core training and educational requirements for:
- countries where tobacco use is widespread or spreading fast, which are planning to introduce regulations in response to the WHO FCTC;
- countries that formerly experienced high prevalence but have succeeded in reducing it through control measures and interventions, with certain groups continuing to use tobacco.

Countries may fall between these two extremes. The NTCP must identify at what stage the country is and how best to tackle the current situation. The models outlined below are only suggestions, and are neither comprehensive nor prescriptive.

Suggested plan for a country with high prevalence and few control measures

- National awareness-raising and advocacy workshop (see Box 4).
- National workshop to build research capacity in order to undertake national prevalence surveys and rapid assessments or social research into:
  - factors influencing tobacco use;
  - obstacles to tobacco control (modification of Box 6);
  - national TOT smoking cessation workshop for health professionals (see Box 5);
  - provincial and district smoking cessation workshops for health professionals (see Box 5);
  - provincial workshops on establishing smoking-cessation clinics and help lines;
  - national workshops to plan media and community-level education and advocacy campaigns;
  - national workshops to build capacity in cost–benefit analysis, economic modelling for pricing and taxation, reduction of smuggling (if relevant) and drafting of legislation;
  - national workshops to build partnerships for legislative change;
  - provincial workshops on planning, monitoring and evaluation of community interventions (see Box 7).

Suggested plan for a country with medium–low prevalence and several control measures

- National awareness-raising and advocacy workshop on legislative weaknesses and other obstacles to reduction (see Box 4).
- National workshop to build capacity in order to conduct rapid assessments and/or social research into:
  - factors influencing tobacco use;
  - obstacles to tobacco control (modification of Box 6).
- Provincial and district smoking-cessation workshops for health professionals working with target populations (modification of Box 5).
- National and provincial dissemination and planning workshops to discuss obstacles identified after second national workshop and develop appropriate strategies.

5. Provincial workshops on planning, monitoring and evaluation of community interventions (see Box 7).

References

1. *Education for health: a manual on health education in primary health care.* Geneva, World Health Organization, 1988: 39–80.

2. Abbatt FR. *Teaching for better learning: a guide for teachers of primary health care staff, 2nd ed.* Geneva, World Health Organization, 1992.

3. *Helping smokers change: a resource pack for training health professionals.* Copenhagen, WHO Regional Office for Europe, 2001.

ANNEX 1

Workshop on strengthening national capacity for tobacco control, held in Brazil in April 2003

AGENDA	
Morning	**Afternoon**
Day 1	
Opening ceremony Presence of Minister of Health, Director of National Cancer Institute and WHO **Presentation** Global and national issues in tobacco control **Exercise** Curbing the Epidemic - identification of key messages of relevance to each country **Presentation** How to make an impact on decision-makers in the area of tobacco control	**Exercise** Completion of country survey questionnaires; discussion on data collected and their importance **Presentation** The experience of Brazil in tobacco control: the country's current situation and how it got there **Presentation** History of tobacco control in Brazil **Presentation** Examples from a state in Brazil
Day 2	
Topic Creating a favourable environment for tobacco control: use of communication tools **Presentations** • Channels & general aspects • Popular mobilization • Assessment of communications work • The media & interviews	**Exercise** Mock interviews on tobacco control issues **Presentations** • Civil society and tobacco control • Social mobilization for tobacco control **Video presentation** Mock interviews with participants **Presentations** • National Tobacco Control Programmes – structural issues, coordination mechanisms, self-sustainability • Experiences from a municipality and three states
Day 3	
Presentations • Agenda of workshop as a model for other national workshops • Epidemiology & tobacco control • Further education activities • Control of tobacco and other risk factors: health units and workplaces • Smoking cessation among health professionals	**Presentations** • Legislation in Brazil • Partnerships with other parts of the Ministry • Economic measures • Municipality presentation • Development of a system of evaluation for tobacco control • Evaluation of tobacco control
Day 4	
Presentation Planning **Exercise** How to prepare funding proposals for tobacco control, based on key issues to be tackled in the country	**Presentation** How to search tobacco industry documents **Closing** Participants given CD ROMS with workshop details and presentations

WHO-sponsored workshop on planning community interventions for tobacco control, held in China in October 2002

AGENDA	
Morning	**Afternoon**

Day 1

Morning

Opening ceremony
Workshop format; self-introduction

1a. What is tobacco control (TC)?
• Health risks of tobacco
• Tobacco control
• Cessation vs. prevention
• Benefits of cessation
• Quitting with and without assistance
• What might work in China?

1b. What is a 'community', an 'intervention'?

Afternoon

1c. Who uses tobacco and why?
Role of social factors

1d. Behaviour change
• How does change happen and what are the typical stages?
• Overcoming challenges

1e. Group work
Pairs exercise: understanding stages of change and decisional balance

Day 2

Morning

2a. Planning an Intervention
The 'Logical Model':
• STEP 1: What are the planning steps?
• Conducting a situation analysis

2b. Group work
• Thinking about the situation analysis
• What information do you need for the baseline?

Afternoon

2c. Interventions: choices and decisions
• Price increase
• Media campaign
• Workplace restriction
• Home restriction
• Behavioural counselling
• Pharmacotherapy
• Healthcare providers

2d. Group work
Decision point:
• Define the target group
• What type of intervention will you choose and why?

Day 3

Morning

3a. Planning a community intervention for TC
STEP 2: Defining objectives and strategies

3b. Group work:
• What objectives are 'reasonable'?
• What specific activities will work best to achieve the objectives?

Afternoon

3c1. A practical model for smoking cessation

3c2. Implementing the programme
Pros and cons of a range of activities in the context of China

3d. Group work
Decision point:
Define strategies and activities clearly linked to the objectives

Day 4

Morning

4a. Introduction to health programme evaluation for tobacco control
• Setting indicators and measures
• Monitoring; process and impact evaluation
• Timing of evaluation

4b. Group work day
Decision point:
Prepare outline: objectives, strategies and activities. Include monitoring and evaluation indicators, if possible.

Afternoon

4c. Plenary discussion of proposed interventions

4d. What happens if the proposal is selected?
Plans for next workshop to present feedback, monitoring, evaluation and dissemination

4e. Workshop evaluation
Closing ceremony

8
Communication and public awareness to build critical mass

*The art of communication is
the language of leadership.*
—James Humes

INTRODUCTION

Tobacco is heavily marketed. By the skilful application of the four principles of commercial marketing – product, place, price and promotion (see Box 1) – the tobacco industry has ensured the social acceptability of tobacco use, and the availability and popularity of tobacco products while generating tremendous profits for its shareholders. The continued consumption of tobacco products, despite the established harm of tobacco, attests to the success of marketing strategies even when the products are known to cause disease and death.

If marketing contributes greatly to the persistence of tobacco use, it stands to reason that the same principles can be applied to achieve the opposite effect. Kotler and Roberto and Andreasen *(1, 2)* were among the first to realize that commercial marketing techniques could be adapted to programmes designed to influence the behaviour of a target audience to enhance their well-being. They defined this as social marketing. The use of social marketing for tobacco control is sometimes also referred to as tobacco counter-marketing, because it aims to reduce tobacco consumption, thus countering the efforts of the tobacco industry to promote tobacco use *(3)* (see Box 2).

Box 1. Using the framework of social marketing for tobacco control

- The **product** is the tobacco control programme and the interventions it intends to implement.
- The **price** refers to both the tangible and intangible costs to engage in action or to participate in the programme; it includes money, time, opportunity costs and even the emotional costs of participation.
- **place** refers to the distribution or the location or mechanism for getting tobacco control interventions to consumers.
- **promotion** involves all strategies to promote tobacco control and to inform consumers about it and its advantages.
- Sometimes, a fifth 'P' – **people** – can be factored into the framework; this refers to the key people who can either ensure a programme's success or block its implementation.

To build a critical mass of public supporters of tobacco control, programme planners of the NTCP need to devise a strategic marketing mix of these 'Ps'. Successful social marketing for tobacco control requires the systematic implementation of a process in which the marketing mix is clearly elucidated in six stages that use decision-based research to provide feedback at every stage. The process is a dynamic one that allows programme adjustments based on continuous feedback (see Figure 1).

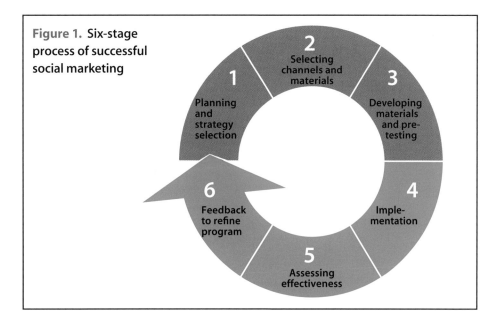

Figure 1. Six-stage process of successful social marketing

1 Planning and strategy selection

2 Selecting channels and materials

3 Developing materials and pre-testing

4 Implementation

5 Assessing effectiveness

6 Feedback to refine program

Box 2. Characteristics of effective counter-marketing efforts

The United States Centers for Disease Control and Prevention, in its review of the evidence on counter-marketing, conclude that the effective counter-marketing efforts:

- use a comprehensive approach, utilizing media, school and community-based activities;

- must have sufficient reach, frequency and duration; this invariably requires the use of paid media placement;

- combine messages on prevention, cessation and protection from second-hand smoke;

- target both young people and adults; and address both individual behaviours and public policies;

- include grass-roots promotions, local media advocacy, event sponsorships, and other community tie-ins to support and reinforce the state-wide campaign;

- maximize the number, variety and novelty of messages and production styles rather than communicate a few messages repeatedly;

- use non-authoritarian appeals that avoid direct exhortations not to smoke and do not highlight a single theme, tagline, identifier or sponsor.

Source: *Best Practices for Comprehensive Tobacco Control Programs – August 1999 (4)*

The social marketing of tobacco control requires strategic communication. Communications strategies are key, not only because they ensure that accurate information is accessible to the population but because well-designed communications campaigns can lead to changes in behaviour that are essential for reducing the prevalence of tobacco use. The experience of several countries like Australia, Canada and Thailand suggests that effective social marketing and communications campaigns can curtail tobacco use. This chapter presents some key strategies and approaches to designing a social marketing and communications campaign for tobacco control. The National Cancer Institute publication *Making Health Communications Programs Work (5)* and the recent *Designing and implementing an effective tobacco counter-marketing campaign (3)* provide a detailed discussion of this issue. An overview of World No Tobacco Day, celebrated every year on 31 May, is provided in this chapter (see Box 3).

THE FIRST STEP: PLAN AND STRATEGIZE

Planning and strategy are the foundation of an effective social marketing and communications campaign. The following are intrinsic to the preparatory phase.

Understand the problem

The basis of any attempt to change knowledge, attitudes or behaviour is a systematic review and understanding of the problem that needs to be addressed. For tobacco control campaigns, this refers to the need to be familiar with the tobacco epidemic as it affects a particular target population within a country. Review existing health and demographic data, survey results, study findings and any other available information. In all cases, search for local data, as this will carry greater weight when preparing the specific messages to communicate. If necessary, seek out and talk to experts, who may be found in academic institutions, tobacco control NGOs or within the community. Your search should include information on the local tobacco industry, which actively promotes the behaviour that needs to be changed.

Be clear about the how the problem relates to the overall plan of action for tobacco control. Describe the problem in specific terms, clearly identifying:

- what the nature of the problem is;
- who it affects, and in what manner it affects the target population;
- how bad the problem is, and what indicators can be used to gauge its severity;
- what and who can enable the resolution of the problem;
- what and who can make the problem worse (e.g. the tobacco industry).

Know the target population

Look for and study the geographical, demographic, economic and social factors that shape the behaviour of the target population. These could include differences in knowledge, attitudes and practices, age, gender, literacy, ethnicity, educational attainment, income, personality and lifestyle, and values. Also consider individual and community variables specific to the locale, which determine the patterns of tobacco use. For example, in some Pacific Islander communities, chewing tobacco is the predominant form of tobacco use, and is as much a social activity as an individual behaviour. In some northern African and eastern Mediterranean countries, the use of water pipes or the *shisha* is very common, while in parts of South-East Asia, clay pipes known as *suipa*, *chillum* or *hookli* are widely used.

The degree of exposure to mass media is another critical factor since this will determine the channels of communication selected. In many developing countries, the Internet and even television are not available in rural communities, but radios are extremely common and popular.

If the target population is large and heterogeneous, identify different target segments within the larger population that would respond to different types of messages and channels. Develop a personality profile for each of the identified population segments. By understanding the audience, you can tailor the marketing mix to best appeal to them.

Tip: Draft a profile of the target audience.

Identify other factors that can affect the campaign

Identify resources, strengths and weaknesses of the NTCP and the sociopolitical environment that relates to the ability to successfully address the problem at hand. Review existing programmes, policies and laws that may have an impact on the intended campaign. Know the key players and stakeholders in the locality. Anticipate the impact of the communications campaign on these stakeholders, and prepare for potential reactions to the campaign. In particular, be ready for potential adverse reactions from the tobacco industry and related organizations. In addition, be aware of the promotional activities of the tobacco industry to increase tobacco use, and possible effects of having a tobacco control campaign while tobacco industry promotional campaigns are ongoing.

Tip: Make a list of all these factors, separating the positive from the negative.

Establish a framework to influence the behaviour of the target population

A theoretical framework that explains why, how and in what order people make changes in their health knowledge, attitudes, intentions and behaviours can guide the selection of objectives, strategies and messages for a social marketing campaign. Several models exist; in practice, many programmes use a combination of these theories. Table 1 summarizes the major theoretical models for behaviour change.

Table 1. Summary of theories: focus and key concepts

	Theory	Focus	Key concepts
Individual level	Stages of change model	Individuals' readiness to change or attempt to change toward healthy behaviours	• Pre-contemplation • Contemplation • Decision/determination • Action • Maintenance
	Health belief model	People's perception of the threat of a health problem and the appraisal of recommended behaviour(s) for preventing or managing the problem	• Perceived susceptibility • Perceived severity • Perceived benefits of action • Perceived barriers to action • Cues to action • Self-efficacy
	Consumer information processing model	Process by which consumers acquire and use information in making decisions	• Information processing • Information search • Decision rules/heuristics • Consumption and learning • Information environment
Interpersonal level	Social learning theory	Behaviour explained via a three-way, dynamic reciprocal theory in which personal factors, environmental influences, and behaviour continually interact	• Behavioural capability • Reciprocal determinism • Expectations • Self-efficacy • Observational learning • Reinforcement • Empowerment
Community level	Community organization theories	Emphasis of active community participation and development of communities that can better evaluate and solve health and social problems	• Community competence • Participation and relevance • Issue selection • Critical consciousness
	Organizational change theory	Processes and strategies for increasing the chances that healthy policies and programmes will be adopted and maintained in formal organizations	• Problem definition (awareness stage) • Initiation of action (adoption stage) • Implementation of change • Institutionalization of change
	Diffusion of innovations theory	How new ideas, products, and social practices spread within a society or from one society to another	• Relative advantage • Compatibility • Complexity • Trialability • Observability

Source: NCI, 1995 *(6)*.

Determine the objectives

Clearly worded objectives are necessary to devise appropriate strategies and messages. Possible general outcomes of tobacco-control social marketing are:

- raise awareness of the problem and/or the tobacco control programme
- enhance knowledge about specific issues
- influence individual attitudes or values, contributing to behaviour change
- shift community norms
- propel people to act (e.g. call a quit line)
- win broad public support for tobacco control issues *(6)*

Set objectives that are **SMART**:
- **S**pecific
- **M**easurable
- **A**ppropriate
- **R**ealistic
- **T**ime-bound

Develop achievable objectives for the target population, and quantify the changes in knowledge, attitudes, behaviour or advocacy that you wish to achieve within a given period of time. If you identified subgroups or segments from within the larger target population, draft specific objectives for each subgroup.

Choose the approaches to achieve the objectives

There are several approaches to tobacco counter-marketing *(3):*
- Advertising: a communication strategy in which messages are repeatedly delivered directly to a mass audience. Advertising permits control over the message's tone, content, placement and amount of exposure.
- Public relations: uses "earned" media coverage to reach target audiences, through cultivating relationships with media gatekeepers.
- Media advocacy: uses media and community advocacy strategically to create changes in social norms and policies.
- Grass-roots marketing: actively involves people in the community in counter-marketing activities.
- Media literacy: develops skills that enable people to assess the use of mass media critically in propagating tobacco use.

Each of these approaches has its inherent strengths and weaknesses. The choice of which approach or combination of approaches to use will depend on the objectives of the social marketing campaign. In general, using a combination of approaches is more effective than using any one approach. The approach chosen must be consistent with the overall strategy and resources of the NTCP.

Design the programme strategy

Every social marketing and communications programme needs a strategic design. This translates the analysis in the preparatory phase into an unambiguous roadmap with clear directions on how to accomplish the project objectives.

Prepare a concise strategy statement that delineates the objectives, target audience profile, the desired behaviour change, potential obstacles, and specific activities and interventions to achieve that change. Clearly indicate how to show the intended audiences a clear benefit from the services or practices promoted, and what is needed to convince them of the benefit.

Create an implementation plan

Set up a plan for implementing the programme. Design all programme tasks, ensuring that each one contributes to the established objectives of the strategy statement. Clearly identify the person or persons responsible for each task. Prepare a budget for each phase of the project. Include a timeline or work schedule with periodic indicators to monitor progress.

Develop the evaluation mechanism

Develop an evaluation scheme before launching the project. Plan to measure the expected changes in the target audience using multiple data sources. Collect baseline data, and ensure that the evaluation scheme is clearly laid out before implementing the interventions.

THE SECOND STEP: SELECT CHANNELS AND MATERIALS

Channels

Channels are the avenues or pathways to deliver programme messages, materials and activities to your target audience. The different channels, and their relative advantages and disadvantages are summarized in Table 2 (see also Tables 3 and 4).

Table 2. Communication channels and activities: pros and cons

Type of channel	Activities	Pros	Cons
Interpersonal channels	• Hotline counselling • Patient counselling • Instruction • Information • Discussion	• Can be credible • Permit two-way discussion • Can be motivational influential, supportive • Most effective for teaching and helping/caring	• Can be expensive • Can be time-consuming • Can have limited intended audience reach • Can be difficult to link into interpersonal channels; sources need to be convinced and taught about the message themselves
Organizational and community channels	• Town hall meetings and other events • Organizational meetings and conferences • Workplace campaigns	• May be familiar, trusted, and influential • May provide more motivation/support than media alone • Can sometimes be inexpensive • Can offer shared experiences • Can reach larger intended audience in one place	• Can be costly, time-consuming to establish • May not provide personalized attention • Organizational constraints may require message approval • May lose control of message if adapted to fit organizational needs
Mass media channels			
Newspaper	• Ads • Inserted sections on a health topic (paid) • News • Feature stories • Letters to the editor • Op/ed pieces • Question and answer articles in magazines or newspapers	• Can reach broad intended audiences rapidly • Can convey health news/breakthroughs more thoroughly than TV or radio • Intended audience has chance to clip, reread, contemplate, and pass along material • Small circulation papers may take print public service announcements (PSAs)	• Coverage demands a newsworthy item • Larger circulation papers may take only paid ads and inserts • Exposure usually limited to one day • Article placement requires contacts and may be time-consuming
Radio	• Ads (paid or public service placement) • News • Public affairs/talk shows • Dramatic programming (entertainment education)	• Range of formats available to intended audiences with known listening preferences • Opportunity for direct intended audience involvement (through call-in shows) • Can distribute ad scripts (termed 'live-copy ads'), which are flexible and inexpensive • Paid ads or specific programming can reach intended audience when they are most receptive; paid ads can be relatively inexpensive • Ad production costs are low relative to TV • Ads allow message and its execution to be controlled	• Reaches smaller intended audiences than TV • Public service ads run infrequently and at low listening times • Many stations have limited formats that may not be conducive to health messages • Difficult for intended audiences to retain or pass on material

Continues…

Table 2 (continued)

Type of channel	Activities	Pros	Cons
Television	• Ads (paid or public service placement) • News • Public affairs/talk shows • Dramatic programming (entertainment education)	• Reaches potentially the largest and widest range of intended audiences • Visual combined with audio good for emotional appeals and demonstrating behaviours • Can reach low-income intended audiences • Paid ads or specific programming can reach intended audience when most receptive • Ads allow message and its execution to be controlled • Opportunity for direct intended audience involvement (through call-in shows)	• Ads are expensive to produce • Paid advertising is expensive • PSAs run infrequently and at low viewing times • Message may be obscured by commercial clutter • Some stations reach very small intended audiences • Promotion can result in huge demand • Can be difficult for intended audiences to retain or pass on material
Internet	• Web sites • E-mail mailing lists • Chat rooms • Newsgroups • Ads (paid or public service placement)	• Can reach large numbers of people rapidly • Can instantaneously update and disseminate information • Can control information provided • Can tailor information specifically for intended audiences • Can be interactive • Can provide health information in a graphically appealing way • Can combine the audio/visual benefits of TV or radio with the self-paced benefits of print media • Can use banner ads to direct intended audience to your programme's web site	• Can be expensive • Many intended audiences do not have access to Internet • Intended audience must be proactive – must search or sign up for information • News groups and chat rooms may require monitoring • Can require maintenance over time

Source: Adapted from DHHS, 2003 *(3)*

Table 3: Pros and cons of different formats for focus groups and individual interviews

Activities	Pros	Cons
Face-to-face Moderator/interviewer and participants are in one room, usually around a table; observers (members of the research team) are behind a one-way mirror	• Can assess body language • If videotaped, can share with others who couldn't attend • Have participants' undivided attention	• Responders lose some anonymity • Higher travel expenses due to multiple locales • Usually excludes people in rural areas or small towns
Telephone Moderator/interviewer and participants are on a conference call; observers listen in	• More convenient for participants and observers • Can easily include people in rural areas, in small towns, and who are homebound • For professional groups, may be easier to gain participation because it is less likely participants will know each other • Relative anonymity may result in more frank discussion of sensitive issues	• Cannot assess nonverbal reactions • More difficult to get reactions to visuals (although they can be sent ahead of time) • Participants can be distracted by their surroundings • Requires technology that allows teleconferencing
Radio Moderator/interviewer and participants are on a conference call, with dialogue broadcast over the radio; observers listen in through radio	• Radio readily available in developing countries • Can easily include people in rural areas, in small towns, and who are homebound • For professional groups, may be easier to gain participation because it is less likely participants will know each other • Relative anonymity may result in more frank discussion of sensitive issues	• Cannot assess nonverbal reactions
Internet chat sessions Moderator and participants "chat"; observers watch	• Complete record of session instantly available • Relative anonymity may result in more frank discussion of sensitive issues	• Requires access to computer technology, the Internet and chat rooms • Only useful for participants • comfortable with this mode of communication • Relatively slow pace limits topics that can be covered • No way to assess if participants meet recruitment criteria • Cannot assess body language or tone of voice • More difficult to get reaction to visuals

Source: Adapted from DHHS, 2003 *(3)*

Table 4: Graphics and audio visual

Strengths	Limitations
• Provides timely reminders • Attracts the attention of the target audience at the place of exposure • Provides basic information on the product and its benefits • Demonstrates steps of behaviour • Provides complex information • Is handy and reusable • Supports interpersonal communication • Provides accurate, standardized information • May be produced locally • Provides instant feedback • Gives confidence and credibility to person communicating messages	• May not be cost effective • Often used out of cultural and educational context • Training necessary for proper use and display

Source: Adapted from NCI, 1989 *(5)*

When deciding on channels:
- Determine the channels most appropriate for the issue and message.
- Decide which channels reach the target audience most effectively. Tailor the channel selected based on the profile of the target audience.
- Select channels that best address the objectives.
- Evaluate the availability, reach and costs of the different channels, based on your time line and budget, and on existing technology.
- Use a combination of channels for maximum impact. When using multiple channels, identify the primary channel and supporting channels.
- Consider the cost effectiveness of the channel.

Materials

Materials are the communication tools that carry the message to your target audience. Materials can come in multiple formats: print materials, such as booklets and posters, videotapes, public service announcements and web-based materials.

When selecting materials:
- Find out if there are existing materials that you can use or adapt. If you are considering the use of existing materials, contact the original producer to discuss:
  – how the messages were developed;
  – whether the materials were tested;
  – how they have been used and by whom;
  – whether they were effective.

Obtain permission to use the materials. This is especially important when using copyrighted materials.

Box 3. World No Tobacco Day, 31 May

1988: Tobacco or Health: Choose Health

1989: Women and Tobacco

1990: Childhood and Youth Without Tobacco

1991: Public Places and Transport: Better Be Tobacco-free

1992: Tobacco-free Workplaces: Safer and Healthier

1993: Health Services: Our Windows to a Tobacco-free World

1994: Media And Tobacco: Get the Message Across

1995: Tobacco Costs More than You Think

1996: Sports and the Arts without Tobacco: Play it Tobacco-free

1997: United for a Tobacco-free World

1998: Growing Up Without Tobacco

1999: Leave the Pack Behind

2000: Tobacco Kills: Don't Be Duped

2001: Second Hand Smoke Kills: Clear the Air

2002: Tobacco Free Sports: Play it Clean

2003: Action: Tobacco Free Films and Fashion

2004: Tobacco and Poverty: A Vicious Circle

World No Tobacco Day (WNTD) is now celebrated in almost all of WHO's 192 Member States. It provides an excellent opportunity to highlight specific tobacco control messages at both national and international levels. Because of the attention given by the international community to WNTD, it has the potential to grab the attention of top national leaders and key decision-makers and media. In past WNTD celebrations, several ministries of health and WHO officially recognized the efforts of individuals and organizations to promote tobacco control within their respective countries, giving legitimacy to the work of these tobacco control advocates. In addition, several ministries of health, some tobacco control NGOs and even the International Federation of Football Associations (FIFA) have timed the launch of specific tobacco control initiatives to coincide with WNTD. For example, on WNTD 2002, FIFA's first tobacco-free World Cup kicked off simultaneously in Japan and the Republic of Korea, coinciding with the WNTD theme of 'Tobacco Free Sports: Play it Clean'. Doing this expands the media mileage for specific initiatives while at the same time strengthening the general social acceptability of reducing tobacco use. Consequently, national tobacco control planners should include the celebration of WNTD into their communications strategy.

Source: http://www.who.int/tobacco/areas/communications/en/

- If you determine the need to produce new materials, be guided by:
  - the complexity, sensitivity, style and objective of the message;
  - the communications preferences of the target audience;
  - the nature of the channels through which the materials will be disseminated;
  - the costs, and availability of resources.

THE THIRD STEP: DEVELOP AND PRETEST THE MESSAGES AND MATERIALS

Message development in public health communications combines science and art. Messages need to be guided by the analysis and strategic design accomplished in the preparatory phase, but they also must be scientifically accurate and emotionally moving to influence the target audience towards some action or change in behaviour (see Box 4).

Begin with message concepts

Based on the results of the analysis and design strategy, develop message concepts by identifying the key words, themes or storylines and the accompanying visual images that reflect the overall strategy. For maximum impact, keep messages clear and simple. Avoid complexity (see Box 5). Highlight benefits and practical solutions that address people's needs.

Work with tobacco control and public health professionals

For public health communications projects, work closely with health professionals to ensure that the technical information is accurate. An additional advantage to working

---

Box 4. Preparing effective messages

1. Establish a personality for the message. Make the message appealing, to make it stand out.
2. Position the message carefully. Carefully delineate how the message fits into the lifestyle and values of the target audience.
3. Highlight a compelling benefit that addresses a real need among the target audience.
4. Create trust. The message should be simple, direct, empathic and credible.
5. Appeal to both heart and mind. Invest the message with emotional as well as intellectual value.
6. Maintain focus. Ensure that the message deals directly with the health issue under consideration.

Box 5. Avoid ineffective messages

1. Non-specific messages – Because of individual differences, as well as differences in age, gender, education and psychological predisposition, people selectively perceive and retain media messages. Messages around a health issue need to appeal to these different subgroups within the target population. 'One size fits all' does not apply to effective communications.

2. Indifferent messages – Unemotional messages are ineffective because most people learn better and respond more positively when their emotions are aroused.

3. Complicated messages – Multiple themes and excessive details distract audiences, who often miss the main point.

4. Messages with no call to action – People need to know what to do with information. Without a specific cue to action, the audience may see, hear and understand, but without effecting a change in their behaviour.

5. Fearful messages – Scare tactics may shock and distract, but their overall effect is often short-lived.

6. Static messages – Different information is needed at each stage of behaviour change. Static messages fail to deliver, because they fail to provide what the target audience needs.

with health professionals is the opportunity to establish an ongoing working relationship with them that facilitates winning their support for the project.

Work with communications professionals

Presenting technically accurate information is not enough to mount a successful public health communications project or campaign. Work closely with experts in mass communications and with other creative talent to produce messages and materials that are packaged to have maximum impact on the audience. In many countries, this type of expertise may not always be found within the ministry of health. Identify professionals and creative talent in the private sector who understand and empathize with the issues being promoted. For ongoing communications programmes, develop a network of contacts in the communications and creative arts fields that can be tapped readily when needed.

Follow the seven Cs of effective communication

1. Command attention; be creative
2. Cater to the heart and the head
3. Create a clear message
4. Communicate a benefit
5. Convey a consistent message
6. Call for action
7. Create trust

Pre-test with pilot audiences

Always pretest and retest message concepts and materials with sample groups of the intended audience, to obtain feedback about their clarity and effectiveness. During these testing sessions, encourage active discussion among the participants to draw out their reactions to the intended messages and materials. Devote special attention to pictures and nonverbal materials that might be misunderstood, or that may convey an idea different from what was intended. For mass media campaigns, which often generate the greatest controversy, solicit the feedback of media professionals and political gatekeepers. Take note of both positive and negative feedback.

Revise as needed

Revise any messages and materials that are not well understood or easily remembered, or that are irrelevant, controversial or offensive to the intended audience. Be prepared for unanticipated changes. Use the feedback from the test audiences to guide the revisions, then retest the new messages and materials, until the feedback is satisfactory.

Produce materials efficiently and promptly

Strive for the best quality when producing materials, within the limits of the resources. High-quality materials are more likely to catch the attention of intended users, hold their value, be reused many times and generate revenue than poorer-quality counterparts. Producing materials in large volumes is often more cost effective than repeated production runs, so ensure that the estimates for materials are accurate. Finally, ensure that materials are available when needed. Late materials mean that a good opportunity to deliver the message was lost.

THE FOURTH STEP: IMPLEMENT THE PROGRAMME EFFICIENTLY

During the implementation phase, the fully developed social marketing programme is introduced to the target audience; promotion and distribution begin through all channels. Programme components are periodically reviewed and revised if necessary. Audience exposure and reaction are tracked to permit alterations if needed.

Introduce the programme

One effective tactic to gain instant visibility for the programme is to use mass media to introduce it to society. This requires preparation, and may involve the steps that follow:

- prepare a directory of media contacts and outlets;
- inform all organizations that should be involved, particularly if they are gatekeepers to important institutional or community channels;
- ensure that the programme staff is ready to respond to inquiries;
- have materials in sufficient quantities for distribution;
- convene a media event, such as a press conference, to launch the programme.

Track progress

In reality, implementation may take longer than anticipated. Problems and issues may arise, which, if not immediately addressed, can lead to further delays. This is why a monitoring system is vital to track progress and identify potential flaws and oversights before they become major obstacles to success. The monitoring system should contain mechanisms to track:

- completeness and timeliness of work performed;
- expenditures;
- participation, inquiries and other responses;
- effectiveness and quality of response systems;
- intermediate indicators of audience awareness, knowledge and actions.

Consider working with others

On many occasions, it may be necessary to work with other individuals, organizations and groups to extend the programme's reach and credibility. For example, many National Tobacco Control Programmes join forces with national cancer societies and associations of health professionals. Partnerships can be crucial when the partners control access to target audiences. Potential partners can enhance the programme's credibility, contribute additional resources and expertise and promote cosponsorship of events. On the other hand, establishing partnerships requires time, flexibility and the willingness to turn over some of the 'ownership' and control over the programme. Weigh the benefits and the drawbacks carefully when contemplating partnerships.

Review and revise programme components as needed

Periodic assessments and progress reports are necessary to determine whether:

- activities are on track and on time;
- target audiences are being reached;

- particular strategies are more effective than others;
- portions of the programme need to be modified or eliminated;
- expenditures are cost effective.

Monitoring feedback to the programme and responding with the necessary revisions are essential to the success of a social marketing campaign. Monitoring should lead to specific improvements, such as rescheduling broadcasting at more popular hours, locating billboards in more visible areas, redrafting specific messages or shifting internal workloads and responsibilities. Alert and train staff members to identify potential problems early, and to respond with the needed revisions quickly.

THE FIFTH STEP: ASSESS EFFECTIVENESS

Evaluating the effectiveness of a tobacco control social marketing and communications campaign is essential to demonstrate whether objectives have been met, knowledge, attitudes and behaviours have been changed to favour a healthier lifestyle and policies have been influenced to support tobacco control. Campaigns that are not evaluated are a waste of time and resources, because they cannot guide future development. The evaluation process, by identifying the effectiveness of different campaign activities on target audiences, can support advocacy initiatives, stimulate programme improvements and guide funding allocations.

Early planning

Plan impact evaluation at the beginning of a campaign or project, not at its end. Design it as carefully as the campaign itself. To demonstrate change, you will need to compare data before and after the interventions are made. This requires the collection of baseline data about the specific parameters you intend to change in the target audience, before implementation of any intervention. In some cases, a comparison group that did not receive the interventions should be identified. Design the tools for evaluation. In many cases, surveys will be required; hence design the survey questionnaire to include all relevant questions. Budget for both internal and external evaluations at a level proportionate to the available resources.

Use multiple evaluation methods

Explore different ways to collect and analyse data for individuals, families, communities, service sites or regions. Use both quantitative and qualitative methods, as appropriate, and the corresponding statistical tools to determine if change occurred and if it can be attributed to the communications interventions. Even with minimal

Table 5. Evaluation options based on available resources

Type of evaluation	Minimal resources	Modest resources	Substantial resources
Formative	Readability of materials	Intercept interviews	Focus groups Individual In-depth interviews
Process	Record keeping (e.g. monitoring activity timetables)	Programme checklist (e.g. review of adherence to programme plans)	Management audit (e.g. external management review of activities)
Outcome	Activity assessments (e.g. number of print ads on smoke-free restaurants published in newspapers)	Monitoring of progress in attaining objectives (e.g. calculation of percentage of public aware of ads)	Assessment of target audience for changes in knowledge and attitudes (e.g. pretest and post-test of change in audience knowledge and attitudes)
Impact	Print media review (e.g. monitoring of content of news articles on tobacco-free restaurants appearing in newspapers)	Public surveys (e.g. telephone surveys of self-reported behaviour – smokers reporting not smoking inside restaurants)	Studies of behaviour change (e.g. measurement of cotinine in air samples inside restaurants, and in breath samples of waiters in restaurants)

Source: NCI, 1995 *(6)*

resources, some form of evaluation is possible. Table 5 illustrates evaluation options based on available resources.

Determine cost effectiveness

Identify the costs of the campaign and measure these against the impact achieved. Study which interventions and which media result in the greatest cost effectiveness.

Disseminate evaluation results

Share the results of the evaluation process with all the appropriate audiences. Use press conferences, reports, publications, meetings, Internet, e-mail and mass media to publicize successful campaigns, tailoring the reporting format to the intended audience. For example, potential donors may be interested in a report, while media professionals would prefer a one-page press release.

MEASURING CHANGE

A communications project or campaign can change knowledge, attitudes or practices. This brief list identifies a number of measurable variables to consider when evaluating the impact of communications.

Knowledge

- Recall of specific messages.
- Understanding of what messages seek to convey.
- Recognition of products, methods, practices or sources of services or supplies that are being promoted (e.g. what number to call for the Quit Smoking line and where to obtain nicotine replacement products).

Approval

- Favourable response to a message (e.g. when surveyed, respondents react favourably to establishing smoke-free areas after a communications campaign on second-hand smoke).
- Discussion of messages or issues with personal networks (e.g. a waitress discusses the issue of work-related second-hand smoke exposure with her co-workers after viewing a communications campaign on second-hand smoke in the workplace).
- Belief that family and friends approve of an issue.
- Approval of a practice (e.g. respondents report that they support a ban on smoking in restaurants and bars after a communications campaign on second-hand smoke).

Intention

- Recognition that specified health practices address a personal need (e.g. after viewing a commercial on the importance of smoking cessation, a long-time smoker recognizes that he or she needs to quit).
- Intention to consult a provider.
- Intention to adopt the practice at some point.

Practice

- Consultation of a provider for help or obtaining more information (e.g. increased visits to doctors for help with cessation).

- Choice of a method or practice and initiation of a health practice (e.g. the life-time smoker who desires to stop chooses NRT to help quit smoking).
- Continuation of a health practice (e.g. non-smoking mothers remain tobacco free).

Advocacy

- Acknowledgement of the benefits of a health practice (e.g. the life-long smoker above who has successfully quit smoking admits to feeling more energetic and coughing less now stopping using tobacco).
- Advocacy of the health practice to others (e.g. people who have quit try to convince smoker-friends to quit too).
- Support for programmes in the community (e.g. joining a support group for smokers attempting to quit).

FINALLY, PLAN FOR CONTINUITY

Communication is an ongoing process. Achieving significant and sustained changes in attitudes, behaviours and community norms requires time, effort and persistence. The communications process is also cyclical – it builds on experience and adjusts to changing conditions and needs. The evaluation process is key to identifying the strengths and weaknesses of a particular communications campaign. Use this process to find out what moves audiences to change, then build on proven strengths while correcting weak areas.

As the campaign proceeds, conduct periodic assessments to determine if policies, programmes and other conditions are changing from baseline as a result of the interventions being implemented. Redefine objectives and adapt the strategies to meet new and evolving needs. Expand successful projects to cover wider geographical areas and new audiences. Build on early successes to maintain the momentum.

Early on, identify and mobilize resources for continuity. Ensure that existing resources will continue, or search for additional and new resources. Outside of government budgets, other potential sources of additional funding include the private sector, bilateral or multilateral donors, philanthropic institutions or commercial sources. However, be aware of tobacco industry efforts to funnel money and assistance to tobacco control activities, including communications campaigns and projects. Refuse all offers of funding and assistance from the tobacco industry because they represent a serious conflict of interest with the ultimate goal of reducing tobacco consumption.

Promote linkages among related services and organizations to improve access. For example, counselling to quit smoking could be integrated into prenatal visits. The national lung association could echo the message for smoke-free public places. By getting messages across at these opportune moments, and through these partner groups, vulnerable populations can be reached more effectively. These linkages also stretch the value of resources considerably.

Finally, support the establishment of coalitions for tobacco control. Train and support staff for communications and advocacy, and work towards attaining a critical mass of skilled communications professionals who can carry the work into the future.

CAMPAIGNING FOR TOBACCO CONTROL

Tobacco control campaigns are among the most challenging in public health. Governments are often ambivalent about tobacco control, particularly when they derive significant revenues from tobacco or when they own or control the domestic tobacco industry. In addition, the tobacco industry is a formidable opponent of tobacco control. They have, and continue to use, their considerable resources, networks and political influence to counter tobacco control efforts. When developing a communications strategy for a tobacco control campaign, a clear vision of what needs to be done to accomplish campaign objectives is critical.

What are we campaigning for?

The tobacco control measures contained in the WHO FCTC should be reflected in the national plan of action for tobacco control. Tobacco control campaigns should work towards mobilizing support for these interventions that have been proven to reduce tobacco consumption, prevent tobacco use among non-tobacco users and reduce the exposure of non-smokers to second-hand smoke.

Where should we campaign?

Many of the measures outlined in the WHO FCTC, ideally reflected in a national plan of action for tobacco control, need government legislation, necessitating a national campaign to garner popular support. In large countries, the regional or provincial government units may be of greater importance in the short term. This level may be the most appropriate to launch or begin a campaign. In contrast, community advocates and NGOs may need to start by building up grass-roots support, working with communities, local governments and businesses. The scope or coverage of the campaign will vary depending on the nature of the tobacco control measure being supported.

Whom should we seek to influence?

In general, the National Tobacco Control Programme (NTCP) seeks to influence governments, decision-makers and key policy-makers. These actors are, in turn, influenced by public opinion. Public opinion is determined by public education and information. Public education consists of programmes aimed at specific target groups, such as school children or women. Public information acts chiefly through the news media. It aims to provide a steady flow of accurate information about tobacco, both for the general public and for target groups such as politicians. To be effective, public information must keep tobacco issues continuously at the forefront of both the selected and general audiences.

How should opinion leaders be approached?

- To begin, make a list of all the key individuals and organizations that are important stakeholders in tobacco control. Keep this reference database and update as needed.
- Identify how, when and through whom these stakeholders could best be contacted.
- Use professional and personal connections and networks as much as possible.
- Look for events that would allow you to meet and make presentations to these important opinion leaders.
- Use mailing lists – both regular and electronic – to reach them.
- If you have no other way to connect with these stakeholders, arrange for a formal meeting and try to establish a rapport.

Approaching politicians

Politicians have the power to decide on tobacco control policies and legislation. Often the best approach is to meet them personally to present the concerns. These meetings tend to be brief, so keep the talking points direct, brief and focused. Identify those actors who can influence politicians and work on them as well. Because politicians are sensitive to public opinion and public pressure, frame the issue to reflect a popular perspective or cause. For example, the need for a policy on smoke-free public places can be framed as a means to protect the health of children, who are vulnerable to the ill effects of tobacco smoke. Politicians are more readily persuaded to support an issue if they perceive it to have popular support. Using letter writing or e-mail campaigns can be effective when you need to attract their attention on a particular tobacco control issue.

References

1. Kotler P and Roberto EL. *Social marketing: Strategies for changing public behaviour.* New York: Free Press, 1989.

2. Andreasen A. *Marketing social change: changing behavior to promote health, social development and the environment.* San Francisco, Jossey-Bass, 1995.

3. *Designing and implementing an effective tobacco counter-marketing campaign.* United States Department of Health and Human Services, Centers for Disease Control and Prevention, Atlanta, National Center for Chronic Disease Prevention and Health Promotion, Office on Smoking and Health, First ed., October 2003.

4. *Best Practices for Comprehensive Tobacco Control Programs – August 1999.* United States Department of Health and Human Services, Centers for Disease Control and Prevention, Atlanta, National Center for Chronic Disease Prevention and Health Promotion, Office on Smoking and Health, August 1999.

5. National Cancer Institute. *Making health communication programs work.* Bethesda, Maryland, National Institutes of Health, National Cancer Institute, 1989.

6. *Theory at a glance: A guide for health promotion practice.* Bethesda, Maryland, National Institutes of Health, National Cancer Institute, 1995.

9
Working with the media

Whoever controls the media...
controls the culture.
—Allen Ginsberg*

THE MEDIA are obviously key players in any tobacco control campaign and, often, the most practical channels through which to disseminate information and tobacco control messages rapidly to a large population. Media is the vehicle that shapes public opinion and influences policy leaders. Frequently, repeated news coverage of an issue can guide a government's policy agenda. Thus, developing good working relationships with media professionals is essential.

Some departments of health are fortunate to have a public information or media relations officer. If this is the case, then the tobacco control programme staff should work closely with this individual when planning, developing, testing, implementing and evaluating media campaigns. However, in developing countries, and in a number of smaller countries, programme staff has to fulfil the liaison role with the media. To work effectively with media professionals observe the following guidelines (and see Boxes 1–4).

> **The more an issue is reported in the news, the more people will be concerned about it, and the more the government will take notice. If you have no direct access to your country's policy-makers, one effective way to reach them is through the media.**
> — Emma Must and Debra Efroymson, PATH Canada, 2002

Develop and maintain a media directory

Have a file of individual journalists and other media professionals that contains detailed contact information, their field of interest, their area of coverage, and the newspapers/magazines/journals/TV stations/radio stations/web sites with which they are affiliated. When searching for media contacts, use the Internet, the yellow pages and the chamber of commerce to identify media outlets in your area. If employing the services of a public relations (PR) firm or consultant, request a media list; most PR companies have access to databases of reporters and editors (1). In countries with diverse populations, develop separate lists of media professionals that reach out to specific ethnic communities and groups.

Know and provide them with what they want

The end goal of the media is to attract more viewers, readers, listeners and advertisers. This prompts them to favour selectively information that is attractive to their audience and to their advertisers. Newsworthy information is:

- new;
- unusual or unexpected;
- entertaining, or has high emotional value;
- related to another emerging trend or breaking news;
- essential information that everyone needs to know;
- accompanied by vivid and graphic visuals;
- supported by scientific evidence.

When providing the media with a news story, ensure that it satisfies one or more of the criteria above. Frame your story so that it has a "hook" that will interest the media. For example, in China, public health professionals used the SARS epidemic to reinforce the message that smoking weakens the lungs and lowers the resistance to respiratory infections. In the United States, having supermodel Christy Turlington speak up about the benefits of cessation grabbed media attention. When new information becomes available, such as through the release of a new study, provide the media with the information immediately. Timing is key.

Keep in mind that most media professionals work on a daily production cycle. This means they usually do not have much lead time when preparing a story. Consequently, requests for information may come on short notice and interviews may have to be done by phone or e-mail, etc. This requires programme officers to:

- be prompt in responding to requests for information on possible stories, a delay in response may mean that the story goes unpublished;
- be flexible about working within the limits of the media's daily production cycle, understanding that it is not the journalist or media professional's lack of organization, but the dynamics of their work that dictates the short lead time and the need for rapid responses *(2, 3)*.

Box 1. Responding to unsolicited media inquiries

Sometimes, reporters will come to you for information when you least expect it. Remember the following:

1. Get all the vital information. This includes:
  - the full and complete contact details for the reporter;
  - the news outlet represented;
  - what story has been planned;
  - what information is needed from your programme;
  - who else will be interviewed;
  - deadlines for submitting the required information.

2. Check out the news outlet that the reporter represents. This can be done by checking your media lists, inquiring from news services in your country and through the Internet. Occasionally, reporters working for tobacco industry-funded publications may contact you for information or opinions. Knowing the affiliation of the news outlet can help prepare you for the encounter, if you choose to respond positively to the request.

3. Be prepared. Have all the relevant information at hand and collect your thoughts before responding.

4. Always call back. Even if you choose to decline an interview or request for information, inform the reporter, respecting deadlines and returning calls promptly.

Source: Adapted from *(1)*

Cultivate good media relationships

Through personal connections, messages and stories can get published. Developing good working relationships with the media can result in free publicity or coverage for the campaign. Remember to:

- treat media professionals with respect and courtesy;
- be prepared with background material, resource people and references;
- respond to their requests for information immediately or as soon as possible;
- respect their deadlines;
- develop an ongoing professional relationship. One strategy to achieve this is to have regular informal meetings with media where new information on tobacco control can be shared. Regular meetings also provide opportunities to tap media expertise on communications strategies. In Brazil, for example, regular breakfast meetings

---

Box 2. Tips for TV interviews

The spokesperson should be comfortable when doing interviews, especially on television. Some helpful hints include the following:

- **Ask a reporter ahead of time what material will be covered in a televised interview, and inform him or her as to what areas you will or will not provide comments on.** If a reporter refuses to provide this information, you can always decline the interview.

- **Dress appropriately.** When dressing for television, colour is fine, but tone it down. Vertical lines, subdued colours and simple jewellery lend authority and seriousness to your remarks. Wear clothing that fits comfortably. Women should be wary of short skirts. Men should avoid short socks.

- **Sit up straight.** If you wear a suit coat or jacket, sit on the tail to prevent it from 'riding up' on your neck.

- **Watch your body language.** Television reporters routinely nod their head during an interview, as if nodding in agreement with the speaker. This can be hypnotic if you are being interviewed, and you may start nodding your head. You may be saying "no," but your head may be saying "yes."

- **Keep yourself focused on the interview.** Avoid getting too 'cosy' with the interviewer or the setting. Some of the most embarrassing mistakes in TV interviews occur not because of tough questions, but because the speaker loses his or her focus and begins to babble. Stay 'on the message'.

- **Be on time.** Unlike an interview with a print reporter, you cannot call back later when it comes to an interview with the electronic media.

- **If possible, speak with the interviewer before going on camera to make sure that you both have the expectations of the material to be discussed.** It may help if you can provide the interviewer with a brief paragraph outlining the subject in question and your viewpoints about it.

- **If possible, find out about other participation, in the event of panel discussions and group interviews.** Check whether the tobacco industry is represented.

Source: University at Buffalo (4)

between tobacco control programme staff and media professionals helped to lay the foundation for an effective channel to relay tobacco control updates and messages to the public.

Have a designated spokesperson

Make it convenient for the media to contact your organization by having a spokesperson. Usually, but not always, the spokesperson is the national focal point. The spokesperson should possess the following:
- capability of representing the message, campaign and programme;
- credibility: to be acceptable to the target audience(s), and capable of commanding respect and projecting sincerity and authority when communicating;
- the ability to be articulate;
- knowledge of the programme;
- the ability to use sound judgment when releasing information, and capability of thinking quickly during unexpected media encounters;
- preferably, experience in working with media;
- accessibility: the spokesperson should be reachable by phone, fax and e-mail;
- discretion;
- the ability to be diplomatic.

Box 3. Tips for radio interviews

Unlike TV interviews, radio interviews do not permit visual feedback to the audience. Hence, your speaking voice will be critical. Here are some tips for an effective radio interview:

- **Study the interview style and personality of the radio host.** Listen to previously recorded interviews to get a 'feel' for the style of interviewing and the types of questions that are likely to be asked.

- **Come prepared.** The benefit of a radio interview over a televised interview is that it allows you to use references, such as cue cards. Write down your key talking points and essential statistics, and keep these in front of you when doing the interview. Use these to stay focused during the interview.

- **Avoid prolonged silences.** Radio hosts will not allow 'dead air' or periods of prolonged silences. By preparing for the interview, you can avoid 'dead air'.

- **Speak clearly.** Sit with your mouth about 2–3 inches from the microphone and speak directly into it. Be careful not to create unpleasant sounds by speaking carefully and enunciating each word. Avoid accentuating your 'Ps' and whistling on your 'Ss'.

- **Use time effectively.** Some radio interviews can be conducted over the phone, saving you time and the need to travel to a radio station. Determine beforehand if this arrangement is appropriate for you.

Box 4. Tips for print interviews

- **Prepare for the interview.** Find out why you were selected for the interview, and who will be doing the interviewing. Read up on any background information or related news stories that may have prompted the request for an interview. Have printed material ready for the reporter to verify facts and figures.

- **Control the environment.** If the interview is to be conducted at your office, rid your table of clutter and ensure that only the relevant documents are on your desk. Keep sensitive material out of sight. Have someone else take your phone calls and ensure that you are not disturbed during the interview.

- **Respond to questions with direct, simple answers.** Use layman's terms, and keep your answers brief.

- **Know your message.** Decide beforehand what key points you wish to emphasize during the interview, and come back to these core messages throughout the conversation.

- **Be honest.** If you are unable to answer the question, say so. Avoid phrases like 'no comment'.

- **Be prudent.** 'Off the record' comments and personal or judgemental opinions should be avoided. Do not say anything to the interviewer that you would not like to see in print.

USING MEDIA INNOVATIVELY

Countries with large budgets for information and advocacy campaigns can afford to use paid media placements. These are often costly because they require a considerable investment in creative development and the sufficient use of paid media space to generate adequate reach and to ensure audience saturation. Many developing countries do not have the resources to conduct paid media campaigns. However, through the use of innovative strategies, free media coverage for tobacco control is possible.

Consider using government-owned media

Many countries have radio and television stations that are predominantly or wholly owned by the government. These stations offer free airtime for government programmes. Using government-owned media channels is one way to obtain media coverage for tobacco control at little or no cost to the department of health. (Note that the cost of materials development should be considered separately.) The drawback to using government-owned media is that there may be limits to the ability to reach all the intended audiences. Moreover, in certain situations, messages from government-owned channels may not be as credible, because individuals may perceive these as overly prescriptive.

Use forms of communication that do not require payment for publication

- **Opinion editorials (op-eds), letters to the editor, and,** in some countries, **press releases** are published in newspapers free of charge. The key is to frame your messages creatively so that they catch the editor's interest. (See the discussion of what is newsworthy in the previous section and see Boxes 6, 7 and 8 below for tips on writing effective op-eds, letters to the editor and press releases.)
- **Some media channels will air public service announcements for free,** usually as a form of public service. It is important to inquire at all potential media outlets if free space or airtime is available for important health messages that need to reach the general public. If you do not ask, you may miss this opportunity.
- **Explore regular features in newspapers, radio and television that solicit contributions from the public.** For example, the *Pacific Daily News* on the island of Guam has a feature called *Islandstyle* that accepts interesting submissions, including photographs, from anyone. Guam's Department of Mental Health and Substance Abuse used *Islandstyle* to announce the start of cessation counselling services, at no cost to the department.

Make news

By creating newsworthy events and activities, free media coverage can be obtained. Make sure that your event has an interesting angle that will capture the interest of journalists and radio and TV newscasters. Announce the event through a press conference, and ensure that all relevant media contacts are invited ahead of time (see Box 5). (Note that sometimes the press conference is in itself an event.) Events can also be announced through a media advisory, which should be sent out to all relevant media contacts ahead of time.

If resources allow, consider using paid media

Ideally, tobacco control programmes should allocate a reasonable budget for paid media placements. Perhaps the media campaign most renowned for decreasing tobacco use in youth recently is Florida's "Truth" campaign, launched in 1998. It has been largely credited with reducing the percentage of youth using tobacco over a 30-day period by 7.4% (from 18.5% to 11.1%) in middle school and 4.8% (from 27.4% to 22.6%) in high school from 1998 to 2001 *(5, 6)*. One key element of this successful campaign was the use of paid media,

> The access to considerable funding had the greatest impact on media. Where traditional anti-tobacco efforts used remainder and public service discount weight, the Florida programme bought media on the open market with a year one budget of more than US$ 15 million. Rather than run for free at midnight or in programming with little teen viewership, "truth" aired on MTV, during the broadcasting of the Super Bowl (the United States football premiership), and in those programmes that youth most wanted to see.
>
> — Jeffrey J Hicks
> Crispin, Porter & Bogusky, Miami, Florida, USA

made possible by a considerable budget for media placements (e.g. US$ 15 million for year one of the campaign) *(7)*.

Most countries, especially those in the developing world, may not have access to large sums of money. However, when resources permit, programme staff should consider the strategic use of paid media space for communicating essential tobacco control messages to the public. The use of paid advertisements, PSAs and news releases in print, broadcast and electronic media, can reinforce the communications campaign for tobacco control.

Box 5. Conducting a press conference [1]

- Choose a location that is accessible, adequately equipped and large enough to accommodate all invited attendees.
- Set the date and time.
- Prepare an agenda and a briefing note. The briefing note should contain a list of speakers with titles and the key points to be covered by the press conference. Have copies of the briefing note available for distribution to attendees.
- Keep the press conference short, usually no more than 30 to 45 minutes. One hour is the absolute maximum time. To ensure availability, reserve the room for one hour.
- Select speakers, assign topics and set time limits for each speaker. In general, have someone make an opening statement, followed by other speakers who can share different perspectives or provide additional information. Limit each speaker to a few minutes each. Apportion most of the time for a question and answer session at the end.
- Assign a moderator to facilitate the open forum and to maintain order.
- Invite public figures. VIPs tend to draw reporters to an event, and having important public figures can enhance your programme's credibility. Because VIPs have busy schedules, be sure to invite them well ahead of time and follow up regularly with their staff to ensure their attendance.
- Choose attractive graphic display materials to convey your message.
- Prepare a news advisory. Include a contact person and phone number. Mail, e-mail and fax this to reporters on your media list at least 1 week before the event.
- Follow up on your invitations to media. Call them and encourage them to attend.
- Prepare media kits and handouts. These should contain a summary of the topic being presented, prepared statements to be read by the speakers, and photos and graphics depicting the topic of the conference.
- Set up the press conference room before the actual date. Check to ensure that equipment (microphones, audiovisual equipment and facilities for recording and translation, if applicable) are working properly. Make sure that there are electrical outlets available for TV cameras at the sides or in the back of the room.
- On the day of the conference, have the members of the media sign in. Provide them with a copy of the media kit, agenda and other handouts.
- Start and end on time.
- Remember to thank the media and guests for attending.
- Follow up and contact reporters who request additional information.

---

[1] Adapted from Department of Health and Human Services, Atlanta, 2002

CREATING MATERIALS FOR THE MEDIA[2]

During important events, such as a programme launch, it is wise to invest in a media kit, which provides key written information to media professionals covering the event. Presenting critical information, and messages, in a convenient manner facilitates a reporter's job, and can increase the likelihood of media coverage.

Public relations firms often refer to the 'media kit' or 'press kit'. Information is organized in a standard way, and materials are created that make it very easy for the media to find and use. A media kit often consists of a major press release, and supporting elements that provide additional information. The information is arranged in order of importance, avoiding redundancy. Media kits are often packaged in folders, which are labelled with the subject matter and details of the organization or programme releasing the information.

The elements of a media kit include:

- Table of contents.
- Pitch letter – This is designed to convince news reporters to cover a specific story. It outlines what your programme is doing and why it is newsworthy. Aim for a short and succinct letter, certainly not longer than one page. Use the programme's official letterhead, and ensure that contact details are included.
- Media advisory – This is a condensed version of information about an upcoming event. It must be very brief, and preferably uses bullet points to describe the 'who, what, when, where, why', contact person, contact details and date. Usually, this is issued in advance of the media kit, but if the materials in it are under embargo, the media advisory can accompany the kit.
- News release.
- Fact sheet or backgrounder on the topic and on the programme or organization
- Appropriate photos with captions.
- Business card or label with contact information for the programme's spokesperson or main media contact.
- Additional information, as available and appropriate, such as:
  - printed brochure;
  - reprints of key speeches or articles by leaders of the organization;
  - biographies of key personnel;
  - press clippings from previous coverage of the organization;
  - other advocacy materials.

Effective media kits contain all the essential information, and present the information in an attractive, direct and interesting manner. If resources permit, have the kits professionally printed. Finally, ensure that the kits are widely disseminated in a timely manner to the proper recipients.

Box 6. Elements of an effective press release

Organizational logo

An organizational logo quickly identifies the source of the news release to the press. It is an important, but often overlooked, element of a press release. Remember that the press often receives many press releases simultaneously from different organizations. Noting the logo of the source of the news item is usually the first thing a journalist or editor does to decide if the press release is worth reading and publishing.

The title

The title provides the focus and must be able to grab attention. It should describe succinctly what the press release is about. It needs to be eye-catching, and interesting but must be kept as short as possible. One strategy to make a title interesting is to use a critical statistic in the title (e.g. "Smoking kills one person every 6 seconds worldwide"). Keep titles to a maximum of two lines, preferably fewer.

Embargo date

An embargo is the earliest date and time at which the press release can be published. Since the press generally have to plan what stories to cover in advance, it is helpful to send them information ahead of time. If you are providing a press release but do not want it published before a certain date and time (perhaps because it is timed to coincide with a specific event), you must include an embargo. Otherwise, the press may use the story at any time.

Bear in mind that the press may not always honour the embargo, although they usually do. The media often will use the information contained in a press release immediately after an embargo, with the aim of being the first to disseminate new information. On the other hand, you may write "For immediate release" at the top of the press release if you do not require a delay before publication, and if the press release is related to a current issue.

Well-structured first paragraph

The first paragraph of a press release should answer the questions 'What?', 'Why?', 'When?', 'Where?', 'Who?' and 'How?' regarding the information you are providing. It should entice the reader to continue reading while conveying all the key information should the reader choose not to proceed any further. It should be written in short, clear sentences, and should be limited to two to three lines.

Contact details

To avoid cluttering up the main body of the press release, provide information for editors at the end of the press release. Contact information should contain the names, e-mail addresses and phone numbers of spokespersons who may be contacted for further information. Be sure to include the hours during which these spokespersons may be reached. If queries from the international media are anticipated, indicate the location and time zone of the spokespersons. List at least two contact persons, and ensure that the phone numbers provided are accurate.

Details such as the full address of a press conference venue (more important for media advisories) or the full title and author names of a report mentioned in the main text are best left to footnotes. Web site addresses where further information about the press release can be found may also be included as a footnote.

Photo opportunity box

This is an optional element in a press release. The 'photo opportunity' box should be situated near the top of the press release. It should be captioned with the day, time, place and brief details about an event or activity. Its presence will indicate to media that they should send a photographer to cover an event. If you include a photo opportunity box, fax the press release to both the copy and photo editors. (For an example of an actual press release sent out by WHO see Annex 1.)

Source: Adapted from *(1)*

Box 7. Creating effective op-eds

Opinion editorials, or op-eds, are short essays written by outside contributors to a newspaper. These essays often provide a unique perspective on a particular issue, and are frequently run opposite the main editorial page *(8)*. Op-eds are more detailed than letters to the editor, express a clear and forceful opinion on relevant issues and often cite several key points documented by scientific research *(1)*.

- **Timing is key.** Op-eds should be strategically published in connection with an important community event, the release of new information from surveys or research, or in response to a recent article. For example, the WHO Director-General and Regional Directors often release op-eds related to the theme for World No Tobacco Day shortly before 31 May of each year.

- **Conform to the newspaper's required format.** Contact the editor to obtain the exact specifications for an op-ed. Most op-eds contain from 500–800 words.

- **Use local data, if available.** Use local data and stories that communicate the message. This strategy ensures that the op-ed is an effective attention-grabber, and increases the likelihood of publication.

- **Choose the author with care.** Carefully select the person whose name will appear as author of the op-ed. Prominent personalities who are credible sources for the message you want to communicate can make the difference in the editor's decision to accept an op-ed for printing.

- **Follow-up.** Call the editor several days after submitting the op-ed to find out if it is being considered for publication.

Source: Adapted from *(1)*

FINALLY, THE MEDIA AS A STAKEHOLDER IN TOBACCO CONTROL

The media should be viewed not only as a channel to communicate messages to the broader audience, but also as a potential partner and stakeholder in tobacco control. Many media personnel are smokers, or reformed smokers, and are aware first hand of the addictive power of nicotine. Non-smoking media professionals are often victims of second-hand smoke exposure. With the proper encouragement and guidance, they could become advocates for cessation services and smoke-free workplaces. Media people are also very much aware of the profit motive of the tobacco industry, and of the tactics the industry can employ; legal and otherwise, to promote their deadly products. Media who are active partners and advocates for tobacco control constitute a formidable presence to counter the tobacco industry's attempts to maintain tobacco use through advertising and marketing and disinformation. Tobacco control programme staff should use every opportunity to educate and motivate media to support effective tobacco control policies and support a smoke-free workplace policy in media facilities such as television, radio and newspaper offices.

Box 8. Writing an effective letter to the editor

Most newspapers devote an entire page to letters from readers. Today, many newspapers even publish electronic letters, making it easier for individuals and organizations to send in their contributions. Using the Letters section of newspapers can be a strategic means to communicate tobacco control messages.

- **Timing is key.** Like op-eds, letters to the editor need to be positioned to respond to recently published news, stories, editorials or other letters.

- **Generate public debate around relevant issues.** Letters can create public debate over issues because other contributors can respond to previously published letters. Thus, a conversation in print can be sustained, and interest in a particular tobacco control topic can mount as the discussion intensifies.

- **Be simple and direct.** Letters have to be shorter than op-eds, and generally are capped at 200–300 words. Some newspapers may edit a letter to maintain certain length requirements; if this is the case, remember that the editing may not be to your liking. To avoid this, keep your message brief, simple and straight to the point.

- **Grab the reader's attention.** Be compelling, even controversial. Keep the letter interesting by using local data, citing local sources or telling local stories.

- **Include contact information.** Some journalists may be interested enough to want to do a follow-up story based on an interesting letter. Having accurate and complete contact information ensures that they can reach you.

- **Follow up.** After submission, follow up with the editorial staff to check on the status of the letter. And never give up. Sometimes, a letter that is not accepted at the first submission just needs revisions to present a different 'hook' or angle. (For an example of a letter to the editor see Annex 2.)

Source: Adapted from *(1)*

References

1. *Designing and implementing an effective tobacco counter-marketing campaign.* United States Department of Health and Human Services, Centers for Disease Control and Prevention, National Center for Chronic Disease Prevention and Health Promotion, Atlanta, Office on Smoking and Health, First ed. October 2003.

2. Goldfarb LMCS et al. *Basis for the implementation of a tobacco control programme.* National Coordination of Tobacco Control and Primary Cancer Prevention, National Cancer Institute, Ministry of Health, Rio de Janeiro, 1996 [In Portuguese].

3. Silva VLC et al. *Practical guidelines to implement a tobacco control programme.* National Coordination of Tobacco Control and Primary Cancer Prevention, National Cancer Institute, Ministry of Health, Rio de Janeiro, 1998 [In Portuguese].

4. UB News Services, University at Buffalo, the State University of New York, Additional Tips for TV Interviews. Available at: http://www.buffalo.edu/news/fast-execute.cgi/wwns-media.html.

5. Bauer UE et al. Changes in youth cigarette use and intentions following implementation of a tobacco control program. Findings from the Florida youth tobacco survey, 1998–2000. *Journal of the American Medical Association*, 2000, 284:723–728[Medline].

6. Sly DF, Heald GR, Ray S. The Florida "Truth" anti-tobacco media evaluation: design, first-year results, and implications for planning future state media evaluations. *Tobacco Control*, 2001, 10:9–15. (Abstract/Full Text at http://tc.bmjjournals.com/cgi/content/abstract/10/1/9, last accessed 1 February 2004).

7. Hicks JJ. The strategy behind Florida's "Truth" campaign. *Tobacco Control*, 2001, 10 (Spring):3–5. (Abstract/Full text at http://tc.bmjjournals.com/cgi/content/full/10/1/3, last accessed 1 February 2004).

8. Must E and Efroymson D. *PATH Canada Guide Using the Media for Tobacco Control.* Dhaka, PATH Canada, August 2002.

ANNEX 1

WORLD HEALTH ORGANIZATION

P O Box 13113   Tel: +27-12-354-8580
Tramshed   Fax: +27-12-354-8551
0126
South Africa

17 October 2003
For immediate release

MEDIA RELEASE

WHO congratulates South Africa on tobacco control efforts

Pretoria - The World Health Organization (WHO) has praised the South African Government for its Bill, which proposes amendments to the Tobacco Products Control Act of 1993, hailing the amendments as visionary and a move forward in protecting the public's health from the impacts of tobacco consumption.

"I am very proud of the country's strong tobacco control efforts, and this Bill raises the bar in terms of tobacco control legislature globally. The country is an example to others in terms of political commitment for the tobacco epidemic," said Dr Welile Shasha, WHO's representative in South Africa.

The amended Tobacco Products Control Act will be in line with the WHO Framework Convention on Tobacco Control (FCTC), a global public health tool to fight the worldwide threat of tobacco.

"South Africa was one of the first signatories of the FCTC in June, and has indicated its intention to ratify it. We wish the country well in the forthcoming legislative process, which will prepare the way for South Africa's early ratification of the FCTC," said Dr Vera da Costa e Silva, head of WHO's Tobacco Free Initiative in Geneva.

The FCTC has provisions on advertising and sponsorship, tax and price increases, labelling, smuggling and second-hand smoke. As soon as 40 countries ratify the Convention, it becomes law for those countries. The FCTC is the first international treaty ever to be negotiated by WHO, the principal health agency of the United Nations.

The Bill proposes substantial increases in fines for those who break the law, particularly with regard to allowing smoking in public places; larger health warnings on packaging, including picture messages; bans on false descriptors such as "low-tar" or "mild"; a ban on duty-free cigarettes; and prohibiting any person under 18 years to be in a designated smoking area in a public place.

The Bill was published today in the Government Gazette, and is open to public comment until 17 November 2003.

E n d s

Issued by the World Health Organization, Pretoria

Enquiries: Greer van Zyl: Health Information & Promotion: 083 647 7045; gvzyl@un.org.za
          Dr Welile Shasha: WHO Liaison Officer: 083 677 7704; wshasha@un.org.za
          Melinda Henry: Information Officer,   09-41-22- 791-2535; henrym@who.int
          Director-General's Office, WHO, Geneva

Updated status of the WHO Framework Convention on Tobacco Control:
http://www.who.int/tobacco/fctc/signing_ceremony/countrylist/en/

Text of FCTC (in 6 languages):
http://www.who.int/tobacco/fctc/text/final/en/

ANNEX 2

Letter to the Editor

Thursday, June 26, 2003
Pacific Daily News
Guam, United States of America

Facts louder than fear in tobacco ban woes

(On June 23) the *Pacific Daily News* published an article from Honolulu, titled "Smoking ban worries businesses". But fears must be separated from facts, and the evidence is clear and compelling: whether in Florida or New York, Hong Kong [SAR] or Australia, smoke-free restaurants do not lose money. In fact, in many cases, they attract more customers, who are happy to enjoy their meals in a healthy, smoke-free environment.

The most recent study I am aware of was published in the June 2003 issue of the *Cornell Hotel and Restaurant Administration Quarterly*. It documented that smoke-free regulations were not associated with adverse economic outcomes in New York restaurants and hotels.

Even on Guam, ask any maitre'd which section is requested and filled, and more often and invariably, they'll point to the non-smoking section. Businesses need to listen to the real voice of the greater majority of their customers, who want breathable, odour-free, non-hazardous, smoke-free air in the establishments they patronize.

ANNETTE M. DAVID, MD, MPH
PO Box XXXXX
Tamuning, Guam 96931
Tel: +1 (671) XXX-XXXX
Fax: +1 (671) XXX-XXXX
e-mail: amdavid@yahoo.com

10

Programming selected tobacco control activities

The pessimist sees difficulty in every opportunity. The optimist sees the opportunity in every difficulty.
—*Winston Churchill*

INTRODUCTION

The community is often the focal point for effective tobacco control activities. The people who live, work and play in a community best understand their area's needs, resources, problems and capacities. Both governments and communities must be willing to collaborate and invest their time and expertise in designing, implementing and evaluating effective tobacco control programmes (see Table 1). The NTCP and its local counterparts should work hand in hand with community partners to promote a long-term, comprehensive approach to tobacco control and to ensure that activities and programmes are culturally appropriate. Whenever possible, they should utilize and support existing facilities, organizations and individuals that have a proven history of effective tobacco control interventions. It is also important that tobacco control activities remain independent of all forms of influence from the tobacco industry.

This chapter is intended to provide an overview of selected programme options that are most often included as part of a comprehensive, integrated action plan for tobacco control. Strategies for community mobilization for tobacco control are also discussed. Future publications by WHO will provide a more detailed discussion of the issues covered. Throughout the chapter, additional references are highlighted for the reader.

Table 1. Selected programme interventions for tobacco control

Programme interventions	Outcomes	Core activities (for all interventions)	Partners (for all interventions)
1. Delivery of school-based tobacco prevention programmes 2. Development of youth peer leaders and networks 3. Treatment to stop smoking and support programmes 4. Implementation of by-laws against smoking in public buildings 5. Creation of smoke-free workplaces 6. Development of training programmes and resources for practitioners 7. Development of tobacco control web sites and/or tobacco control clearing houses to disseminate best practices	1. Fewer young people taking up smoking 2. Young people actively involved in tobacco control activities 3. More smokers quitting 4. Reduced exposure to second-hand tobacco smoke in homes, schools, and other public places 5. Reduced exposure to second-hand smoke in workplaces 6. Individuals and communities better equipped and able to deliver programmes 7. a) Information on best practices widely available b) Improved health in the population c) Savings in the health-care system	– Sustained programme funding – Research to determine best practices – Needs assessments to determine priorities, gaps, etc. – Public consultations – Gathering, analysis and dissemination of knowledge – Technical assistance for capacity-building – Monitoring and assessment of impact, effectiveness and cost effectiveness of interventions – Effective communication of successes via newsletters, workshops and conferences	The commitment and expertise of national and regional governments, health professionals, educators, young people, parents, researchers, employers, workers, the media, voluntary associations and others is necessary for the delivery of effective tobacco prevention, cessation and protection programmes

PREVENTION

Supporting tobacco prevention activities

Efforts to prevent and reduce smoking among young people, if successful, can have a significant impact on tobacco-related mortality and morbidity in the future.

Schools are an ideal setting for tobacco control interventions. Of the world's 6 billion people, about 1 billion are enrolled in schools. Of the developing world's children, 80% now enrol in school, and 60% complete at least 4 years. There are more than five times as many teachers in the developing world as there are health workers, and those teachers often have regular and long-term contact with pupils. Thus, the formal education system is an important channel for disseminating information about tobacco control.

WHO's 'health-promoting schools' concept under the Healthy Settings and Global School Health initiatives offers many opportunities to promote prevention of tobacco use in the school setting. The *Guidelines for school health programs to prevent tobacco use and addiction* of the United States Centers for Disease Control and Prevention, Atlanta (CDC), identify some of the crucial elements of a school-based tobacco prevention programme:

- developing and enforcing a school policy on tobacco use;
- providing information about the short- and long-term adverse physiological effects and social consequences of tobacco use, peer norms regarding tobacco use and refusal skills;
- providing education to prevent tobacco use from kindergarten until 12th grade; this instruction should be especially intensive in junior high or middle school and should be reinforced in high school;
- providing programme-specific training for teachers;
- involving parents or families in support of school-based programmes to prevent tobacco use;
- supporting cessation efforts among students and all school staff who use tobacco;
- assessing the programme on prevention of tobacco use at regular intervals.

Two further important aspects of school-based programmes on tobacco prevention that should be taken into consideration are (a) partnership between the health and education sectors; and (b) involvement of students in policy and programme development, implementation and evaluation.

School-based prevention programmes should start in primary grades and continue through secondary school, with reinforcing or booster sessions. Educational interventions should be age-appropriate, and should take into consideration the specific developmental issues that predominate in specific age groups. The transition from primary to secondary school is particularly important. During this time, students broaden their peer groups and come in contact with older students who may use tobacco. For these reasons, interventions need to be especially intensive in early secondary school. The main goal of these interventions is to equip younger adolescents with specific skills and resources that would help them resist direct and indirect social pressure to try smoking.

The effectiveness of school programmes which aim to prevent the onset of smoking appears to be enhanced by coordinated community-wide programmes. The success of efforts to prevent and reduce tobacco use through schools relies on the awareness and commitment of parents and other members of the community. Representatives of local government and NGOs, businesses, religious leaders, community youth agencies, health service providers, sports personalities, the media and other members of the community can play an active role in preventing the use of tobacco.

A community advisory committee could be set up to coordinate efforts with members of the school team. It is important that young people be involved at all stages of the planning. A situation analysis should be considered in order to identify target areas and priorities for action. If the aim is to reduce youth smoking through mass communication programmes, then focus groups, surveys, or even unstructured interviews with young people will provide useful information to create more effective campaigns.

The community, rather than helping young people refrain from using tobacco, might actually be creating an environment in which tobacco use is encouraged, whether through pervasive tobacco advertising, easy access to tobacco for minors or widespread smoking in public places. Community action to remove these incentives to smoke will strongly enhance educational efforts in schools.

Unfortunately, school-based programmes that have not been backed up by community programmes and policies show limited results. Even early modest success has dissipated over time. However, when placed in the context of strong, coherent community tobacco control policies and programmes, and supported by schools that are completely smoke-free, school-based programmes can be a useful part of comprehensive tobacco control.

Characteristics of effective school-based educational campaigns for tobacco control

Ideally, school-based campaigns should be linked to anti-tobacco activities in the local community and in the mass media. Effective school-based educational campaigns will:

- Cover faculty, staff, students and school visitors alike.
- Emphasize that tobacco use is harmful to all smokers, young and old.
- Teach that most young people do not smoke.
- Promote peer leadership and leading by example.
- Provide training in refusal skills.
- Teach media literacy.
- Discuss the social influences on decisions to smoke.
- Emphasize the short-term effects of smoking, such as yellow teeth, bad breath and shortness of breath.
- Stress the advantages of remaining a non-smoker.
- Tackle issues related to addiction, second-hand smoke and the deceitful behaviour of the tobacco industry.

An effective 'tobacco-free' school policy

The effective policy:

- begins with a rationale for preventing and reducing tobacco use, based on current evidence, and a description of the situation in the school;

- requires coordination between health and educational authorities at local levels;

- enumerates procedures for communicating the policy to students, school faculty and staff, parents, visitors and community members;

- includes interventions to raise awareness of the effects and consequences of tobacco use on both young and old;

- prohibits tobacco use by students, faculty, other school staff, parents and visitors on school property, in school vehicles and at school-sponsored activities outside school property;

- totally bans tobacco advertising in school buildings, school surroundings, school publications and other school property;

- prohibits the sale or trade of tobacco products on school property;

- prohibits tobacco company sponsorship of school activities;

- requires that education to prevent tobacco use be provided at school, integrated in the school curriculum, complementing other relevant school health activities;

- shows teachers, student leaders and school personnel how to implement tobacco use prevention;

- provides all students and school staff with access to help for quitting smoking;

- specifies mechanisms for enforcing the policy (sanctions, complaints procedures, etc.);

- determines methods to monitor progress and evaluate impact;

- designates one or more individuals or a committee responsible to oversee the policy's implementation and evaluation.

CESSATION

Tobacco cessation programmes

Helping smokers to quit can result in significant health and economic benefits to individuals and societies (see Figure 1).

WHO recently published the monograph *Policy recommendations for smoking cessation and treatment of tobacco dependence*, based on the results of a global consultation of experts and country representatives from developed and developing countries in June 2002. The monograph contains a set of recommendations that can be adjusted to available resources and the level of political support for smoking cessation within countries. This handbook can be used to shape the cessation component of a national action plan for tobacco control that suits the country's circumstances.

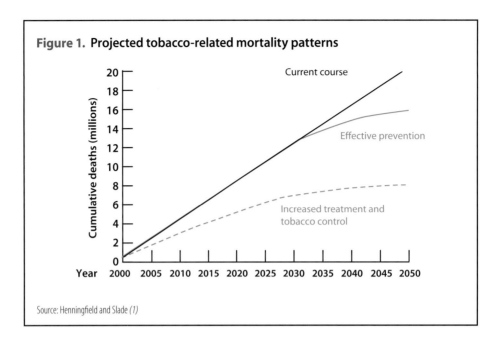

Figure 1. Projected tobacco-related mortality patterns

Source: Henningfield and Slade *(1)*

The following recommendations, known as the 'Mayo Clinic Recommendations', provide a framework for governments and health professionals to jointly tackle nicotine addiction:

• Make treatment a public health priority;

• Make treatment available;

• Assess and monitor tobacco use and provide proven interventions;

• Set an example for peers and patients by ceasing tobacco use;

• Fund effective treatment;

• Motivate tobacco users to quit;

• Monitor and regulate tobacco processing, marketing and sales;

• Develop new types of treatment.

Source: *(2)*

There are several behavioural and pharmacological interventions for cessation of tobacco use. Their efficacy has been assessed among smokers, although users of other tobacco products will also find them helpful. Chapter 3 of WHO's *Policy recommendations for smoking cessation and treatment of tobacco dependence* reviews the evidence of the efficacy of these cessation strategies. Clinical practice guidelines to assist clinicians and others in delivering and supporting effective forms of treatment of tobacco use are presented in *Treating tobacco use and dependence*, a publication of the United States Department of Health and Human Services. Another useful tool is *Helping smokers quit,* a publication of the WHO Regional Office for Europe.

National Tobacco Control Programme staff and their local counterparts need to assess the applicability and feasibility of the different approaches to cessation in the light of the country's needs and resources. As with school-based prevention programmes, cessation programmes must be part of a comprehensive package that integrates policies with interventions. Within this integrated framework, one should select appropriate cessation interventions, train the members of staff chosen to carry them out, disseminate the interventions using the NTCP infrastructure and other networks, and establish a monitoring and evaluation system to measure impact.

One effective strategy to make smoking cessation interventions more widely available and sustainable is to incorporate them into other basic community health care services. For instance, the risks of smoking during pregnancy are well known and documented. Programmes to assist pregnant women and their families to stop smoking during and after pregnancy provide opportunities to intervene when tobacco users are more receptive to messages encouraging them to quit smoking. These might be integrated into a programme for pregnant women. Canada has used this strategy effectively, and the programme of the Canadian Public Health Association, Asking to listen, provides a training video and written guidelines to assist health professionals in providing effective advice to pregnant women.

Similar opportunities to integrate smoking cessation activities into health care exist for specific groups of people, such as those recovering from a heart attack or stroke. Recruiting other health care professionals to take advantage of these opportunities and deliver cessation messages and assistance can enhance the efforts to reduce tobacco consumption.

GYTS, a collaborative project of WHO and the CDC, indicates that many young people who smoke, wish to quit, but are unsuccessful: many do not know how to change their ways. Smoking cessation programmes designed specifically for young people should be considered for inclusion in community and school-based programmes when tobacco use rates are high.

The Quit 4 life/Une vie 100 fumer self-help programme, which can be found on the Health Canada site, www.gosmokefree.ca, provides ideas for a smoking cessation programme aimed at young people. It is based on cognitive behavioural principles that teach young people to practice being non-smokers. The programme also focuses on building motivation to quit, the importance of a strong social support network and on problem-solving skills.

PROTECTION

Promoting smoke-free environments

Policies that create smoke-free environments are needed to protect the health of non-smokers. In addition, smoke-free policies in workplaces and public spaces have been shown to promote a reduction or cessation of tobacco use among smokers. The widespread implementation of smoking bans in public places leads to:
• better health for non-smokers and smokers;

- fewer cigarettes smoked daily by smokers (often a first step towards quitting);
- greater public awareness of the seriousness of exposure to second-hand tobacco smoke;
- the emergence of societies and environments where non-smoking is viewed as the norm.

Governments can provide strong leadership to reduce exposure to second-hand tobacco smoke by banning smoking in all official buildings, and by ensuring compliance with non-smoking policies and regulations at both national and local levels. For example, the Non-Smokers Health Act in Canada restricts smoking in federally regulated workplaces, on airline flights, on intercity buses and trains, inside transport terminals and in hospitals that are under federal jurisdiction.

Exposure to tobacco smoke is a major health threat in the workplace, responsible for some 25–35% of all employee absence from work. To assist employers and employees in creating non-smoking workplaces, a number of guides exist, including the booklet *Tobacco in the workplace: Meeting the challenge. A handbook for employers* produced by the WHO European Partnership Project To Reduce Tobacco Dependence.

Smoke Free Americas was launched in 2001 by the Pan American Health Organization to support efforts to reduce exposure to second-hand tobacco smoke in the Americas. The initiative provides technical cooperation to governments that wish to implement smoke free environments, and a wide range of resources to assist advocates,

Table 2. Expanding the number of smoke-free public places

	Phase 1 Preparation (1–2 years)	Phase 2 Action (6–8 months)	Phase 3 Maintenance (1 year intensive and then ongoing)
Objectives	Increase public knowledge of the dangers of second-hand smoke and building support for smoke-free spaces in the community, homes and cars	Maintain strong public & political support for smoke-free legislation; smoke-free legislation (by-laws) approved by government	Compliance with smoke-free legislation greater than 80%
Activities	Establish a team; determine costs and sources of funding Recruit 'champions' to promote smoke-free spaces Develop advocacy, communication and enforcement plans Launch public education programmes to build support; working with local schools and businesses to implement voluntary non-smoking policies Develop draft legislation	Meet the local media to highlight the problems of second-hand smoke and gain their support Hold public consultations and meetings with politicians Meet with local businesses to advocate implementation of smoke-free workplaces	Establish and implement the enforcement process Work with businesses to ensure compliance with new smoke-free legislation Educate parents and caregivers regarding the new smoke-free policies Monitor public support and compliance Celebrate success!

parents, communities and the public in creating smoke free environments where they live and work. It can be accessed at the web site www.smokefreeamericas.org.

Table 2 gives a brief extract from *Smoke-free public places: You can get there,* produced by Health Canada *(3)*, which provides step-by-step guidelines to implementing smoking bans, including sample by-laws and community surveys, economic information, evaluation strategies, promotion and communication plans, information on enforcement strategies and detailed case studies. The table highlights the importance of developing partnerships and using targeted media, education and advocacy campaigns to expand the number of smoke-free public places where non-smokers are protected from the insidious effects of second-hand smoke.

HIGH-RISK POPULATIONS

The poor and less educated

According to the World Bank, today, the poor and less educated are more likely to smoke than the wealthy and better educated. Overall, the smoking epidemic is spreading from its original focus among men in high-income countries, to women in high-income countries and men in low-income regions.

In general, smokers in these high-risk populations do not benefit so much from more traditional approaches to tobacco prevention and cessation. Many poor and less educated smokers do not have regular contact with physicians or other health professionals and as a result do not benefit from clinical interventions. A significant proportion of young smokers do not attend school, and are not covered by school-based programmes. It is critical to reach out to those populations and involve them in programmes, which are culturally appropriate, easily accessible, geared toward their socioeconomic realities and delivered by individuals with whom they are comfortable.

Integrating tobacco control interventions into existing programmes for poverty alleviation is one way of reaching out to the high-risk smokers. Smoking cessation can be incorporated into public health programmes for the medically indigent. This should include ensuring social insurance coverage for cessation services. Educational and advocacy campaigns should specifically target these groups with effective messages. Other strategies should be developed as appropriate.

Women and girls

Tobacco use is also one of the greatest threats to the health and well-being of women and girls around the world. As women acquire greater independence in society, their spending power increases. The tobacco industry is aware of this, and is increasingly targeting women in its advertising campaigns. In countries without high rates of smoking among women, they are often exposed to second-hand tobacco smoke throughout their lives, which makes them vulnerable to smoking-related diseases and death. Certain forms of tobacco use fall within the realm of accepted female social activities in several cultures. In India, for example, betel quid chewing is widespread among women. Already, oral cancer has surpassed breast cancer as the leading cause of cancer death among these women.

One should consider strategies and policies that specifically address rates of smoking among women, and the need to prevent tobacco use among women.

Some of these strategies are listed below:

- fostering awareness of the various motivational factors of women at different stages of their life cycle, and utilizing this information when developing advocacy messages;
- including media literacy skills in relation to tobacco advertising in activities for women's empowerment;
- broadening the tobacco control network to include organizations concerned with women's rights, and urging women's organizations to refrain from accepting tobacco sponsorship;
- asking leading women to speak up against the deceitful marketing practices of the tobacco industry.

COMMUNITY MOBILIZATION

When approaching community mobilization, careful consideration should be given to the following issues.

The individual and the community

- While tobacco control is traditionally assigned to the health sector, in reality, it is successful only when different sectors and groups work in partnership to promote a reduction in tobacco use. This is true at the national, local and community levels.
- All national health programmes are intended to reach out to people. If they are run effectively, some individuals will pick up, process and use what a programme disseminates.
- If more than one person in a group or community picks up an idea, there is a greater likelihood that the larger group or community will be influenced. To make families, groups and communities change, a critical threshold must be reached.
- How families, natural groups and communities process the information received affects any changes in their attitude and behaviour. The power of the opinion of others in the community is often unrecognized or underestimated in public health work. A message about the consequences of tobacco use can be lost on a group where the dominant attitude tends to dismiss it. For example, an immediate reac-

tion by an influential group member saying sarcastically, "Wow, they seem to have discovered that smokers die. Those who don't smoke live forever, I guess", trivializes for the group the idea that is being transmitted.

The importance of the milieu

- The prevailing attitude or milieu then influences how each person responds to messages from a given programme. Any tobacco control programme must consider this perspective, and aim to influence the social settings in which people live and learn as much as people's smoking behaviour.
- Changes in milieu can occur at the community level as well as at the global level. The best examples come from countries and states that run successful tobacco control programmes. In California, USA, for example, smoking has shifted from being a socially acceptable behaviour to one that is generally frowned upon.
- Rather than waiting for such changes to occur spontaneously, planners of tobacco control programmes should aim deliberately to influence social attitudes. This requires thoughtful consideration of the factors that contribute to social change when designing programme interventions. These factors include the way opinion is created in communities and groups, and the key opinion leaders. For instance, a cartoon with a smoking character in it will have a greater impact on children and they are more likely to start smoking if the character appeals to the 'influential' kids in the group. These young 'opinion leaders' who determine what other children say and do are the likely targets in tobacco advertising. A tobacco control programme can target such children and use their ability to influence their peers to disseminate interventions designed to counteract tobacco industry marketing.

Bringing about changes in milieu

- Given the importance of social settings, tobacco control efforts should aim to change attitudes and habits in the community, focusing on ways to make it more aware of and interested in tobacco control. The term 'community mobilization' is sometimes used to refer to this process.
- The influential members of a community should be identified and initially targeted, so that they can influence and recruit others to support tobacco control.
- Communities are not homogeneous: besides influential individuals, there are also influential subgroups. In mobilizing a community, one should determine how different subgroups relate to each other, and how best to reach and influence each one of them. Tobacco industry marketing is often designed to appeal to specific subgroups within a community, such as ethnic minorities, special interest groups or young executives. Hence, tobacco control programmes also need to tailor some of the approaches and messages to those subgroups.
- In smaller, well defined settings, such as schools, workplaces and villages, direct outreach efforts yield good results. Other communities may be more difficult to

access because they are more vague, and have large populations. To reach these broader, more diffused communities, several intensive visits or remote means are needed.

Outreach or direct contact

When working with communities, a facilitator can considerably enhance effectiveness. Candidates for working directly with communities include:

- health workers
- other outreach or field staff
- teachers
- groups of young people
- any club, organization or community-based organization
- trade unions.

What should communities try to achieve?

A clear understanding of our objectives is essential for community action, as for anything else. People who want to stop the spread of tobacco-related harm are generally aware of the final goals. They would like to prevent people from starting to use tobacco, encourage current users to quit and, in the interim, protect non-users from harm.

We must also consider how to achieve these goals and look for contributing factors at community level. Each community will have to discover how best to encourage quitting and discourage initiation. A few examples are given below:

- understanding of the full range, and concern about the extent, of harm caused by tobacco;
- the attractiveness or unattractiveness of the image of tobacco use and users;
- understanding of, and resistance to, overt and covert promotion of tobacco use by the industry and by others;
- respect and concern for clean, uncontaminated and pleasant environments;
- encouragement and support of those who still use tobacco, to quit or continually reduce tobacco use;
- pros and cons identified by the smokers for smoking;
- ease of access to, acceptability and affordability of tobacco products at community level;
- advocacy for the establishment and enforcement of good public policies in the field of tobacco.

The actions we need to take to reduce initiation, promote quitting and protect the community are implicit in the items listed above.

A society or community that wants to reduce the harmful consequences of tobacco use should take steps according to each of the suggestions above.

A practical example

A member of a savings and loan club in a semi-urban community shares his experiences during one of the club meetings. Since he was suffering from acute tuberculosis (TB) and was bedridden for several months, the club gave him a loan to help his family. It also supported him to go through all the steps of the treatment without defaulting. He is now cured from tuberculosis. His family members were also screened for TB, and fortunately found to be free from the disease. However, he is still coughing a lot. The doctor at the primary health care facility has strongly advised him to stop smoking. He has been smoking for the last 15 years and although he wishes to quit, he is unable to do so. He has tried a couple of times but could not keep away from smoking.

This revelation initiates a lively discussion in the group. Smokers, users of chewing tobacco and others who feel disturbed by tobacco smoke or are concerned about family members share their views on the subject. The participants of the meeting conclude that they need to know more about the harmful effects of tobacco as well as how they can help those who wish to quit. They decide to approach a community nurse who is widely respected for her counselling skills. She agrees to help and consults with the general physician and the medical social worker at the primary health care facility. Together with them, she manages to collect relevant information and educational material on the subject, which she shares with the club members.

As a result, some 15 smokers who want to quit decide to form a support group. They meet once every week, to share their experiences on how they cope with their urge to smoke or chew tobacco, and keep up each other's motivation to remain tobacco free. The community nurse meets the support group once a month. Upon her initiative, the primary health care facility also introduces counselling sessions for tobacco users who want to quit, and family members who want to support them. The primary health care facility also adopts a smoke-free policy on its premises. The savings and loan club decides that their club meetings will be smoke-free.

A youth club and two local schools get involved in informing young people on the risks of using tobacco or being exposed to tobacco smoke, and motivating them to stay free from tobacco. In their group discussions, boys and girls discover that the glamorous image of smoking, as depicted in advertisements and promotions, is grossly misleading. Smoking is no longer considered as "cool" among the young people in the community.

The community has a Health Committee consisting of elected community leaders, administrators and health professionals. This committee has the mandate from the government and the local authorities to design a community health development plan. After several rounds of heated discussions, the Health Committee decides to integrate support for cessation of tobacco use and prevention of uptake into the proposed plan. These include provisions for counselling and public information to support cessation of tobacco use, prevent its uptake and protect people in public places from involuntary exposure to tobacco smoke.

This example shows that a combination of local initiative and support through existing formal and informal structures is needed to address the tobacco problem at the community level.

Facilitators should be trained to identify:
- the objectives to be reached in the community;
- the indicators that will help people assess progress in the desired direction;
- how to get members of a community interested and moving towards the desired objectives;
- how to assess their progress in moving in the desired direction.

> **Reaching wider communities**
>
> Mass media are an obvious resource. We can look for the best content to bring about the changes that were listed in the earlier box entitled *What should communities try to achieve?*
>
> The production of small training kits covering issues required for good community action is another option. This kit should be based on practical proven steps and should tackle all the aspects listed in the section on community objectives mentioned above. Ideas arising from within the community can be added as well.
>
> The involvement of people or structures that have a wide network of community connections is another possible approach. In many countries there is a network of field health staff who can be informed and mobilized. Schools or teachers are another potential resource. Many agencies and organizations outside government structures have good grass-roots connections and it may be possible to involve them in disseminating responses from communities to efforts aimed at reducing the harmful effects of tobacco.

Consolidating progress and maximizing impact require a few other steps. These include the following:

- Ensuring sustained progress and preventing burnout to help communities deal with tobacco control effectively. Keep expectations realistic and space out activities so that they are easy to sustain.
- Including more formal evaluation than the community measures listed above. This ensures that progress is tracked systematically, and gaps and weak areas in programme interventions are easily identified and addressed. The impact on selected indicators can also be objectively measured.

Remote interventions

Direct contact is not always feasible when dealing with large communities; in such cases more cost-effective means need to be found. Other less expensive methods – which still aim to bring about change in a community – should be developed. Several strategies are possible. Examples are listed below.

Conclusions

A brief outline of possible approaches has been given here; they are intended mainly as examples and stimuli for community discussion and mobilization. The key to success is community participation in the process of understanding tobacco more clearly and responding in an appropriate way.

A more detailed booklet entitled *Prevention and cessation of tobacco use – a manual for clinic and community-based interventions* has been published through the WHO Regional Office for South-East Asia *(4)*. It explains in much greater detail the community process and how it should be set in motion, monitored and guided. Publications that tackle the different programme interventions for tobacco control will be produced by WHO in the near future.

References

1. Henningfield JE, Slade J. Tobacco-dependence medications: public health and regulatory issues. *Food Drug and Law Journal,* 1998, 53, suppl:75–114.

2. World Health Organization. *Mayo report on addressing the worldwide tobacco epidemic through effective, evidence-based treatment: Report of an expert meeting.* March 1999, Rochester (Minnesota), USA. Geneva, World Health Organization, 2000.

3. Health Canada, *Smoke-Free Public Places: You Can Get There.* Ottawa, Health Canada (www.hc-sc.gc.ca/hecs-sesc/tobacco/facts/blueribbon/sfpp.html).

4. *Prevention and cessation of tobacco use. A manual for clinic and community based interventions.* World Health Organization, Regional Office for South-East Asia, New Delhi, 2003.

Resources

This section contains links to sites that will provide additional information to assist governments and others in establishing and evaluating effective tobacco control programmes.

- The World Health Organization Tobacco Free Initiative (TFI) web site www.who.int/tobacco/en provides information about various areas of policy development for tobacco control. Web sites of the Regional Offices of TFI can also be accessed.

- The Australian government web site, www.quitnow.info.au, offers an on-line quit book in eight languages as well as other tobacco-related information of help to smokers and health professionals.

- The Campaign for Tobacco Free Kids is dedicated to protecting children from tobacco addiction and from exposure to second-hand smoke. Its web site, www.tobaccofreekids.org, offers up-to-date information related to tobacco industry misinformation and manipulation.

- The site of the Canadian Cancer Society, www.cancer.ca, provides information on smoking cessation, the adverse effects of smoking and smokers' behaviour.

- The tobacco control web site of the Centers for Disease Control and Prevention, Atlanta (USA), www.cdc.gov/tobacco, covers best practices, research, smoking cessation standards, media campaigns, educational materials, surveillance and evaluation data for comprehensive tobacco control programmes designed to prevent tobacco use among young people, promote smoking cessation and much more.

- The UICC GLOBALink web site, www.globalink.org, provides information relating to tobacco control initiatives around the world. It also contains fact sheets on such topics as second-hand tobacco smoke, youth and cigarettes, the Campaign for Tobacco-Free Kids and fact sheets from the World Bank.

- The Health Canada web site, www.gosmokefree.ca, contains information on all aspects of tobacco control, including a self-help, interactive cessation programme; electronic 30 day cessation messages; a self-help tobacco cessation programme for teenagers; guides for planning and establishing smoke-free buildings; guidelines for establishing smoke-free workplaces; data on smokers' behaviour; tobacco prevention information and resources; training resources for service providers; media literacy resources for teenagers; research and best practice information; and Canadian statistics on smoking and tobacco use. Information is available in English and French.

- The web site of the Massachusetts Department of Health (USA), www.trytostop.org, gives advice to smokers who would like to quit and provides an on-line service at registration. Some basic information is available in Cambodian, Chinese, Haitian Creole, Italian, Korean, Portuguese, Russian and Spanish.

- The web site of the National Clearinghouse on Tobacco and Health (Canada), www.ncth.ca, serves the information needs of health intermediaries. It is an information provider, knowledge broker and facilitator of networking. It also contains information related to best practices, smoking prevention, cessation and protection.

- www.wiredforhealth.gov.uk is the site supported by the Department of Health and the Department for Education and Skills (United Kingdom); it offers health information for teachers and students. The site covers a number of issues, including smoking, and it offers guidelines for integrating tobacco control in the school curriculum. It also provides links to other interactive sites suitable for classroom resources.

11
Legislative and regulatory measures

Good laws derive from evil habits.
—*Macrobius*

COMPREHENSIVE TOBACCO CONTROL LEGISLATION is a crucial component of a successful tobacco control programme. Since the 1970s WHO has endorsed successively stronger resolutions calling on governments to adopt legislative measures to curb the tobacco epidemic. This process culminated in the WHO FCTC, which requires parties, according to their capabilities, "to adopt and implement effective legislative, executive, administrative and/or other measures … in developing appropriate policies for preventing and reducing tobacco consumption, nicotine addiction and exposure to tobacco smoke". *(1)* In implementing tobacco control legislation, governments acknowledge that tobacco use is a significant public health issue and initiate cultural changes to bring about a tobacco-free society.

THE WHO INTRODUCTORY GUIDE TO TOBACCO CONTROL LEGISLATION

WHO developed *Tobacco control legislation: an introductory guide* ("the guide"), comprehensive document that aims to equip policy-makers, legislators and stakeholders with the skills to develop and implement effective tobacco control laws *(2)*. The guide presents international experience, from both developed and developing countries, identifying tobacco industry tactics and potential legislative pitfalls. While recognizing that there is no universal formula for enacting effective tobacco control laws, the guide explains the legislative process and provides model legislation that can assist countries in drafting laws that are appropriate to their particular national situation, system of government and legislative process.

The guide examines in detail each of the following steps to implement effective tobacco control legislation:

- tailoring legislation to a country's legal and political framework
- advocating for legislation
- policy development
- drafting legislation
- passing legislation
- monitoring and enforcing legislation
- evaluating legislation.

The guide provides valuable advice for all parties involved in the legislative process and should be the main reference work for those seeking to initiate new tobacco control legislation or amend existing laws. A publication from the Pan American Health Organization, *Developing legislation for tobacco control: template and guidelines,* complements the guide. It contains a legislative template for a comprehensive tobacco control law and details the evidence on which each proposed legislative measure is based *(3)*. The aim of this chapter is not to repeat what is contained in those publications, but rather to build on them, offering practical advice of relevance to countries seeking to develop and implement tobacco control legislation.

LEGISLATIVE MEASURES ON TOBACCO CONTROL

The legislative measures on tobacco control recommended by WHO as part of a comprehensive tobacco control programme are summarized in Box 1. The guide provides detailed explanations of each of those measures and examples of jurisdictions where they have been implemented. It is recognized that the particular situation of a country may not be conducive to the adoption of a comprehensive programme and that it may be more appropriate for that country to develop its legislation step by step.

Box 1. Summary of legislative measures on tobacco control

Measures that influence demand and consumer behaviour:

- raising taxes and prices of cigarettes;
- banning cigarette advertising, promotion and sponsorship;
- health warnings and statement of tar and nicotine contents;
- smoke-free public places, workplaces and transport;
- public information and school-based education programmes.

Measures that affect supply:

- agricultural policies, such as crop diversification and elimination of subsidies;
- trade policies and smuggling;
- restricting access of young people to tobacco;
- product regulation.

Legislation enabling litigation[1] by:

- allowing class actions in tobacco control suits;
- allowing for litigation in the public interest;
- waiving legal costs in tobacco control litigation.

Source: Resolution WHA39.14. Tobacco or Health *(4)*; Resolution WHA56.1. WHO Framework Convention on Tobacco Control *(5)*

INFLUENCING LEGISLATORS

More and more countries are implementing strong tobacco control laws. However, despite the success of laws in jurisdictions such as Canada and South Africa, legislators in many other countries have failed to address the tobacco pandemic, even in the light of an ever growing body of evidence showing the damage to health and the enormous social and economic costs of tobacco use. Furthermore, in many jurisdictions,

---

[1] WHO Tobacco Free Initiative has developed a document on the role of litigation in tobacco control *(6)*.

tobacco control legislation has failed to keep pace with changing public attitudes to tobacco use, particularly in relation to smoke-free laws. The tobacco industry is a powerful constituency, with highly developed and effective lobbying techniques and it is unlikely that a government will choose to enact tobacco control legislation without a strong foundation being laid by tobacco control advocates. Therefore, in addition to scientific and economic evidence of the need for tobacco control measures, the community must be able to press legislators to act on this serious issue.

To facilitate the enactment of tobacco control legislation, the following steps are recommended:

- identify leaders who can mobilize support for tobacco control;
- establish an NCTC with broad membership from governmental and nongovernmental agencies to coordinate all tobacco control actions;
- gather tobacco-related information including data on smoking prevalence, morbidity and mortality from tobacco-related diseases, social and economic costs of tobacco use, existing legislation and stakeholders;
- build alliances and partnerships at both national and international levels;
- inform policy-makers, political leaders and the general public about the extent of the tobacco problem.

The effective mobilization of public support for tobacco control legislation is illustrated below with an example from Thailand.[2]

In 1992, Thailand enacted two progressive pieces of tobacco control legislation, the Tobacco Products Control Act, which bans all forms of tobacco advertising and promotions, and the Non-Smokers' Health Protection Act, which prohibits smoking in public buildings. These laws were passed in extraordinary circumstances by an unelected government following a military coup, but that does not diminish their standing as an example of the successful outcome of a coordinated strategic approach to influencing legislators.

At the time those laws were passed, the Thai tobacco control movement was still in its infancy. In 1986, the Thai Anti-Smoking Campaign Project (currently ASH Thailand) was established by a group of prominent medical professionals, with the support of a number of nongovernmental health organizations. With a limited budget, ASH Thailand used the media to promote anti-smoking messages and garner widespread support for tobacco control measures. One particularly successful strategy was to

"Through active social marketing, activities using media specialists and involving key figures from just about every walk of life, [Thai] NGOs turned the anti-smoking movement into a form of social mobilisation which had a lasting impact on the consciousness of the whole society concerning the subject matter of smoking control." (7)

[2] This discussion draws on Vaughan J, Collin J, Lee K (8).

team physicians with people who had media experience, combining medical and communications expertise to convey health messages with maximum media impact. National petitions were also used to raise public awareness of tobacco issues, and 6 million Thais signed one such petition in 1987.

Strong strategic alliances ensured that the Thai anti-tobacco movement had an influential and long-term impact on the whole society. Key alliances were formed with government, NGOs, health organizations, businesses, academic institutions and religious bodies. Support was also garnered from anti-smoking advocates around the globe, including the Asia Pacific Association for the Control of Tobacco (APACT) and WHO.

Other key strategies used by the Thai anti-smoking movement were (9, 10):
- highlighting the experience of countries with successful tobacco control legislation (the Tobacco Products Control Act was modelled on Canadian legislation);
- relying on populist sentiment (strengthened by a 1990 GATT[3] ruling that Thailand's ban on imported cigarettes was illegal);
- using the debate over the import of foreign cigarettes to raise health concerns;
- establishing direct links with ministers and government officials;
- understanding the political climate and using the system to best advantage, for example by relying on the 'guilt' of members of an unelected government;
- using highly influential public figures as advocates.

The Thai experience stands as an example of how, with limited resources, the anti-tobacco movement can raise public awareness and motivate legislative action, through effective communication and alliance building.

TOOLS AND STRATEGIES TO IMPLEMENT AND ENFORCE LEGISLATION

By enacting tobacco control legislation, a government demonstrates a certain degree of commitment to reducing the harmful effects of tobacco use on its citizens. However, enacting a law is not enough. It will have no impact unless those concerned know and abide by it, and sanctions are provided for in case of non-compliance. Legislation should be designed to be self-enforcing and should be supported by a commitment to adequately maintain an information, implementation, monitoring and enforcement programme.

These issues are discussed in more detail below.

---

[3] General Agreement on Tariffs and Trade, now the World Trade Organization.

Implementation

To facilitate compliance with a law, those concerned must be aware of it and know how to comply. Thus, where a new tobacco control law is enacted, a communication campaign is essential, particularly where a law affects a large section of the public (e.g. smoke-free laws) or businesses (e.g. laws on advertising and display of tobacco products). A successful communication campaign can reduce expenditure on active enforcement activities by increasing voluntary compliance with the law.

The extent of the communication campaign will depend on the type of law and the resources available. Box 2 outlines the key components of an AU$ 200 000 communication campaign conducted by the state government of Victoria, Australia, when it introduced smoke-free bars and gaming legislation in September 2002. While it is recognized that not all governments have the ability to conduct such a comprehensive campaign, strategic use of the media (which is discussed in more detail in Chapter 9) and dissemination of information through existing business networks can be cost-effective ways of informing both businesses and the public about new laws. For example, one way in which information was effectively disseminated in Victoria was through an advisory group with broad membership including major employers, industry groups, health bodies, unions, enforcement officers and other key government departments. As well as providing advice about how the government could meet the communication needs of both businesses and the general public, the members

---

Box 2. Key components of the communication campaign on introducing smoke-free bars and gaming legislation, conducted by the State Government of Victoria

- Establishment of an advisory group consisting of key stakeholders.
- Distribution of fact sheets (in English and five community languages) summarizing the law for members of the advisory group and the general public as soon as the laws were passed.
- Publication of a comprehensive booklet explaining the laws and how to comply with them. This was mailed free of charge to all affected businesses (approximately 5000), six weeks before the laws came into force.
- Provision of material or support to industry groups to enable them to conduct training for members.
- Availability of training sessions conducted by government officers for industry groups and businesses.
- Community and industry radio and press advertising campaign in both mainstream and multicultural media.
- Workshops to educate enforcement officers about the new laws. Enforcement officers were funded to visit affected premises and provide education about the laws.
- Maintenance of a telephone information line and web site http://www.tobaccoreforms.vic.gov.au/.

of that group played an important role in disseminating information about the laws through industry seminars and newsletters. One vital function of that group was to provide feedback on potential implementation issues, enabling these to be tackled at an early stage.

The success of the Victorian communication campaign was confirmed by pre- and post-campaign surveys, which showed a high level of awareness of the laws among businesses and the community in general. In particular, the communication campaign in Victoria was shown to significantly increase awareness of the details of the new laws, including what businesses needed to do to comply with them.

Communication campaigns can also be successful in developing countries. For example, a campaign conducted in Fiji in 1999 applied many of the techniques used in Victoria. The Fiji campaign consisted of television and radio advertisements in three languages, posters about the consequences of smoking, a pocket-size publication summarizing tobacco control legislation and stickers with smoke-free and no-sales to minors slogans. The material was distributed through Ministry of Health outlets, schools, public transport and retail outlets *(11)*.

Enforcement

In jurisdictions where tobacco control legislation has contributed to changes in social norms about the acceptability of tobacco use, many types of tobacco control legislation appear to be self-enforcing. For example, in Canada, New Zealand and the United States, smoke-free laws enjoy widespread community support and have led to a change in community behaviour, with people voluntarily refraining from smoking in smoke-free areas. However, the experience with smoke-free laws in Mozambique and Côte d'Ivoire was quite different: in the absence of enforcement, the laws were widely ignored. Other types of law, such as those prohibiting the sale of tobacco products to minors, have been almost universally unsuccessful in the absence of enforcement *(12, 13)*. There are a number of strategies that jurisdictions can adopt to ensure that legislation is both enforceable and enforced. These strategies are summarized in Box 3.

Tobacco industry efforts to frustrate the effective implementation of tobacco control legislation should not be underestimated. Those involved in the legislative process should consider the experience of other jurisdictions in attempting to enact and enforce tobacco control legislation, with the aim of predicting some of the obstacles that the tactics of the tobacco industry will raise. For example, a ban on billboards in Venezuela resulted in the industry using mobile billboards. Recently in South Africa, tobacco companies have taken advantage of ambiguous wording in legislation intended to allow a single sign advertising tobacco products at each point of sale to erect multiple signs at each point of sale. These examples show the importance of monitoring the legislation in operation, including industry responses to it, and taking follow-up action where necessary, such as amending the legislation. Of course it would be best to avoid these pitfalls altogether, and the following section discusses how this can be done, by drawing on international expertise and experience.

Box 3. Tips for effective enforcement of legislation

When drafting the legislation:

- Clearly identify offences, and penalties for breaches.*

- Penalties should be sufficient to deter non-compliance, and should be proportional to the offence. Consider graded penalties and incentives to comply, such as loss of licence to sell tobacco.*

- Consider using on-the-spot fines for breaches to save time and money in launching prosecutions.

- Clearly identify who will enforce the law. Select the enforcement authority carefully (the police may have other priorities). Consider the establishment of an enforcement agency. The use of community volunteers may increase community involvement in enforcement action.

- Consult with enforcement officers when drafting the law in order to identify potential enforcement pitfalls.

- Clearly define the powers of enforcement officers, such as the right to seize products.

- Make the law easy to comply with: require, for example, the display of no-smoking signs and the removal of ashtrays in no-smoking areas.*

- Draft legislation in clear language.*

- Avoid or minimize exemptions. Any exemptions should be easy to apply.*

- Take into account tobacco industry tactics to get around legislation.

When devising the enforcement policy:

- Ensure adequate funding of enforcement officers (consider innovative funding sources such as tobacco tax, licence fees or legal action against the tobacco industry).

- Train enforcement officers in all aspects of the law (e.g. evidence collection) and other relevant laws. A written enforcement protocol may be useful in ensuring a consistent approach to enforcement.

- Provide for an introductory phase focusing on education before strict enforcement.

- Provide funding for education of concerned parties, such as businesses, members of the public and smokers. Enforcement officers should have an educational as well as an enforcement role.

- Involve the community in enforcement action by, for example, maintaining a telephone complaint line.

- Provide for active regular compliance checks in addition to responding to complaints.

- Keep abreast of industry responses to the law.

* This symbol indicates measures, which, if well explained to businesses and the public, will contribute to a law being self-enforcing.

Source: Karugaba P *(15)*; Barnsley K, Jacobs M *(16)*

HARNESSING INTERNATIONAL LEGISLATIVE EXPERIENCE

Each jurisdiction seeking to introduce legislative measures on tobacco control faces unique challenges stemming from its culture, system of government, legislative process and other individual circumstances. Tobacco-growing countries such as Zimbabwe, for instance, face different tobacco control obstacles to countries such as Japan, where government has full or partial ownership of tobacco companies. Nevertheless, jurisdictions seeking to pass tobacco control legislation often face similar problems, such as tobacco industry attempts to prevent and subvert the law. Those jurisdictions will, therefore, find it useful to look at the experiences (both successful and unsuccessful) of other countries.

The case of tobacco control advocates is significantly strengthened if they are able to point to the successful introduction of a similar legislative measure in another jurisdiction. As pointed out earlier, Thai advocates emphasized that proposed Thai legislation was modelled on successful Canadian legislation. The success of legislative measures in Thailand has subsequently been used to press for similar laws in other countries of South-East Asia. The comparison of one jurisdiction's tobacco control legislation with another may also result in healthy competition, with jurisdictions 'leapfrogging' each other, introducing successively more comprehensive tobacco control initiatives *(14)*. This has happened in Australia, where state and territory governments have successively brought in more stringent legislation, such as the law concerning point-of-sale advertising. In the United States, the task of comparing legislation across the nation is facilitated by two indicators devised by the National Cancer Institute, which aim to measure the extent of youth access and smoke-free laws in each state (http://www.scld-nci.net/state_tobacco_control_law_rating.htm).

Legislative databases are a useful starting point for examining legislative tobacco control measures in force around the globe. There are a number of databases that can be used to access detailed information about tobacco control legislation; the most useful are:

- Globalink (http://www.globalink.org/tobacco/docs/): this is indexed by geographical region and provides links to many specific pieces of legislation.
- TobaccoPedia (http://www.tobaccopedia.org/): indexed by subject matter, this gives examples of legislation used to tackle different tobacco control issues such as advertising and smoke-free areas.

Currently, WHO with its partner agencies is developing a global database with access to regional databases as well as to other international sources of tobacco control information, including legislation. This will be accessible from the web site http://www.who.int/tobacco/en.

There are also a number of databases summarizing subnational tobacco control legislation, such as:

- American Non-smokers' Rights Foundation (http://www.no-smoke.org/lists): database of local tobacco control ordinances.

- State Cancer Legislative Database Program, Tobacco Use Laws (http://scld-nci.net/): it contains summaries of US legislation.
- Canadian Law and Tobacco Database (http://www.ncth.ca/CCTCLAWweb.nsf): it contains major federal, provincial and territorial laws. It also has case studies and information on new developments and lessons learned.

However, the written words that form legislation tell only half of the story. Beyond the acts, regulations and ordinances lies practical experience with implementation, enforcement, tobacco industry opposition and legislative provisions, which did or did not achieve the desired outcome. It is, therefore, essential that jurisdictions seeking to enact tobacco control legislation communicate with key players in jurisdictions that have already implemented such reforms, and harness their experience.

CONCLUSION

The WHO FCTC recognizes that legislation is a significant component of any jurisdiction's tobacco control programme and urges parties to adopt legislative measures to tackle the tobacco epidemic. The legislative process can be lengthy, arduous and fraught with hidden obstacles, particularly in the light of the tactics used by the tobacco industry to prevent, weaken or undermine legislation. It is hoped that, through use of the tips in this chapter and the comprehensive material outlined in the guide, jurisdictions around the globe will be able to overcome the many challenges and implement effective tobacco control legislation as a component of their tobacco control programme.

References

1. WHO Framework Convention on Tobacco Control. Geneva, World Health Organization, 2003 (http://www.who.int/tobacco/en/).

2. *Tobacco control legislation: an introductory guide.* Geneva, World Health Organization, 2003.

3. Pan American Health Organization. *Developing legislation for tobacco control: template and guidelines.* Washington, DC, PAHO, 2002 (http://www.paho.org/English/HPP/HPM/TOH/tobacco_legislation.pdf).

4. Resolution WHA39.14. Tobacco or health. In: *Thirty-ninth World Health Assembly, Geneva, 5–16 May 1986. Volume I. Resolutions and decisions, and list of participants.* Geneva, World Health Organization, 1986 (WHA39/1986/REC/1).

5. Resolution WHA56.1. WHO Framework Convention on Tobacco Control. In: *Fifty-sixth World Health Assembly, Geneva, 19–28 May 2003. Volume I. Resolutions and decisions, and list of participants.* Geneva, World Health Organization, 2003 (WHA56/1986/REC/1).

6. *Towards health with justice. Litigation and public inquiries as tools for tobacco control.* Geneva, World Health Organization, 2002 (http://www.who.int/tobacco/en/).

7. Chantornvong S, McCargo D. Political economy of tobacco control in Thailand. *Tobacco Control,* 2001, 10:54.

8. Vaughn J, Collin J, Lee K. *Case study report: global analysis project on the political economy of tobacco control in low and middle-income countries.* London, London School of Hygiene and Tropical Medicine, 2000.

9. Vateesatokit P. Thai tobacco control development through strategic alliances. *Development Bulletin,* 2001, 54: 63–66 (http://devnet.anu.edu.au/db54.htm).

10. Chantornvong S, McCargo D. Political economy of tobacco control in Thailand. *Tobacco Control,* 2001, 10:48–54.

11. Cornelius M. Tobacco control: The Fiji experience. *Development Bulletin,* 2001, 54:69–71 (http://devnet.anu.edu.au/db54.htm).

12. Forster J, Wolfson M. Youth access to tobacco: policies and politics. *Annual Review of Public Health,* 1998, 19:203–235.

13. Ohmi H et al. The centenary of the enactment of the law prohibiting minors from smoking in Japan. *Tobacco Control,* 2000, 9:258–260.

14. Wakefield M, Chaloupka FJ. Improving the measurement and use of tobacco control 'inputs'. *Tobacco Control,* 1998, 7:333–335.

15. Karugaba P. Issues characterizing effective tobacco control legislation. Paper presented at the 2nd National Consensus Building Workshop on the Review of the Control of Smoking Act 1992, Francistown, Botswana, 25 April 2002 (http://tean.globalink.org/BotswanaIssues.html).

16. Barnsley K, Jacobs M. World's best practice in tobacco control. *Tobacco Control,* 2000, 9:228–236.

Bibliography

Chollat-Traquet C. *Evaluating tobacco control activities: experience and guiding principles.* Geneva, World Health Organization, 1996.

Curbing the epidemic: governments and the economics of tobacco control. Washington, DC, The World Bank. 1999 (Development in practice).

Developing legislation for tobacco control: template and guidelines. Washington, DC, Pan American Health Organization, 2002 (http://www.paho.org/English/HPP/HPM/TOH/tobacco_legislation.pdf).

Efroymson D. *PATH Canada briefing paper: Tobacco control law.* PATH Canada, 2001 (http://wbb.globalink.org/public/Law_briefing.pdf).

Guidelines for controlling and monitoring the tobacco epidemic. Geneva, World Health Organization, 1998.

Jacobson P, Wasserman J, Raube K. The politics of antismoking legislation. *Journal of Health Politics, Policy and Law*, 1993,18:4:787–819.

Jacobson P, Wasserman J, Raube K. *The political evolution of anti-smoking legislation.* Santa Monica, CA, RAND, 1992.

Jha P, Chaloupka FJ, eds. *Tobacco control in developing countries.* New York, Oxford University Press, 2000.

Roemer R. *Legislative action to combat the world tobacco epidemic.* Geneva, World Health Organization, 1993.

12

Exploring economic measures and funding initiatives

No tax is ever value-free, ethically neutral, or morally indifferent.
—Anon.

INTRODUCTION

The tobacco epidemic is unique among public health problems. Tobacco and tobacco products are extensively traded and highly valued legitimate consumer products, and tobacco use is considered acceptable in many cultures. Several governments own or subsidize their local tobacco industry, and revenues from tobacco form a significant part of the economy of many countries. The economic aspects of tobacco production and consumption must therefore play a critical role in the development of strategies for the reduction of tobacco use. The WHO Framework Convention on Tobacco Control (WHO FCTC) highlights comprehensive and synergistic economic measures that have proven effective in curbing tobacco use, and it shows how developing countries need financial resources if they are to put tobacco control measures into effect.

This chapter presents basic information about the key economic issues in tobacco control. It shows the evidence on price and tobacco consumption; describes key steps to introduce or increase tobacco taxes and prices, which countries may adapt to their specific socioeconomic and political situation; and deals with funding initiatives for tobacco control. More details on these economic issues can be found in the following publications and web sites:

- *Curbing the epidemic: Governments and the economics of tobacco control.* Washington, DC, The World Bank Development in Practice series, 1999 (http://www1.worldbank.org/tobacco/reports.asp).
- Jha P, Chaloupka FJ, eds. *Tobacco control in developing countries.* Oxford, Oxford University Press, 2002 (http://www1.worldbank.org/tobacco/tcdc.asp).
- World Bank. Economics of tobacco control toolkit (http://www1.worldbank.org/tobacco/toolkit.asp).

EVIDENCE ON TOBACCO PRICE AND CONSUMPTION

Increasing the price of tobacco and tobacco products is the single most effective way to reduce consumption. A 10% increase on cigarette prices reduces consumption by approximately 4% in high-income countries and 8% in low- and middle-income countries. Low- and middle-income countries are more responsive to price increases *(1)*.

Key fact:

Increasing the price of tobacco and tobacco products is the single most effective measure to reduce consumption.

Despite this, governments are often reluctant to increase taxes on tobacco and tobacco products because they mistakenly believe that doing so will lead to reduced revenues. Experience has demonstrated that increasing cigarette taxes will not lead to lower tax revenues in the short and medium term. Tax increases that raise the price of cigarettes by 10% worldwide would actually increase revenues by about 7% on average *(2)*. In China, a 10% increase in cigarette tax would cut consumption by 5% and increase revenues by 5% – this is enough to finance a package of essential health services for one-third of China's poorest 100 million people *(3)*. Recently, Palau reinstated its tax increase on cigarettes, after discovering that lowering the taxes on cigarettes led to a considerable decrease in government revenue *(4)*. Table 1 shows the potential impact of a 10% tobacco price increase on tobacco consumption, leading to an estimated reduction of 42 million in the number of smokers worldwide, and saving 10 million lives. In contrast, non-price efforts that decrease smoker prevalence by 2% have only half the effect of a 10% price increase, reducing the number of smokers by 23 million and saving only 5 million lives. Clearly, increasing prices of tobacco as part of a comprehensive approach to tobacco control is very effective in reducing consumption while augmenting government revenues.

Evidence shows that cigarette prices tend to be higher in wealthier countries, especially in those with strong tobacco control programs *(5)*. This has apparently contributed to considerable reductions in tobacco consumption, despite lower price elasticity in these established economies. However, in many developing countries, tobacco and cigarette prices have failed to keep up with increases in the general price level of goods and services, and this has made tobacco and cigarettes more affordable. For example, in Indonesia, the Philippines and Venezuela, the number of minutes of labour required to purchase a pack of cigarettes is significantly less than that needed to purchase a kilogram of bread *(5)*. Furthermore, taxes account for less than half of the retail price of cigarettes in most developing countries, while in developed countries, at least two-thirds of the retail price of cigarettes is accounted for by tax. Not surprisingly, developing and transitional economy countries account for 84% of the world's smokers *(6)*.

Table 1. Potential impact of a price increase of 10%, and a set of non-price measures (for smokers alive in 1995)

Countries	Number of smokers (million)		Number of deaths (million)	
	10% price increase	Non-price measures that reduce smoking prevalence by 2%	10% price increase	Non-price measures that reduce smoking prevalence by 2%
Low/middle-income	-38	-19	-9	-4
High-income	-4	-4	-1	-1
World	-42	-23	-10	-5

Source: Jha & Chaloupka *(1)*

There is definitely a lot of room for tax increases on tobacco products in the developing world. A small but growing body of evidence indicates that smokers in developing countries are more responsive to price increases than those in developed countries. In addition, studies from developed and several developing countries indicate that young people and the poor are more responsive to price increases than older and wealthier and better-educated individuals. This means that increasing cigarette prices through tax increases would be more likely to protect the young and economically disadvantaged from the harms of tobacco use.

Another argument used against tax increases on tobacco and tobacco products is that higher prices would result in increased smuggling. However, studies by the World Bank *(7)* stress that the determinants of smuggling go beyond price. Using indicators of corruption, based on the Transparency International's Index, the World Bank demonstrated that the level of tobacco contraband tends to increase with the degree of corruption in a country. For example, Scandinavian countries have some of the highest taxes on cigarettes. Despite the high cigarette prices, smuggling is almost non-existent. In contrast, cigarettes are relatively cheap in Italy, Spain and several of the central and eastern European countries, yet smuggling is rampant.

Smuggling is believed to account for around 6% to 8.5% of the world's total consumption of cigarettes. In some countries such as Bangladesh, Cambodia, Colombia, Latvia, Lithuania, Myanmar and Pakistan, smuggling accounts for 30% to 53% of domestic sales (1995 estimates) *(1)*. There is some evidence that the tobacco industry may be involved in the smuggling of cigarettes in a number of countries *(8)*. The tobacco industry also benefits from smuggling indirectly. Trade barriers are effectively bypassed when tobacco products enter into markets illegally *(9)*. Also, smuggled cigarettes are often less expensive than their legal counterparts. The availability of lower-priced, smuggled cigarettes increases consumption and augments the tobacco industry's total sales *(10)*. Moreover, smuggling deprives governments of revenue. For example, it is estimated that a single truckload of smuggled cigarettes could evade US$ 1.2 million of taxes in the European Union *(11)*. It is therefore in the interest of governments to control smuggling by adopting policies that make it "less profitable, more difficult and more costly to engage in smuggling," including the use of prominent tax stamps, serial numbers, special package markings, health warning labels in local languages, better tracking systems and good governance *(1)*. This represents the key supply side measure to reduce smoking. However, even in the presence of smuggling, a rise in cigarette tax results in higher tax revenues and lower consumption *(1)*.

USING ECONOMIC MEASURES TO CONTROL TOBACCO USE

Assessing and establishing evidence

While the tobacco control community is familiar with the evidence in support of economic measures to control tobacco use, many government leaders and policy-makers

Myths and facts about tobacco and taxes

MYTH: Cigarette taxes are already high in most countries.

FACT: In most high-income countries, taxes account for two-thirds or more of the retail price of a pack of cigarettes. In low-income countries, taxes generally account for less than half the retail price of a pack of cigarettes. This means there is still ample room to increase cigarette tax levels in many low-income countries.

MYTH: Governments will lose revenues if they increase cigarette taxes, because people will buy fewer cigarettes.

FACT: Even substantial cigarette tax increases will reduce consumption while increasing tax revenues, because smokers respond relatively slowly to increases in price. Actual experience in several countries demonstrates that raising tobacco taxes generates additional revenue for the government.

MYTH: Smuggling negates the beneficial effects of tobacco tax increases.

FACT: Even in the presence of smuggling, evidence from a number of countries shows that tax increases still increase revenue and reduce cigarette consumption. Furthermore, governments can adopt effective policies to control smuggling.

Source: Jha & Chaloupka *(12)*

may not be aware of this information. To obtain the support of these key players, the technical evidence needs to be linked to specific policies. Using local data is extremely critical, as these decision-makers need to be convinced that economic measures such as tax increases will result in good outcomes for their economies as a whole.

The relative importance of tobacco to a country

Basic information is essential to influence agenda and policy formulation for tobacco control. Technical capacity is required to compile and analyse health and economic data and statistics, to determine the current status of tobacco taxation and price, the economic consequences of tobacco related illnesses and deaths, and the relative benefits of tobacco control measures on the economy. In addition, for countries that have instituted economic measures to reduce tobacco consumption, technical expertise is needed to evaluate and refine existing control strategies.

Tobacco trade and agriculture statistics reflect the size of the tobacco industry in a country. A net exporter (of cigarette or tobacco leaf) with significant foreign earnings from exports and many people employed in the tobacco manufacturing sector might face difficulties when proposing tobacco control measures.

From the basic information on the tobacco industry, it is possible to determine the government's vested interest in tobacco. For example, if local tobacco production is monopolized by the government and generates significant revenue for the national economy, mobilizing support from the government for tobacco control may be more challenging. On the other hand, anecdotal evidence indicates that governments that control the production and distribution of tobacco are able to implement certain tobacco control interventions more readily, such as increasing tobacco taxes to generate greater revenues. Mobilizing these governments to institute tobacco control measures to protect people's health may be more difficult. However, the evidence of the long-term financial burden of tobacco related illnesses, which may offset any income generated by the continued production of tobacco, may persuade some of the key decision-makers to consider tobacco control as a sound investment for the country's future well-being. This analysis is essential, and results should be publicized.

Table 2 indicates how much governments of developing countries rely on tobacco revenue for their annual budget *(13)*.

Table 2. Tobacco tax as a percentage of total government revenue

Country	% of total government revenue
Democratic Republic of the Congo/Zaire	26.0
Malawi	17.0
United Republic of Tanzania	16.0
China	9.0
Kenya	9.0
Nigeria	8.0
Tunisia	6.0
Egypt	6.0
Zimbabwe	5.0
Ethiopia	4.0
South Africa	2.0
Algeria	0.2

Source: Townsend *(13)*

The following information will be essential to the formulation of strategic approaches for tobacco control:

- cigarette imports and exports;
- tobacco leaf imports and exports;
- cigarette production;
- tobacco leaf production;
- land devoted to tobacco growing as a percentage of agricultural land;
- total employment in tobacco agriculture and manufacturing;
- status of local manufacturing: private company, state enterprise, monopoly or competitive market;
- sales volume of domestic brands;
- annual revenue generated, disbursement to the government by state enterprise, corporate tax in addition to excise tax and other tariffs.

Tobacco excise tax

Excise taxes on tobacco and tobacco products determine how much the country earns from cigarettes and other tobacco products. Tobacco excises are a significant source of revenue for many countries (see Table 3). For example, tobacco excise tax represent over 5% of total tax revenues in Brazil, Greece and Nepal *(14)*. Cigarettes are the major tobacco product and generate over 90% of the total tobacco excise revenues. A comparison of the retail price of a typical pack of 20 cigarettes across countries reveals room for tax increases in many countries, especially in the developing world.

The critical data needed to fully understand how tobacco excise taxes work include:

- total government revenue from tobacco (excise tax, sales tax, import duties, other duties and special taxes and tariffs);
- total revenue from tobacco, and percentage of total government revenue;
- breakdown of excise tax generated from domestic production and imports;
- domestic and foreign brand retail prices;
- comparison of the consumer price index of tobacco products with other basic commodities – this information can be obtained by searching the general consumer price index, often produced by Ministries of Trade or Commerce.

There is a real need for a thorough understanding of how current national laws and regulations regarding tobacco excise tax are interpreted and practiced. Almost all countries have either an *ad valorem* tax (excise tax based on the value of the product, determined by the post-production or retail prices) or specific tax (based on the number or weight of cigarettes). Some countries use a combination of *ad valorem* and specific taxes on tobacco products *(15)*.

Ad valorem versus specific tax *(16)* – what is the rationale for a country's decision to use a particular type of excise tax on tobacco and tobacco products? The answer to this question could help with the formulation of strategies to revise the tax rate and ceiling so that retail prices keep pace more closely with inflation.

Tip: Usually, a proposed revision of the tax rate and ceiling undergoes a rigorous legislative review process, necessitating either amendments of a ministerial regulation or decree, or an amended national act. You need to familiarize yourself with, and thoroughly understand the political dynamics of the legislative process if an amendment of the tobacco excise law to raise tobacco prices is being contemplated.

Table 3. Tobacco excise tax, selected European countries

No.	Country	Excise tax	Sales tax	Import duty
1.	Albania	8.5 LCU/20 cigs	22%	25%; 1% customs fee - Bosnia & Herzegovina imports
2.	Armenia	4.3 US$/1000 filter cigs; 2.2 US$/1000 plain cigs	20%	10%
3.	Austria	246 LCU/1000 cigs or 42% of retail price	20%	---
4.	Azerbaijan	50%	20%	15%
5.	Belgium	521 LCU/1000 cigs; 47.36% of RP	21%	---
6.	Bosnia and Herzegovina	0.88 − 2.3 LCU/pack based on tar content	20%	15%, other import duties 1%
7.	Bulgaria	30% and 2000 LCU/1000 filter cigs; 10% and 1000 LCU/1000 plain cigs	20%	68% (min 13.1 ECU/1000 cigs) other import duty 2% (preferential import duty for Turkey and CEFTA)
8.	Cyprus	6.38 LCU/kg; 27 LCU/kg luxury tax. Preferential excise tax for EU and Locally produced cigs	8%	68.4%
9.	Denmark	606.8 LCU/ 1000 cigs; 21.22% of RP	25%	---
10.	Estonia	5.5 LCU/pack	18%	---
11.	Finland	90 LCU/ 1000 cigs; 50% of RP	22%	---
12.	France	54.5%RP; 38 LCU/1000 cigs	20.60%	0.74%
13.	Germany	92.2 LCU/1000 cigs; 21.96% of RP	16%	---
14.	Greece	53.86% of RP; 1182 LCU/1000 cigs	18%	---
15.	Hungary	75% of RP; 1725 LCU/1000 cigs	25%	63%; other import duty 17%; 2%; 3%
16.	Italy	54.3% of RP; 7280 LCU/1000 cigs	20%	63%
17.	Moldova	20 LCU/1000 luxury cigs; 12.5 LCU/1000 cigs over 81 mm; 5 LCU/1000 cigs under 81 mm	---	5LCU/ 1000 cigs under 81 mm
18.	Netherlands	21.05% of RP; 96.35 LCU/1000 cigs	17.5%	---
19.	Norway	1580 LCU/1000 cigs	23%	17 LCU/ kg, import duty exemption for EFTA and Portugal
20.	Poland	63.6 - 97.4 LCU/1000 cigs based on import status	22%	63; other import duty 90%- within quota (min 9 ECU/ 1000 cigs); 253.8% over quota (min 25.7 ECU/ 1000 cigs)
21.	Republic of Belarus	1.8 ECU/1000 filter cigs; 0.8 ECU/1000 plain cigs; 0.5 ECU/1000 papirossi cigs	20%	30% (min 3 ECU/1000 cigs), Former Soviet and LDC exempted. Other import duties : 0.15%; 22.5% on imports from developing countries
22.	Romania	2 ECU/1000 cigs; 8 LCU/cig; 25% of RP	22%	98%; other import duty; 6%; -0.25 to 0.5% customs fee based on EU status

	Retail price of 20 cigs with tax				
	Domestic brand		**Foreign brand**		
Source	**USD**	**Local**	**USD**	**Local**	**Source**
ERC, 1999	1.38	10.00	2.20	16.00	EIU, Autumn 1999
ERC, 1999	0.17	89.00	3.75	2000.00	TMA International Tobacco Guide (September 1999 data)
ERC, 1999	3.26	42.9	3.49	45.90	EIU, Autumn 1999
ERC, 1999	0.25	1000.00	0.25	3500.00	EIU, Autumn 1999
ERC, 1999	2.89	111.20	3.14	121.00	EIU, Autumn 1999
ERC, 1999	0.21	1.70	0.38	3.00	ACS/WHO survey, 2000
ERC, 1999	0.43	0.686	1.14	2.30	ACS/WHO survey, 2000
TMA- inter Tobacco guide	1.38	0.65	2.13	1.00	EIU, Autumn 1999
ERC, 1999	4.3	30.50	4.37	31.00	EIU, Autumn 1999
ERC, 1999	0.43	7.00	1.21	19.50	EIU, Autumn 1999
ERC, 1999	3.68	20.90	3.96	22.50	EIU, Autumn 1999
ERC, 1999	2.76	17.3	3.26	20.40	EIU, Autumn 1999
ERC, 1999	2.79	5.21	2.87	5.37	EIU, Autumn 1999
ERC, 1999	1.86	580.00	2.18	680.00	EIU, Autumn 1999
ERC, 1999	0.89	215.00	1.01	245.00	EIU, Autumn 1999
ERC, 1999	2.16	4000.00	3.03	5600.00	EIU, Autumn 1999
ERC, 1999	0.19	2.35	1.07	13.50	ACS/WHO survey, 2000
ERC, 1999	2.61	5.48	2.93	6.15	EIU, Autumn 1999
ERC, 1999	7.28	57.00	7.28	57.00	EIU, Autumn 1999
ERC & USDA, 1999	0.99	3.99	1.21	4.89	EIU, Autumn 1999
ERC, 1999	---	290.00	---	1200.00	ACS/WHO survey, 2000
ERC, 1999	0.80	1300.00	1.53	2500.00	EIU, Autumn 1999

Continues…

Table 3 Tobacco excise tax, selected countries in European Union (continued)

No.	Country	Excise tax	Sales tax	Import duty
23.	Russian Federation	4.8–30 LCU/1000 cigs, Based on filter and length	20%	33% (min of 3 ECU/1000 cigs) other import duty: 2 ECU/1000 cigs
24.	Slovakia	9.5 LCU/ pack cig < 70 mm; 17.9 LCU/ pack cig > 70 mm	23%	58.3% on all cigs from EU and MFN, other import duty: 10% surcharge on Czech imports
25.	Slovenia	45% of RP		53%; preferential rate for EFTA and CEFTA
26.	Spain	500 LCU/1000 cigs; 54% of RP	16%	---
27.	Sweden	39.2% of RP; 200 LCU/1000 cigs	25%	---
28.	Switzerland	59.89 LCU/1000 cigs; 1.3 LCU/1000cigs; 25%	7.5%	---
29.	Turkey	0.4 USD/pack of 20 cigs	15%; 2% applied before VAT, after VAT 15% education, 2% veterans fund, 100% additional tax, 10%–defence fund	68.40%
30.	Ukraine	2.5 ECU/1000 plain cigs, 3 ECU/1000 filter cigs,	---	2.5 ECU/1000 cigs Former Soviet countries exempted from import duties
31.	United Kingdom	---	---	---
32.	Uzbekistan	750% of RP	30%	30%
30.	Serbia and Montenegro	40% and 0.6 LCU/pack-standard quality; 50% and 0.7 LCU/pack extra class; 70% and 1 LCU/ pack foreign licensed and imports	21%	---

Source: Tobacco Control Resource Center *(15)*

| Source | Retail price of 20 cigs with tax | | | | Source |
| | Domestic brand | | Foreign brand | | |
	USD	Local	USD	Local	
ERC, 1999	0.49	13.90	0.81	23.20	ACS/WHO survey, 2000
ERC, 1999	0.71	30.5	1.35	58.00	ACS/WHO survey, 2000
ERC, 1999	1.41	175.00	2.23	290.00	EIU, Autumn 1997
ERC, 1999	1.26	200.00	2.30	365.00	EIU, Autumn 1999
ERC, 1999	4.20	34.50	4.32	35.50	EIU, Autumn 1999
ERC, 1999	2.88	4.40	2.94	4.50	EIU, Autumn 1999
ERC, 1999	0.99	450.00	1.32	600.00	EIU Autumn 1999
ERC, 1999	---	---	0.55	1.00	WHO/EURO survey, 1997
---	6.27	---	6.27	---	EIU, Autumn 1999
ERC, 1999	1.57	980.00	5.12	3200.00	EIU, Autumn 1999
ERC, 1999	0.40	4.00	1.25	12.50	EIU, Autumn 1999

Yurekli and de Beyer *(16)* provide a comprehensive tool kit for designing and administering tobacco taxes. Table 4 summarizes the effects of specific and *ad valorem* taxes on consumer choices in relation to the quality and variety of tobacco products, on government revenues and on domestic tobacco producers. When deciding on a specific excise tax structure for tobacco and tobacco products, a country should consider all factors relevant to its particular situation. The purchasing power of local consumers, rates and tax structure in neighbouring countries, the ability of tax and customs authorities to enforce compliance, the need for revenue and the need to tackle the growing burden of tobacco-related illnesses are important considerations.

Table 4. Effects of specific and *ad valorem* taxes on tobacco industry stakeholders

Stakeholders/concerns	Specific tax	*Ad valorem* tax
Consumer: quality and variety		
Provide an incentive for higher quality and greater variety of products	Yes (upgrading effect) [1]	No [2]
Effect of tax increase on prices	Higher prices (over-shifting) [3]	Lower prices (under-shifting)
Government: revenue and administration		
Maintain revenue value under high inflation	No (should be adjusted by CPI)	Yes
Minimize tax evasion or avoidance and realize expected revenues	Manufacturer can manipulate cigarette length or pack size to reduce tax payment	May need to set minimum price to counter abusive transfer pricing [4]
Administration and enforcement	Easy [5]	Must define the base for *ad valorem* in a way that minimizes the industry's ability to avoid taxes [6]
Domestic producer: profits and market share		
Protect domestic brands against international brands	No	Yes (the higher the price, the higher the absolute amount of tax paid per unit since tax is a percentage of price) [7]

Source: Yurekli & de Beyer *(16)*

---

[1] Per unit taxes are the same for all cigarettes. This reduces the price differential between high and low quality/price cigarettes and may lead consumers to switch to higher quality/price cigarettes (assuming that more expensive cigarettes are considered to be of higher quality).

[2] *Ad valorem* tax adds the same percentage to the price of high and low quality versions of the product and thus keeps relative prices the same.

[3] Faced with a tax increase, an oligopolist or a monopolist producer tends to increase the consumer price by more than the amount of a specific tax increase, but will increase the price less than the full amount of an *ad valorem* tax increase.

[4] If the *ad valorem* tax is a percentage of the manufacturer's price, the manufacturer may sell cigarettes to a related marketing company at an artificially low price in order to reduce its excise liability.

[5] Specific taxation is easier to administer, particularly in countries where tax administration is weak. Tax administrators can easily determine and verify liability by counting goods and marking or affixing stamps to taxed units.

[6] In developing countries, a tax based on value (*ad valorem*) can be difficult to administer if market prices of the excise goods are not established or are undervalued due to the non-existence of formal markets. This can cause a substantial loss of tax revenue.

[7] With *ad valorem* taxation, part of any increase in the consumer price goes to the government as tax revenue.

Cost of tobacco-related illnesses

The cost of the tobacco epidemic, in terms of tobacco-related illnesses and premature deaths and lost productivity, is a key point for mobilizing political and public support for tobacco control measures. Usually, the burden of proof falls on the Ministry of Health. However, this type of analysis requires technical expertise in the field of health economics. Collaboration with economists who have this type of expertise is highly recommended.

Methods to estimate tobacco consumption are discussed in Chapter 15. Lightwood et al *(17)* have developed a detailed methodology to estimate the cost of tobacco use. The following data are required for this estimation:

- disease burden in terms of prevalence and incidence, and time trend of three important tobacco-related illnesses: chronic obstructive lung disease, lung cancer and cardiovascular diseases;
- direct per capita medical and non-medical costs, and indirect costs due to illnesses and premature deaths;
- the total estimated financial burden of tobacco use on the government and households;
- the proportion of government and household expenditure on tobacco related illnesses.

Tobacco smuggling

Because smuggled cigarettes can represent a significant proportion of domestic cigarette sales that bypass government revenues, one must estimate the extent of contraband, its political dimensions and the political will of governments to suppress smuggling.

It is necessary to assess:

- products smuggled, including brand and country of origin;
- volume of smuggled cigarettes;
- estimated losses in revenues from uncollected taxes;
- government capacity to crack down on smuggling;
- level of good governance versus corruption related to smuggling;
- confiscation incentive for police and customs officers;
- financial incentives for informers;
- effective management of illicit products.

Translating evidence into political agenda

Once the evidence has been collected, it must be translated into policy messages that will persuade decision-makers to support economic measures in tobacco control. The NTCP under the Ministry of Health or its equivalent must take the lead in this endeavour.

To influence decision-makers, data must to be translated into powerful and moving messages, and disseminated to the intended target audiences. Working with economic experts and media and communications professionals can facilitate this process.

Packaging policy messages to specific audiences requires familiarity with what messages or 'hot buttons' will move decision-makers to act. For example, ministers of finance need to know that increasing taxes on tobacco products will lead to increases in government revenue, and that discretionary income previously spent on tobacco will likely be shifted to purchase other goods. Ministers of labour need to be convinced that tobacco control measures will not result in rampant unemployment.

> ✸ **Tip:** Economic data are often highly technical. This information will need to be translated into simple language that is easily understood and communicated.

Once the appropriate messages have been crafted (refer to Chapter 8), ensure that they reach the intended audience. Choose the right media (refer to Chapter 9), and the right messengers to reach the targets. Remember that in many cases, the informal and personal networks of decision-makers are more influential than official networks. Try to identify personal contacts of key policy leaders who may be supportive of tobacco control and willing to deliver your message about the economics of tobacco control. In Thailand, for example, the passage of a law earmarking tobacco taxes for health promotion was positively influenced by the efforts of a physician–advocate whose patients included important leaders in the legislature.

Stakeholder analysis

Tobacco control strategists need analytical skills to identify all stakeholders involved in tobacco taxation and to determine their positions (supportive, neutral or resistant) through research, interviews of key informants and analysis of contents of press interviews by each stakeholder, etc. In addition, they need to assess each stakeholder's relative power and influence over other stakeholders.

On the basis of this analysis, strategists from the tobacco control programme should facilitate an alliance between the supportive and the neutral groups by emphasizing common interest and goals, highlighting shared benefits of a tobacco tax increase and minimizing conflict over minor issues. Keep in mind that neutral groups will also be courted by those resisting the tax increase; a majority against tax increase can result if conflicting issues with the supportive groups are exaggerated.

Chevalier *(18)* identifies three key attributes to be examined in stakeholder analysis:
- power (refers to authoritative, command and control and legislative power);
- legitimacy (righteousness, impartiality or technical credibility);
- sense of urgency or interest with regard to the subject matter.

Definitive stakeholders possess all three attributes. Dependent stakeholders have keen interest and legitimacy but have no power. Dominant stakeholders have power and legitimacy but have no sense of urgency or interest. Dangerous stakeholders have power and keen interest but not legitimacy: they are potentially dangerous as they do not possess technical expertise and wisdom and could do more harm than good in the attempt to increase tobacco taxes (see Figure 1).

The possible combinations of the three attributes in Figure 1 give rise to different types of stakeholder who can be classified as follows:

- Category 1. Dormant stakeholders
- Category 2. Discretionary stakeholders
- Category 3. Demanding stakeholders
- Category 4. Dominant stakeholders
- Category 5. Dangerous stakeholders
- Category 6. Dependent stakeholders
- Category 7. Definitive stakeholders

Figure 1. Stakeholder typology

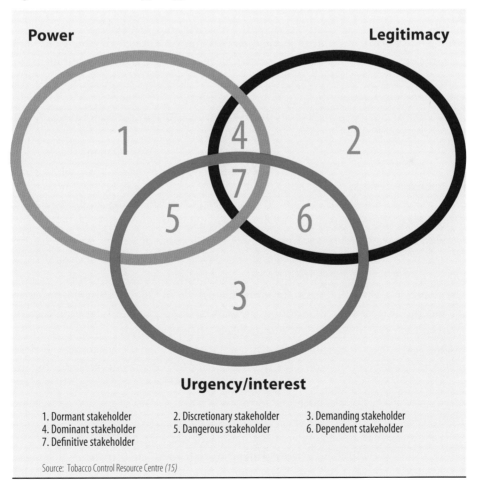

1. Dormant stakeholder
2. Discretionary stakeholder
3. Demanding stakeholder
4. Dominant stakeholder
5. Dangerous stakeholder
6. Dependent stakeholder
7. Definitive stakeholder

Source: Tobacco Control Resource Centre (15)

Which of the stakeholders are likely to support, and which are likely to oppose, an increase in excise tax for tobacco products? The major groups to be considered include:

Group 1: Bureaucrats

- Excise Department within the Ministry of Finance
- Ministry of Health and the National Tobacco Control Office
- local governments

The Excise Department within the Ministry of Finance is usually keenly interested in revenue generation, and is likely to support tobacco tax increases. The Customs Department officers and the police may overestimate the effect of tobacco tax rise on smuggling, and may assume that these tax increases may generate more work for their staff. Unless they are brought on board through incentive schemes and advocacy, they may be against tax increases. However, if confiscation incentives are attractive, they might be persuaded to support increased excise taxes on tobacco and tobacco products. The Fiscal Policy Office and the Bureau of Budget might have a more conservative view about tax increases in general, but they would be likely to support an increase in tobacco excise tax.

The Ministry of Health and the National Tobacco Control Office are usually strongly supportive of decreasing tobacco consumption through economic and non-price measures. They are the most legitimate agencies with keen interest but no power to amend the law. They have to form an alliance with the Excise Department and other stakeholders to ensure the adoption of a tax increase on tobacco.

Local governments generally support an excise tax increase because it usually means more revenue for their particular local government unit.

Group 2: Tobacco industry

- local manufacturers
- transnational tobacco industry
- importers, who are the proxies of the transnational tobacco industry
- tobacco growers' groups and associations, and the local tobacco-growing industry

Understandably, the tobacco industry resists any and all increases of excise tax, because this results in a lower profit margin for its shareholders. The tobacco industry's own documents prove that they are willing to resort to dishonourable tactics to persuade governments to maintain the lowest possible retail price for their products. When *ad valorem* taxes (based on the declared value of the product) are used, for example, manufacturers have been known to sell their cigarettes to a related marketing company at an artificially low price, reducing their tax liability. This situation led the government of the Philippines to abandon *ad valorem* taxes in favour of specific excise taxes in 1996.

In the absence of good governance, the tobacco industry may provide direct and indirect incentives (bribes) to government officials to block, impede or delay serious action to raise tobacco excise taxes. In this situation, the role of NGOs is critical.

NGOs can bring unethical practices to the attention of the public and apply pressure on government officials and agencies to remain accountable to the population. Never underestimate the powerful and unethical lobbying strategies employed by the tobacco industry and its representatives. This alliance can be categorized as dangerous, as it has money, power and a keen interest in fighting tobacco tax increases. The proxies of the tobacco industry (e.g. tobacco leaf growers, importers, etc.) can and have played a very damaging role against tobacco price increases. Industry-supported smokers' rights groups are weaker stakeholders who also rally against tobacco tax increases.

Group 3: NGOs and the media

- community-based organizations
- civic organizations
- other special interest groups
- media

The NGO community can be characterized as a demanding stakeholder, since it has a strong interest in protecting health and the environment against tobacco; hence, NGOs usually support measures, including tax increases, to reduce tobacco use. When, in addition to interest, they are equipped with knowledge on the subject matter, they become legitimate dependent stakeholders. The crucial role of NGOs acting as society's 'watch dogs', and working together with the NTCP is well documented in many countries.

The media's role is to inform the public about the issues surrounding the debate on tobacco tax increases. At the same time, the media can influence and shape public opinion on the subject matter. It is essential that the media are thoroughly briefed on the benefits of tax increases to reduce tobacco consumption. This transforms them into legitimate stakeholders who support increasing tobacco taxes. Do not underestimate the ability of the tobacco industry to apply pressure on the media, through direct bribes or the threat of withholding advertising revenue, in order to discredit the value of tobacco tax increases.

Group 4: Academia and professional associations

- economists
- physicians' groups
- other health professionals' groups
- health associations (national cancer society, heart association, etc.)

The academic community and the professional associations mentioned above are best characterized as dependent stakeholders, since they have legitimacy and interest in the subject matter. They can play a significant role as credible experts in validating the evidence provided to the media and the general public. Government tobacco control officers should seek close collaboration with this group.

Regional cooperation

Harmonizing taxes among countries can lead to reductions in smuggling of contraband cigarettes and increases in government revenues. Regional cooperation to harmonize prices and minimize disparities in excise taxation has been successful among members of the European Union and countries in other regions such as the Gulf States *(5)*.

However, regional trade agreements can work against tax increases as an effective tobacco control measure. Several regional economic cooperation agreements, notably the Association of Southeast Asian Nations (ASEAN), the American Free Trade Area (AFTA), and the North American Free Trade Agreement (NAFTA) include provisions to lower tobacco excise taxes to zero when tobacco is traded among their member nations. The impact of these provisions on public health is potentially deleterious, and will lead to poorer health and countless lives lost in the affected countries.

FUNDING INITIATIVES FOR TOBACCO CONTROL

A central issue for all national tobacco control programmes is establishing adequate funding for programme activities and personnel. Government allocations for public health are usually meagre. Thus, depending solely on the Ministry of Health's budget to fund a national tobacco control programme is unrealistic.

However, there are other possible sources of support for tobacco control. The experience of Australia, Canada, Guam, French Polynesia, New Zealand, Thailand and the United States demonstrates that earmarked tobacco taxes, funds accruing from tobacco industry litigation, surtaxes on tobacco products, and grants and donations from international agencies and philanthropic institutions can be viable sources of financial support for tobacco control programmes. Of these, the greatest potential for sustained funding arises from the first three options. Grants and donations usually are neither adequate nor sustainable over time.

Sustained government funding for national tobacco control, through its regular budgetary allocation, requires political will. Government programme budgets are decided through a political process. In countries where tobacco control advocacy has succeeded in raising tobacco control to a national priority, this avenue can be a viable source of programme support. A sizable budget for tobacco control will likely be opposed by the tobacco industry, which usually exerts considerable influence over politicians and political parties. Counteracting this opposition is one of the main responsibilities of the national tobacco control programme and its allies.

Sin taxes – taxes levied on 'sin' products such as tobacco and alcohol – are potentially the best source of sustainable funding for a national tobacco control programme. These taxes can be earmarked directly from excise taxes into a specific fund, without going through the general government revenue. The funds are therefore not subject to the annual process of determining the government's budget, which can be influenced by political whim. Several countries have successfully used this model to fund their anti-tobacco campaigns, including Australia, Egypt, Iran and Thailand, and the states of California and Massachusetts in the United States *(5)*.

In Thailand, 2% of tobacco and alcohol excise taxes goes to a Health Promotion Fund for comprehensive health promotion activities, including tobacco control, occupational safety, and HIV/AIDS prevention. Legislation passed in 2001 *(19)* ensures sustained funding of these programmes for as long as people continue to consume (and pay taxes on) cigarettes and alcohol. The guaranteed funding, in turn, enables those health promotion programmes to implement comprehensive strategies over prolonged periods of time.

Table 5 summarizes three models of organization and funding for tobacco control in Australia (Victoria), New Zealand and Thailand *(19)*.

Table 5. Three models of organzation and funding for tobacco control

	Victorian Health Promotion Foundation (VicHealth)	**New Zealand Health Sponsorship Council (HSC)**	**Thai Health Promotion Fund**
Legal framework	Tobacco Act 1987	Smoke-Free Environment Act 1990	Health Promotion Fund Act 2001
Responsible agency	Quasi-governmental organization, with independent status	National quasi-public agency	Governmental non-profit agency having corporate status but independent from bureaucracy; own governing board, chaired by the prime minister
Objectives and missions	• Funding activities related to health promotion, safety and disease prevention • Building up positive attitude among community members toward health promoting healthy life style through community programme activities • Promoting research and development to support these programme activities	• Acting as a national service provider • Providing financial support to sports, cultural events and IEC activities, to foster norms and attitudes leading to good health	• Promoting and supporting a holistic approach to health promotion • Raising awareness about healthy behaviour and risks from consumption of tobacco, alcohol and other hazardous substances • Researching and supporting research and development of health promotion activities • Capacity-building for health promotion in the community • Supporting and promoting health campaigns
Management	One governing body: the Executive Board. The director is in charge of the fund administration	Two governing bodies: the Executive and the Advisory Boards. The director serves as secretary and reports to the Executive Board	Two governing bodies: the Executive and the Evaluation Boards. The director serves as secretary and reports to the Executive Board
Administrative cost	10% to 15%	No data available	No more than 10%
Sources of revenue	No more than 1/15 of tobacco tax and tobacco sales license	General budget support	2% of excise tax on tobacco and alcohol

Source: Siwarak *(19)*

CONCLUSION

Economic issues are central to tobacco control, giving rise to effective interventions to reduce tobacco consumption (by increasing tobacco prices through higher taxes), and providing potential sources of sustainable funding for tobacco control programmes. Understanding the critical role of economics in controlling tobacco consumption is essential for the successful management of national and local tobacco control programmes.

References

1. Jha P, Chaloupka FJ, eds. *Tobacco control in developing countries*. Oxford, Oxford University Press, 2002.

2. Sunley EM, Yurekli A, Chaloupka FJ. The design, administration, and potential revenue of tobacco excises. In: Jha P, Chaloupka FJ, eds. *Tobacco control in developing countries*. Oxford, Oxford University Press, 2002.

3. WHO Public Information Office. Tobacco facts 1. In: *Tobacco control in developing countries – Media information kit*. Geneva, World Health Organization, 2002.

4. Scott Radway. Sin taxes to help fund SARS work. *Pacific Daily News,* 6 July 2003.

5. Guindon GE, Tobin S, Yach D. Trend and affordability of cigarette prices: ample room for tax increases and related health gains. *Tobacco Control,* March 2002,11: 35–43.

6. Guindon GE, Boisclair D. *Past, current and future trends in tobacco use*. HNP Discussion Paper no. 6, Economics of Tobacco Control Paper no. 6. The World Bank, 2003.

7. *Curbing the epidemic: governments and the economics of tobacco control*. Washington, DC, The World Bank Development in Practice series, 1999 (http://www1.worldbank.org/tobacco/reports.htm).

8. *Surveying the damage: cut-rate tobacco products and public health in the 1990s*. Ottawa, Canada Cancer Society, 1999.

9. Market Tracking International. *World Tobacco File 1996*. London, DMG Business Media, 1996

10. Thursby JG, Thursby MC. Interstate cigarette bootlegging: extent, revenue losses, and effects of federal intervention. *National Tax Journal*, 2000, 53(1):59–78.

11. Joossens l. Tobacco smuggling: an optimal policy approach. In: Abedian I et. al, eds. *The economics of tobacco control*. Cape Town, Applied Fiscal Research Centre, 1998.

12. Jha P, Chaloupka FJ, eds. *Tobacco control in developing countries – media information kit*. Geneva, World Health Organization, 2000.

13. Townsend J. The role of taxation policy in tobacco control. In: Abedian I et al., eds. *The economics of tobacco control: towards an optimal policy mix*. West Cape, Edson-Clyde Press, 1998.

14. Sunley EM, Yurekli A, Chaloupka FJ. The design, administration and potential revenue of tobacco excises. In: Jha P, Chaloupka FJ, eds. *Tobacco control in developing countries*. Washington, DC, The World Bank, 2000: Chapter 17.

15. Tobacco Control Resource Centre (http//tcrc-profiles.globalink.org).

16. Yurekli A, de Beyer J, eds. *Design and administer tobacco taxes – Tool 4: design and administration*. Washington, DC, The World Bank, 2002 (Economics of Tobacco Toolkit).

17. Lightwood J et al. Estimating the costs of tobacco use. In: Jha P, Chaloupka FJ, eds. *Tobacco control in developing countries*. Oxford, Oxford University Press, 2002.

18. Chevalier J. *Stakeholder analysis and natural resource management*. Carleton University, Ottawa, June 2001 (http://www.carleton.ca/~jchevali/STAKEH2.html).

19. Siwarak P. *The birth of the Thai Health Promotion Fund: a case study*. Bangkok, Desire Publishing, 2001.

20. Chantornvong S, McCargo D. Political economy of tobacco control in Thailand. *Tobacco Control*, 2001, 10:48–54.

13

Countering the tobacco industry

Pick battles big enough to matter,
small enough to win.
—*Jonathan Kozol*

INTRODUCTION

Tobacco is unique among the risks to health in that it has an entire industry devoted to the promotion of its use, despite the known adverse health impact of tobacco consumption. Predictably, the tobacco industry aggressively blocks any attempt to effectively reduce tobacco use. Chapter 2 describes some of the global strategies employed by the industry to impede effective tobacco control interventions.

This chapter focuses on strategies to counter the tobacco industry. Building capacity to face the greatest opponent of successful tobacco control must be a priority for national and local tobacco control officers. In many cases, tobacco control advocates and NGOs are more experienced in this area, and much can be learned from them.

THE FIRST STEP TOWARDS COUNTERING THE INDUSTRY – KNOW IT WELL

The tobacco industry documents – a rich source of information

Chapter 2 provides background information on the tobacco industry documents. Because valuable insights can be gained from the tobacco industry documents, tobacco control programme officers should ensure that the analysis of the country scenario includes an initial assessment and regular analysis of industry documents with local relevance (Annex 1).

As rich as the information provided by these documents is, the documents have limitations. There are missing pages, often it is difficult to place the information within the proper context and there are incomplete sets in correspondence exchange, to name a few of the problems. In addition, not many of the BAT documents at the Guildford depository are available online, and access to the paper archives is often difficult, which adds complexity to the search strategies *(1–3)*. Nevertheless, the availability of these documents for public and academic analysis has been interpreted by many as the most significant outcome of the litigation against the tobacco companies.

OTHER APPROACHES TO COUNTERING THE TOBACCO INDUSTRY

After searching tobacco industry documents for specific references to your country, and becoming familiar with the local tobacco industry, proceed with the following steps to monitor and counter the industry:
- keep an eye on the local tobacco industry;
- inform and involve the public;

- obtain and use evidence strategically;
- use champions to speak the truth about tobacco;
- apply lessons learned from international experience;
- expose the myths: refute the industry's arguments;
- build strong anti-smoking coalitions;
- communicate and strictly enforce tobacco control measures;
- make the industry accountable;
- regulate the industry.

Keep an eye on the local tobacco industry

In addition to learning about industry practices, monitoring the local tobacco industry's daily activities can alert tobacco control programme officers about possible interference with national tobacco control efforts. WHA Resolution 54.18 "calls on WHO to continue to inform Member States on activities of the tobacco industry that have negative impact on tobacco control efforts". Reports produced pursuant to this resolution provide countries with information on their tobacco companies' activities based on the analysis of the international media (4). The industry's own web sites are often good sources of press releases and other industry-related news.

At the national level, monitoring the tobacco industry might involve activities such as:
- noting media coverage of industry-related issues regularly;
- reviewing industry publications as well as marketing and economics publications that may report on tobacco issues, and taking note of authors (and their institutional affiliations) of pro-industry reports and publications;
- accessing local company web sites frequently;
- searching for and identifying organizations and activities sponsored by the industry;
- undertaking political mapping, which includes reviewing speeches and declarations of legislators and performing interviews with key ministry officials to identify those who promote industry views, and those who support tobacco control measures;
- reviewing reports on the enforcement of tobacco-related laws and of court cases that resulted from their infringement.

Sources of information include the Internet, national and local media, and documents stored in public libraries (e.g. minutes of parliamentary meetings, legal documents of groups likely supported by the industry, collections of industry publications and industry commissioned research papers). Agencies responsible for enforcing rules related to tobacco and smoking might provide information on the industry's compliance with these rules. In many cases, tapping personal networks can be invaluable.

Inform and involve the public

Results of efforts to monitor the industry can be used to raise the awareness of the public about the industry's attempts to deter and derail tobacco control. Choose the appropriate means of publicizing information on the industry based on the nature of the information and the target audience whose attention must be secured. Some possibilities include press conferences, press releases, presentations at scientific meetings, publications, scientific articles and letters to editors of influential newspapers, letters to key actors in the political arena such as members of legislative bodies, testimonies in legislative forums and public hearings. If necessary, obtain legal counsel before releasing sensitive or controversial information.

Involve the public in monitoring the tobacco industry. Well-informed citizens can demand that the tobacco industry be held accountable for actions that undermine public health. This can be done through public hearings, public inquiries and the strategic use of channels of communication through which the public may inform NTCP of tobacco industry efforts to disrupt or sabotage tobacco control interventions. In Brazil, for example, the Minister of Health initiated the use of telephone 'hotlines' that enable members of the public to report to NTCP on suspicious activity by the industry. The Minnesota Smoke-free Coalition maintains a web site that encourages individuals to inform local policy-makers of the tactics the industry uses to oppose proposals for tobacco control ordinances during public hearings. Other possible channels include the use of e-mail, text messaging or designated mailboxes, which the public can use to reach the NTCP.

Presenting the public and key decision-makers with the facts about the tobacco industry, when done effectively, can reinforce tobacco control efforts greatly. As the United States Advocacy Institute puts it: "tobacco control advocacy flourishes best in an environment of fresh public outrage at the tobacco industry's wrongful behavior".

Obtain and use evidence strategically

Tobacco industry documents can reveal evidence of industry interference in tobacco control in the past. This information needs to be strategically coupled with up-to-date local data on the magnitude, patterns, determinants and impact of tobacco consumption and exposure to tobacco smoke, to enable policy change. The legislative agenda influences the pattern of data sets needed. For example, to regulate tobacco marketing a variety of information and evidence is needed. Such data could include:

- information on industry advertising and promotional expenditures;
- evidence of the significant impact of advertising on motivating young people to smoke;
- information on how valuable the industry regards advertising;
- past industry efforts to block advertising bans, including attempts to get governments to agree to the use of deceptive voluntary marketing codes.

To achieve smoke-free public places, current data on the impact and magnitude of second-hand smoke exposure on the population is vital. Also essential is information on how the industry covered up the adverse health effects of second-hand smoke and how it uses the hospitality industry to promote a culture of accommodation through its 'Courtesy of choice' programme. Proper surveillance for data gathering and a thorough search of the industry documents as part of national tobacco control strategies are crucial to obtaining these types of information. In addition, data on public knowledge, attitudes and beliefs on planned measures (e.g. does the population support a ban on tobacco advertising?) can be helpful in persuading decision-makers to support effective interventions to curb tobacco use.

Use champions to speak the truth about tobacco

Champions are individuals who have high visibility and/or high credibility in society. Their presence is usually enough to attract the media's attention. They wield immense influence over the general population. When they speak the truth about tobacco, people pay attention. In Kiribati, the Ministry of Health tapped the country's young athletic stars to promote a tobacco-free lifestyle, with good results. In the Republic of South Korea, a popular comic actor who was struck with a tobacco-related malignancy, became a vocal critic of smoking during the final days of his life. His advocacy is credited with having helped lower the smoking prevalence among Korean adults in recent years.

Apply lessons learned from international experience

The experience of nations with more advanced tobacco-control policies provides valuable insight for countries struggling to establish sound tobacco control policies and interventions. Likewise, international tobacco control organizations can advise and assist local advocates in developing and implementing tobacco control strategies. Lessons learned from the international community can be adapted to address local needs, guiding the development of policy measures. Health departments and tobacco control organizations should seek out information on which tobacco control measures have already worked elsewhere, particularly in countries with similar political, economic and sociocultural attributes to their own, learning from successes and failures in other countries, and applying these insights to their efforts.

Expose the myths: refute the industry's arguments

Tobacco companies often disseminate economic and scientific arguments, to oppose attempts to legislate tobacco. These arguments are frequently concocted by industry-sponsored economists, scientists and media consultants and unsubstantiated by evidence. Health departments and tobacco control groups should have responses to

Box 1. Common myths in tobacco control

Myth 1: Tobacco is only an issue for affluent people and affluent countries.
Reality: Smoking is declining among males in most high-income countries. In contrast, it is increasing in males in most low- and middle-income countries and in women worldwide. Within individual countries, tobacco consumption and tobacco-related disease burdens are usually greatest among the poor.

Myth 2: Governments should not discourage smoking other than making its risks widely known. Otherwise, they would interfere with consumers' freedom of choice.
Reality: First, many smokers are unaware of their risks, or they simply underestimate or minimize the personal relevance of those risks, even in high-income societies where the risks are relatively widely known. Second, most smokers start when they are children or adolescents – when they have incomplete information about the risks of tobacco and its addictive nature – and by the time they try to quit, many are addicted. Third, smoking imposes costs on non-smokers. For these reasons, the choice to smoke may differ from the choice to buy other consumer goods and governments may consider interventions justified.

Myth 3: Smokers always bear the costs of their consumption choices.
Reality: Not necessarily so. They do impose certain costs on non-smokers. The evident costs include health damage, nuisance and irritation from exposure to environmental tobacco smoke. In addition, smokers may impose financial costs on others (such as bearing a portion of smokers' excess health care costs) . However, the scope of these costs is difficult to measure and they vary in place and time, so this report makes no attempt to quantify them. In high-income countries, smokers' health care costs on average exceed non-smokers' in any given year. It has been argued that, because smokers tend to die earlier than non-smokers, their lifetime health care costs may be no greater than those of non-smokers; however, recent reviews in high-income nations conclude that smokers' lifetime health care costs do indeed exceed non-smokers', despite their shorter lives. If health care is paid for to some extent by the public sector, smokers will thus impose their costs on others.

Myth 4: Tobacco control will result in permanent job losses for an economy.
Reality: Successful control policies will lead to only a slow decline in global tobacco use (which is projected to stay high for the next several decades). The resulting need for downsizing will be far less dramatic than many other industries have had to face. Furthermore, money not spent on tobacco will be spent on other goods, generating alternative employment. Studies for this report *(5)* show that most countries would see no net job losses and that a few would see net gains if consumption fell.

Myth 5: Tobacco addiction is so strong that simply raising taxes will not reduce demand; therefore, raising taxes is not justified.
Reality: Scores of studies have shown that increased taxes reduce the number of smokers and the number of smoking-related deaths. Price increases induce some smokers to quit and prevent others from becoming regular or persistent smokers. They also reduce the number of ex-smokers returning to cigarettes and reduce consumption among continuing smokers. Children and adolescents are more responsive to changes in the price of consumer goods than adults – that is, if the price goes up, they are more likely to reduce their consumption. This intervention would therefore have a major impact on them. Similarly, people on low incomes are more price-responsive than those on high incomes, so there is likely to be a bigger impact in developing countries where tobacco consumption is still increasing. Models developed for this report show that tax increases that would raise the real price of cigarettes by 10% worldwide would cause 40 million smokers alive in 1995 to quit and prevent a minimum of 10 million tobacco-related deaths.

Myth 6: Governments will lose revenues if they increase cigarette taxes, because people will buy fewer cigarettes.
Reality: Wrong. The evidence is clear: calculations show that even very substantial cigarette tax increases will still reduce consumption and increase tax revenues. This is in part because the proportionate reduction in demand does not match the proportionate size of the tax increase, since addicted consumers respond relatively slowly to price rises. Furthermore, some of the money saved by quitters will be spent on other goods that are also taxed. Historically, raising tobacco taxes, no matter how large the increase, has never once led to a decrease in cigarette tax revenues.

Myth 7: Smuggling and illicit production will undermine the effects of raised tobacco taxes.
Reality: Smuggling is a serious concern. But even in the face of smuggling, the evidence from a number

of countries shows that tax increases still increase revenues and reduce cigarette consumption. Furthermore, governments can adopt effective policies to control smuggling. Such policies include prominent tax stamps and local-language warnings on cigarette packs, as well as the aggressive enforcement and consistent application of tough penalties to deter smugglers.

Myth 8: Governments should not raise cigarette taxes because such increases will have a disproportionate impact on poor consumers.

Reality: Existing tobacco taxes do consume a higher share of the poor consumers' income than of rich consumers'. However, policy-makers' main concern should be over the distributional impact of the entire tax and expenditure system, and less on particular taxes in isolation. Poor consumers are usually more responsive to price increases than rich consumers, so it is likely that their consumption of cigarettes will fall more sharply, and their relative financial burden may be correspondingly reduced.

Myth 9: In response to higher cigarette taxes, smokers will switch to cheaper brands or cheaper tobacco products and thus there will be no reduction in overall tobacco consumption.

Reality: This behaviour, which is also known as 'substitution', establishes a legitimate concern. However, not all smokers will engage in this behaviour. Price increases will discourage non-smokers from taking up smoking and induce many smokers to quit or reduce consumption. Consequently, there will be reductions in overall consumption and prevalence. Only a certain portion of smokers will not be affected and some of them manage to maintain their levels of tobacco consumption through substitution. Non-price measures, NRT and other cessation interventions can help curb tobacco use among this group.

Myth 10: Tax rates for cigarettes are already too high in most countries.

Reality: The question of what the 'right' level of tax should be is a complex one. The size of the tax depends in subtle ways on empirical facts that may not yet be available, such as the scale of the costs to non-smokers, income levels, and also on varying societal values, such as the extent to which children should be protected. It also depends on what a society hopes to achieve through the tax, such as a specific gain in revenue or a specific reduction in disease burden. For the time being, a useful yardstick may be the tax levels adopted as part of the comprehensive tobacco control policies of a number of countries where cigarette consumption has fallen. In such countries, the tax component of the price of a pack of cigarettes is between two

thirds and four fifths of the retail cost. Currently, in high-income countries, taxes average about two thirds or more of the retail price of a pack of cigarettes. In lower-income countries, taxes amount to not more than half the retail price of a pack of cigarettes, which are still very much below the level in high-income countries.

Myth 11: Measures to reduce tobacco supply are effective ways to reduce consumption.

Reality: While interventions to reduce demand for tobacco are likely to succeed, measures to reduce its supply are less promising. This is because if one supplier is shut down, an alternative supplier gains an incentive to enter the market. The extreme measure of prohibiting tobacco is unwarranted on economic grounds, unrealistic and likely to fail. Although crop substitution is often proposed as a means to reduce the tobacco supply, there is scarcely any evidence that it reduces consumption, since the incentives to farmers to grow tobacco are currently much greater than for most other crops. However, it may be a useful strategy where needed to aid the poorest tobacco farmers in transition to other livelihoods, as part of a broader diversification programme. Similarly, the evidence so far suggests that trade restrictions, such as import bans, will have little impact on cigarette consumption worldwide. Instead, countries are more likely to succeed in curbing tobacco consumption by adopting measures that effectively reduce demand, and applying those measures symmetrically to imported and domestically produced cigarettes. However, there is one supply-side measure that is key to an effective strategy for tobacco control: action against smuggling. Control of smuggling will improve governments' revenue yields from tobacco tax increases.

Myth 12: Tobacco controls will simply compound the poverty of rural economies that are heavily dependent on tobacco farming.

Reality: The market for tobacco is likely to remain substantial for at least the next several decades and, while any future gradual decline in consumption will clearly cut the number of tobacco-farming jobs, those jobs will be lost over a decade or more, not overnight. Adopting sound agricultural and trade policies can help farmers in poor countries compete fairly for the world market. Governments are justified to prudently help the poorest of tobacco farmers with the adjustment costs of a gradual decrease in demand for their product. Many governments have helped with such adjustment costs for other industries.

Source: (5)

these arguments ready to refute the industry. The responses should be factual, and based on the best available scientific evidence. References need to be documented carefully, and data selected from the most credible sources. Common myths in tobacco control with appropriate responses to refute them are summarized in Box 1.

Ensure that the key target audiences get the facts straight by disseminating information widely. When refuting the industry's arguments, remain in control of what issues are discussed, and where, when, how and with whom these are broadcast to the public. Be aware that the industry and its representatives may try to catch tobacco control spokespersons unawares, especially on live radio and television programmes. Consider all invitations to publicly discuss tobacco control issues head to head with industry representatives very carefully, and avoid all circumstances where you are unable to control the agenda and flow of discussions.

Perhaps one of the biggest myths the industry has perpetuated about itself is that it has reformed and now seeks to be socially responsible. This is best illustrated by BAT's CSR programme discussed in Chapter 2. As a public relations strategy to polish the tobacco industry's tarnished image, BAT has launched a new series of social dialogues in 24 countries around the world. To date, however, the only outcome of these dialogues is a report, widely publicized in the media and on the net, which BAT uses to portray itself as a reformed and socially responsible corporation. Yet, the promotion of its lethal products continues.

Box 2. Coordinated action for preventing a university–industry partnership in Turkey

Philip Morris documents show that in 1992, during discussions on the second tobacco bill in the Turkish Parliament, Philip Morris's Turkish headquarters planned to defeat the bill they called the "ad ban proposal". Their plan included measures to enhance the company's image as a socially responsible company to mask their intentions on the ad ban. The major strategy was to offer the Ministry of Education a youth smoking prevention programme. While Philip Morris did not succeed in preventing the passage of the anti-tobacco law by Parliament in 1996, it still continued to launch its 'youth smoking prevention' initiative to improve its image. It found its partner in the Faculty of Education of Bosphorus University, one of the oldest universities of Istanbul. In 2000, the University announced it was starting a project in schools with the slogan 'The power is yours'. Newspapers reported that Philip Morris provided funding – US$ 100 000 – for project-related costs. The project's focus was allegedly to teach students how to make lifestyle decisions. Tobacco use was never discussed. The National Committee on Tobacco and Health wrote to the University, to warn them about the hidden agenda behind the donation. The university leaders lacked information about the tobacco industry's real intentions. The Committee worked with the media, denouncing the use of tobacco money, which would allow Turkish teenagers to be continuously exposed to an industry promoting a deadly product. The internal documents of Philip Morris indicating the company's plans to influence the legislature in 1992 were made public. Additional pressure from the international tobacco control community and from the university students themselves eventually led the Ministry of Education to intervene to stop the initiative *(6)*.

Build strong anti-smoking coalitions

The involvement of the widest possible range of stakeholders in developing and implementing tobacco control interventions is necessary to generate public support for comprehensive tobacco control programmes. Collaboration between the public and private sectors is critical. In addition, individuals and groups who are required for the implementation of future tobacco control measures need to be involved in the policy development process from the outset.

Box 3. Advice from the experts: examples of activities that government and NGOs should avoid

- Do NOT partner with the tobacco companies on activities that are not tobacco-related. The true, but hidden, aim of these activities is to "buy" good will for the tobacco companies and to portray the companies as responsible corporate citizens. For example, governmental agencies and NGOs should not partner with tobacco companies on:
  - domestic violence-prevention programmes, as has been the case in the Australia, Panama and the Republic of Korea;
  - immunization programmes, as has happened in Malawi;
  - education and sports programmes focused on youth, as has been the case in Argentina and Thailand.

- Do NOT participate in industry-initiated dialogues – the industry portrays participation in these dialogue sessions as endorsement for its programmes, as has been the case in Chile, Peru, Uganda and Venezuela.

- Do NOT accept compromises in smoke-free spaces initiatives that include utilization of ventilation technology and/or separate smoking and non-smoking areas as an alternative to smoke-free areas. These compromises are ineffective health measures.

- Do NOT endorse the tobacco companies "accommodation" and "courtesy of choice" programmes, which are NOT health protection measures.

- Do NOT endorse, participate or partner with the tobacco companies' youth smoking prevention programmes. These programmes have proven to be ineffective and often exclude measures of proven effectiveness, such as telling the truth about the tobacco industry's strategies. Instead, tobacco companies use these programmes to leverage governments to opt for weaker legislation that do not effectively reduce tobacco consumption.

- Do NOT focus all tobacco control activities on school-based programmes, often paid for by the tobacco companies. School-based programmes are only useful within the context of a comprehensive tobacco control programme.

- Do NOT accept compromises on tax increases because of the tobacco companies' arguments that it will lead to an increase in smuggling. Instead, tax increases should be coupled with measures to tackle smuggling.

- Do NOT compromise on a comprehensive advertising ban. Any compromise that limits legislative and regulatory measures to ban advertising and promotion to places, events, and activities attended by minors should not be accepted because they are very difficult to enforce.

Political decision-makers and the media are key to the policy-adoption process. The media can shape public debate: it also can influence decision-makers by publicly highlighting the expectations of their constituencies, and emphasizing their accountability to the public. Legislators sympathetic to tobacco control can be found in every political party: they need to be identified and given the necessary support. In several instances, tobacco control interventions can be packaged to appeal to those areas to which political decision-makers are sensitive. For example, bills to ensure smoke-free public places can be promoted as interventions to protect the safety and health of children. Well-designed coordinated media and political advocacy strategies are essential to achieve success (see Box 2 for a successful strategy used in Turkey to stop a tobacco industry led youth smoking prevention programme).

Communicate and strictly enforce tobacco control measures

The general public must be well informed of the expected positive impact of tobacco control measures taken by governments. If communication of policy measures to the public is neglected, people might mistakenly perceive certain tobacco control measures as infringing on personal freedoms. Communication campaigns are therefore crucial before the measures are actually approved and implemented. In addition, designating and preparing enforcement agencies to monitor the compliance with tobacco control measures is critical in ensuring the effectiveness of legislative measures. Coupled with serious penalties for non-compliance, effective public information campaigns can contribute significantly to high enforcement rates.

Make the industry accountable

Litigation and public inquiries generate international interest and contribute to decreasing the social acceptability of the tobacco industry. Over time, these can lead to a sociopolitical environment supportive of tobacco control policies. Countries can explore the feasibility of utilizing litigation to assist in their efforts to curb tobacco use. Anti-smoking organizations could take up the role of 'social watch dogs', monitoring the tobacco industry's compliance with tobacco control legislation. For example, in France the *Comité National Contre le Tabagisme* (CNCT) orchestrates liability actions against companies that fail to comply with the country's tobacco control laws, especially related to tobacco advertising *(2)*.

Regulate the industry

While monitoring the industry's activities, every opportunity to regulate its actions should be explored and acted upon. Specifically, regulation should seek to address the manufacture, sales and presentation of tobacco products, including:
- setting acceptable levels of tar, nicotine and other components;

- using effective strategies for packaging and labelling to communicate health messages;
- implementing measures to counter smuggling, through the use of serial numbers on all packs of cigarettes for tracking, and standard chain-of-custody protocols, among others.

Finally, certain activities, such as the examples listed in Box 3, should be avoided by those engaged in developing and implementing tobacco control programmes.

THE WHO FCTC: INTERNATIONAL HELP FOR NATIONS TO COUNTER THE TOBACCO INDUSTRY

The WHO FCTC *(7)* recommends specific interventions to offset the tobacco industry's efforts to derail the development of national tobacco control programmes.
- The preamble states that countries "need to be informed of activities of the tobacco industry that have a negative impact on tobacco control efforts".
- Article 2 states that the public should have access to a wide range of information on the tobacco industry relevant to achieving the objectives of this treaty.
- Article 10 states that companies should disclose information on all toxic constituents of tobacco products and their emissions, information hidden by companies for years.
- Article 12 requests agencies involved in tobacco control not to have any liaison with tobacco companies.
- Article 13 recommends tobacco companies should not be left to advertise or promote their products in any way, or to sponsor any socially accepted activities.
- Article 19 directs Parties to consider taking legislative action or promote existing laws to deal with civil or criminal liability, including compensation. (Note: This is a novel feature of the WHO FCTC, because it represents the first time ever of the inclusion of liability issues in an international treaty.)
- Article 20 states that research and information exchange among Parties should also focus on industry practices, including establishing a global system for collecting and disseminating information on various aspects of tobacco production and control and the activities of the tobacco industry that might have an impact on national tobacco control efforts.

SUMMARY

The tobacco industry continues to thrive. Effective measures to reduce tobacco consumption are available and have been proven to work. Developing national capacities to monitor the tobacco industry and neutralize its efforts to impede or delay tobacco control interventions is necessary. The evidence already accumulated on the tobacco companies' methods of interfering with tobacco control efforts, as well as international experience in propagating the tobacco control movement, can provide technical support for this work.

References

1. Enstrom JE, Kabat GC. Environmental tobacco smoke and tobacco-related mortality in a prospective study of Californians, 1960–98. *British Medical Journal*. 17 May 2003, 326:1057 (http://bmj.com/cgi/reprint/326/7398/1057.pdf, accessed 27 May 2003).

2. http://www.cnct.org/, accessed 29 May 2003.

3. Resolution WHA 56.1. WHO Framework Convention on Tobacco Control. In: *Fifty-sixth World Health Assembly, Geneva, 19–28 May 2003. Volume 1. Resolutions and decisions, and list of participants*. Geneva, World Health Organization, 2003 (WHA56/1986/REC/1).

4. *Tobacco industry monitoring report*. October 2002–December 2002. Geneva, World Health Organization, 2002 (http://tobacco.who.int/repository/stp91/tob-ind-monitoring02.pdf, accessed 22 May 2003).

5. *Curbing the epidemic: governments and the economics of tobacco control*. Washington, DC, The World Bank Development in Practice series, 1999 (http://www1.worldbank.org/tobacco/faq.asp#7.

6. Dagli E, Lawrence S. Tobacco companies and youth projects. *Filter Online*, June 2001, 1(2). (http://filter.tobinfo.org/archives/200102/).

7. Resolution WHA 56.1. WHO Framework Convention on Tobacco Control. In: *Fifty-sixth World Health Assembly, Geneva, 21 May 2003* (http://www.who.int/tobacco/en/, accessed 27 May 2003).

Bibliography

Tobacco companies and their expansion

Van Liemt, G. *The World Tobacco Industry: Trends and Prospects*. Geneva, International Labour Office, 2002 (http://www.ilo.org/public/english/dialogue/sector/papers/tobacco/wp179.pdf).

Guindon GE, Boisclair D. Past, *Current and Future Trends in Tobacco Use*. HNP Discussion Paper. Geneva, Tobacco Free Initiative, World Health Organization. February 2003 (http://www1.worldbank.org/tobacco/pdf/Guindon.pdf).

Internal tobacco industry documents and tobacco industry practices

Tobacco Industry Conduct. Selection of resources on the topic on the site of the Tobacco Free Initiative at http://www.who.int/tobacco/en (case studies on the interference of the tobacco industry with legislative efforts in various countries).

Compilation of materials on *"dirty tricks and real truth about what goes on inside the tobacco industry"* on the site of Action on Smoking and Health UK. URL: http://www.ash.org.uk/.

Tobacco Explained. The truth about the tobacco industry... in its own words. Adapted for the World No Tobacco Day 31 May 2000. Tobacco Free Initiative. World Health Organization 2000. Available online at http://www.who.int/tobacco/en/ (excerpts and quotes from internal industry documents).

Tobacco Industry Activities to Market Cigarettes and Undermine Public Health in Latin America and the Caribbean. In: Pan American Health Organization. *Profits over people.* Washington, DC, PAHO, November 2002 (http://www.paho.org/English/HPP/HPM/TOH/profits_over_people.pdf) (with summary sheets at http://www.paho.org/English/HPP/HPM/TOH/profits_over_people-ss.pdf).

Smoke and Mirrors. How the Tobacco Industry Buys & Lies Its Way to Power & Profits. The Advocacy Institute, Washington, DC. August 1998. (Excellent overview of strategies and tactics used by tobacco companies to maintain their profits.)

Countering the tobacco industry

A movement rising. *A strategic analysis of U.S. tobacco control advocacy.* The Advocacy Institute, Washington, DC, March 1999 (http://www.advocacy.org/publications/pdf/amovementrising.pdf) (useful resource for the development of countries' anti-tobacco movements).

Pan American Health Organization. *Developing Legislation for Tobacco Control. Template and Guidelines.* Washington, DC, PAHO, May 2002 (http://www.paho.org/English/HPP/HPM/TOH/tobacco_legislation.pdf) (provides guidance for developing a legal framework to control tobacco).

Communicating the Evidence for Tobacco Control. Myths & Facts. Penang, Malaysia, Clearinghouse for Tobacco Control, National Poison Centre, 2002.

Blanke DD. *Towards health with justice. Litigation and public inquiries as tools for tobacco control.* Geneva, World Health Organization, 2002 (http://tobacco.who.int/repository/stp69/final_jordan_report.pdf) (overview of the use of litigation in particular countries).

ANNEX 1:

Accessing and searching internal tobacco industry documents

There are a number of web sites available that provide access to documents and document collections. Key online resources include:

General search tools

Stella Aguinaga Bialous & Stan Shatenstein, WHO – TFI Workshop: Internet 101: Following the tobacco trail on the web, World Conference on Tobacco or Health, Helsinki, Finland, August 2003.

News and information

Google News: http://news.google.com/
Yahoo! News: http://news.yahoo.com/
Moreover [Client Log In]: http://w.moreover.com/
World News: http://www.worldnews.com
[Advanced search: http://www.worldnews.com/s/worldnews/adv_search.html]
Tobacco Factfile [BMA]: http://www.tobaccofactfile.org/
Tobacco.org: http://www.tobacco.org/articles/edition/9999/
Globalink: http://www.globalink.org/

Medical journals

Medline [Abstracts]: http://www.ncbi.nlm.nih.gov/PubMed/
Bioscience [Journals links]: http://bioscience.org/urllists/jourlink.htm

Tobacco company sites

Philip Morris International: [PMI] http://www.philipmorrisinternational.com/
British American Tobacco: [BAT] http://www.bat.com
Japan Tobacco International: [JTI] http://www.jti.com/english/

Selected national & international companies (several have a news page as well):

Altadis: [France-Spain] http://www.altadis.com/home_en.php3
Austria Tabak: [German-language. See Gallaher] http://www.austriatabak.at/new/
Brown & Williamson: [US. See BAT] http://www.bw.com/home.html
ETI: [Ente Tabacchi Italiani] http://www.etispa.it/index.asp?linid=1
Gallaher: [UK] http://www.gallaher-group.com/
Hongta: [People's Republic of China] http://www.hongta.com/ehtml/hongta.html
ITC: [India] http://www.itccorporate.com/sets/cigarette_frameset.htm
Imperial Tobacco: [IT, UK] http://www.imperial-tobacco.com/
Imperial Tobacco Canada: [See BAT] http://www.imperialtobaccocanada.com/
KG&T: [Korea Ginseng & Tobacco] http://www.ktg.or.kr/
Reemtsma: [Germany. See IT] http://www.reemtsma.com/uebergang/index.php?lang=en
RJ Reynolds: [US] http://www.rjrt.com/home.asp

Souza Cruz: [Brazil. See BAT] http://www.souzacruz.com.br/
Swedish Match: http://www.swedishmatch.com/eng/
Links to several companies: http://www.geocities.com/Paris/Villa/2913/companie.htm

Tobacco industry trade journals
These contain useful information on current industry issues and news, including some free features. Other current material requires subscriptions, but they can be accessed freely once archived.

Tobacco Journal International: http://www.tobaccojournal.com/
Tobacco Reporter: http://www.tobaccoreporter.com/
Tobacco Asia: http://www.tobaccoasia.com/

Tobacco industry documents available online

Industry-maintained sites
Brown & Williamson: [B&W] http://www.bwdocs.com/
Lorillard: http://www.lorillarddocs.com/
Philip Morris: [PM] http://www.pmdocs.com
RJ Reynolds: [RJR] http://www.rjrtdocs.com/rjrtdocs/index.wmt?tab=home
Council for Tobacco Research: [CTR] http://www.ctr-usa.org/ctr/index.wmt?tab=home
Tobacco Institute: http://www.tobaccoinstitute.com/
Tobacco Archives: [Access to all 6 sites above] http://www.tobaccoarchives.com/
Gallaher: http://www.gallaher-docs.com/subindex.htm

Industry document sites maintained by governments, universities and private parties
On many of these, you can access all industry sites through a single search. The search is convenient in many ways, but not always the most current, e.g. Philip Morris's newest documents.

CDC: Industry Documents: http://www.cdc.gov/tobacco/industrydocs/index.htm
Legacy Tobacco Documents Library: http://legacy.library.ucsf.edu/
Tobacco.org: http://www.tobacco.org/Documents/documents.html
TDO [Tobacco Documents Online]: http://tobaccodocuments.org/
TDO: Anne Landman collection: http://tobaccodocuments.org/landman/
Tobacco Industry Document Gateway (U. Sydney):
http://tobacco.health.usyd.edu.au/site/gateway/docs/other.htm
United States House Committee on Commerce Tobacco Documents [Bliley Set, also available on TDO]: http://www.house.gov/commerce/TobaccoDocs/documents.html

Guildford documents (as available on the Internet – limited collections and some overlap)
British Columbia: http://www.healthplanning.gov.bc.ca/guildford/index.html

CDC: http://outside.cdc.gov:8080/BASIS/ncctld/web/guildford/sf
Health Canada: http://www.ncth.ca/Guildford.nsf
NCTH [National Clearinghouse, Canada]: http://www.ncth.ca/Guildford.nsf
TDO [Tobacco Documents Online]: http://tobaccodocuments.org/
UCSF: http://www.library.ucsf.edu/tobacco/batco/

Research and tobacco industry monitoring reports based on industry documents

Americans for Nonsmokers' Rights Tobacco Industry Tracking Database: http://www.no-smoke.org/tidbase.html
Globalink: http://www.globalink.org/tobacco/docs/
ICIJ [International Consortium of Investigative Journalists]: www.icij.org/dtaweb/report.asp?ReportID=62&L1=10&L2=70&L3=10&L4=0&L5=0
London School of Hygiene and Tropical Medicine: http://www.lshtm.ac.uk/cgch/tobacco/
[Search handbook by the LSH&TM: http://www.lshtm.ac.uk/cgch/tobacco/industry_docs.htm]
Non-Smokers' Rights Association [NSRA, Canada] http://www.nsra-adnf.ca/
The cigarette papers: [1996, full text online] http://ark.cdlib.org/ark:/13030/ft8489p25j/
Tobacco Control Supersite: (University of Sidney) http://dev.health.usyd.edu.au/tobacco/
Tobacco Scam [Smokefree public places and restaurants]: www.tobaccoscam.ucsf.edu
Tobacco Control [Journal]: http://tc.bmjjournals.com/
University of California San Francisco: http://www.library.ucsf.edu/tobacco/
World Health Organization: [WHO & regional offices] http://www.who.int/tobacco/en/

GLOBALink – The International Tobacco Control Network – maintains a discussion list of those interested in tobacco industry document searches. In addition, it developed an automatic searching and archiving tool, which assists searching and downloading of documents. For more information contact help@globalink.org

The Tobacco Industry Documents: an Introductory Handbook and Resource Guide for Researchers
Ross MacKenzie, Jeff Collin and Kelley Lee
http://www.lshtm.ac.uk/cgch/tobacco/industry_docs.htm
This handbook is designed as an introduction for those interested in searching the online industry document collections. Among the topics covered are a brief history of the industry documents, how to search the online collections (with examples) and an extensive listing of online resources, including document-based publications, online information sources and articles and reports on various aspects of tobacco control.

Further reading on how to search the tobacco industry documents database
Searching tobacco industry documents: information and hints. In: Hammond R, Rowell A. *Trust us: we're the tobacco industry.* Campaign for Tobacco-Free Kids (USA), Action on Smoking and Health (UK), May 2001 (http://www.ash.org.uk/html/conduct/html/trustus.html#_Toc514752798).

Searching tobacco industry documents: basic information, steps and hints. In: *Tobacco Fact Sheets*. 11th World Conference on Tobacco or Health (http://tobaccofreekids. org/campaign/global/docs/searching.pdf).

The tobacco industry documents. *What they are, what they tell us and how to search them. A practical manual.* World Health Organization, Regional Office for the Eastern Mediterranean. Cairo, 2002.

Glantz, Stanton A et al., eds. *The cigarette papers.* Berkeley University of California Press, 1996 (http://ark.cdlib.org/ark:/13030/ft8489p25j/).

Balbach, ED, Gasior R and Barbeau E. Tobacco Industry Documents: Comparing Depository and Internet Searching. *Tobacco Control*, 2002, 11: 68–72.

14
Forming effective partnerships

You cannot clap with one hand.
—*Chinese proverb*

Politicians make laws, and they decide which ones to introduce and when. Citizen and business groupings can have an important influence on the law-making process. They can accelerate or delay the development of laws, broaden or narrow their scope, and assist or hinder their effective implementation.

In every country with successful tobacco control legislation, NGOs have played a major role in campaigning for change. The WHO FCTC recognizes that the "participation of civil society is essential in achieving the objectives of the Convention" and encourages the participation of NGOs in national and international tobacco control efforts.

This chapter focuses on how associations can contribute to tobacco control efforts in the legislative field. In particular it:

- highlights the role and responsibilities of civil society;
- focuses on how to build and strengthen national tobacco control movements;
- provides guidelines for working with the private sector.

ROLE OF NGOS

Governments cannot be neutral in tobacco control. When a government has no, or poor, policies in this field it allows the tobacco industry to operate unhindered, and this leads to increased tobacco sales and health hazards. When a government adopts comprehensive tobacco control policies, it prioritizes health, and tobacco use falls. By agreeing on the text of the WHO FCTC, WHO Member States have shown willingness to supplant policies which sustain tobacco use with policies which promote health.

Local and global NGOs have a crucial role in encouraging and assisting governments to create a policy environment that supports tobacco control. NGOs can support governments to adopt, ratify and enact laws to implement the WHO FCTC. "Educate, mobilize and challenge" should be the watchwords of the NGO tobacco control movement. Creating awareness of the WHO FCTC, mobilizing allies and supporters, and challenging the propaganda of pro-tobacco groupings are the main responsibilities of these NGOs. They should:

- **Create a national climate of opinion that favours action to control tobacco use** – This requires widespread societal understanding of the relative importance of tobacco as a major health, social and economic problem and of the need to take political action. It means working with the media, organizing promotional events, encouraging community initiatives, and producing and distributing information on the WHO FCTC.
- **Support the government to do what is needed in tobacco control** – This requires submitting reports, recommendations and proposals on tobacco control issues to government and parliament. The best way to obtain political support is to provide politicians and society with convincing answers to the question – what interventions work and at what social and economic cost? If clear health benefits can be

achieved at a reasonable cost, most politicians will support health legislation. Influencing politicians also means showing them that tobacco control is well accepted in the community. National surveys regularly find that in most countries a substantial majority of both smokers and non-smokers support tobacco control measures *(1)*.

- **Identify national legislative priorities for tobacco control and help develop a workable legislative package by presenting the different options for political consideration** – Give an informed opinion on existing legislation and propose cost-effective new laws and policy initiatives that are relevant to your country and its customs *(2, 3)*.

- **Make the case that tobacco control measures are a reasonable and effective response to the epidemic** – Set the public agenda so that the focus remains on health and keeping young people free of addiction. Do not allow the tobacco industry to side-track the debate into issues of "personal choice" or "freedom of speech". In all democracies it is accepted that restrictions to protect public welfare are legitimate. The utilitarian philosopher, JS Mill, noted, "The rights of the individual must be thus far restricted, he must not make a nuisance of himself to other people" *(4)*.

- **Increase awareness that the tobacco industry has acted and continues to act irresponsibly** – The cigarette manufacturers try to portray themselves as responsible companies in a controversial industry. The reality remains that the tobacco industry is a "rogue industry" that peddles addiction for profit. The industry's claim to be a legitimate stakeholder in drafting legislation should be challenged. As one Kenyan advocate stated, "Asking the tobacco industry for input on tobacco legislation is like asking a thief where to build the police station" *(5)*.

- **Provide a powerful and respectable public image for the tobacco control campaign** – Health professionals usually enjoy a special position of trust in the community. They bring with them intrinsic assumptions about healing, caring and serving the public interest rather than being motivated by commercial gain. Acting individually and through their professional associations they can provide a strong public image for the campaign.

At a glance: six tasks of NGOs

- create a national climate of opinion that favours action to control tobacco use;
- support the government to do what is needed in tobacco control;
- identify national legislative priorities for tobacco control and help develop a workable legislative package by presenting the different options for political consideration;
- make the case that tobacco control measures are a reasonable and effective response to the epidemic;
- increase awareness that the tobacco industry has acted and continues to act irresponsibly;
- provide a powerful and respectable public image for the tobacco control campaign.

WHAT NGOs CAN DO

The following groups are the main targets of NGO advocacy for tobacco control, because their decisions and actions ultimately determine the long-term viability of the marketplace for tobacco:

- political decision-makers;
- the public (smokers and non-smokers), the business sector, trade unions, and many others potentially sympathetic to tobacco control;
- the mass media.

For effective tobacco control, NGOs should:

- regularly brief key legislators on important tobacco control issues;
- persuade politicians to place their support for tobacco control laws on record;
- provide health ministers and other key politicians with evidence for various legislative options;
- meet with and brief officials from all relevant ministries;
- be aware of the political dynamics within the government.

Political decision-makers

Briefings for key legislators should be developed. These briefings provide opportunities to inform them of the real issues surrounding tobacco use, and enable them to meet the leaders of the tobacco control movement (6). Effective briefings should primarily focus on the benefits of regulating tobacco but must also dispel the myths that cloud the issue. Clear and concise policy statements need to be disseminated on topics such as cost–benefit analysis of tobacco production and consumption, environmental and occupation-related effects, relative costs of health and loss of productivity, and the benefits derived from established tobacco control policies. Regular briefing papers and meetings with government ministers and opposition politicians are essential to gain their interest and maintain their commitment to protect the public from tobacco.

In the initial stages of the campaign it is important to get politicians to officially support tobacco control laws. Ideally, this should take the form of a statement to Parliament, but it could also be a speech at a public meeting or a press statement following a meeting with health groups. The public commitment of senior politicians to tobacco control helps build support for the campaign.

Once the decision to develop legislation is made, the key issue then becomes what to include in the law. The WHO FCTC provides an excellent starting point on which to base legislation, but Article 2.1 of the treaty states, "all Parties are encouraged to implement measures that are stronger than the minimum standards required by the treaty". Providing health ministers and other key politicians with solid evidence for various legislative options allows them to select the best options rationally and to defend their policy choices.

Although the Health Ministry is the lead ministry for tobacco control, it is also important to meet with finance, agriculture, trade, sports, cultural and other government ministries, as their support will be needed. Both the governing and opposition political parties should be briefed. Health is not usually a party political issue and political diversity is an asset for a public health movement.

In addition, be aware of the political dynamics within the cabinet. Some cabinet members are 'more equal than others', and have the confidence of the prime minister or president, regardless of their portfolios. Obtaining the support of these influential ministers is vital.

Public support

Direct political lobbying alone cannot stop the industry. Public support must be enlisted through a comprehensive programme of communications and mobilization to reach out to the smoking and non-smoking public and other allies. It should be remembered that smokers are not the problem, the industry is. Most smokers want to quit, do not want children to smoke, recognize the benefits of not smoking in public and support tobacco control legislation. A vocal minority of smokers may fiercely challenge the laws, but it is unfair to marginalize the majority because of a small minority.

The principal resources for mass mobilization are media advocacy and a database of supporters. The database should include all the individuals and organizations with whom regular communications will be necessary. As political opportunities arise, these groups are vital partners in communicating with decision-makers and the media. A campaign newsletter and e-mail are the most visible communication vehicles for this group.

It is important to remember that the health hazards of tobacco are so great and the case for regulation so compelling that there is no need to overstate the evidence. The evidence is best presented in a calm, rational manner and without exaggeration.

The opportunity to generate public support through either paid advocacy advertisements or public service announcements in the media should also be investigated. In South Africa, industry arguments against a ban on tobacco advertising were elegantly refuted with a counter-advertisement on radio using an ex-smoker with laryngeal cancer. The ad asks, "The tobacco industry claims that a ban on tobacco advertising and promotions is an attack on freedom of speech. We asked a former smoker what he thinks?" A tinny voice replies, "When you have lost your voice to cancer of the larynx, you don't have much freedom of speech". The advertisement not only made an important advocacy point but greatly increased calls to a 'Quit Line' from smokers wanting to quit.

Mass media

It is vital for the media to receive accurate information on key tobacco issues. Although public opinion is formed over time, it can change quite rapidly under the influence of hostile media *(7)*. NGOs, professional bodies, academics and government can join to make and maintain a compelling case for legislation that appeals to all sectors of society.

The communications programme should generate media articles and academic pieces on the benefits of excise taxation, the case for banning advertising or restricting smoking in public places, the economics of tobacco, the ill effects of inappropriate policy, the benefits of quitting and tobacco industry disinformation. Ask different individuals and groups to provide these media articles and press releases, as the press prefers not to publish a series releases from a single source over an extended period.

A monitoring system should be established to track articles and editorials about tobacco on radio, television, in daily newspapers and in periodicals throughout the country. This allows emerging themes in the debate to be detected. It is particularly important that no claim from the tobacco industry goes unchallenged. Responses to the media include: rebuttal pieces; letters to the editor; meetings with editorial boards or journalists; and media briefings.

The media monitoring system can be formal or informal. Commercial media monitoring groups can be employed – these are usually thorough and fast but can be expensive. An informal system would consist of friends and colleagues who fax or e-mail news items to a central office on a daily basis.

The media may be divided on the tobacco issue. Some will support tobacco control laws but others may be openly hostile to them, particularly if they stand to lose advertising revenues. While it is necessary to challenge inaccurate information, it is unwise to harangue reporters or editors. The rule that one should not argue with 'people who buy ink by the gallon' holds – journalists will always have the last word.

THE STRUCTURE OF THE TOBACCO CONTROL MOVEMENT

There is a truism in tobacco control which states that "No one can do everything but everyone can do something". A successful tobacco control movement has to be able to call upon the expertise of many individuals and groups:

- scientists to provide solid expertise in support of tobacco control efforts;
- advocates and voluntary associations to mobilize communities and lobby for action;
- strategists who can anticipate and meet the tobacco industry's tactics head-on;
- journalists and other media professionals willing to tell the truth about smoking and also ready to challenge the indirect censorship imposed by tobacco advertising revenues on the media;

- economists able to estimate the monetary costs of tobacco to society and the alternative employment that could be created in a tobacco-free society;
- lawyers to assist in drafting and analysing proposed laws;
- advertising agencies to develop creative campaigns in support of the cause;
- trade unions to debunk myths about tobacco and employment and to protect workers from active and passive smoking;
- business leaders willing to support tobacco control activities financially and to introduce smoke-free policies in the workplace;
- researchers to provide accurate information on smoking prevalence and public beliefs, knowledge and attitudes;
- celebrities, religious leaders, doctors, nurses and sports personalities to lend their distinctive authority and support;
- parents to join in letter-writing campaigns and non-smokers to demand tobacco-free air;
- friends to gather and share critical intelligence, including tracking government policy initiatives and the reactions of the industry.

Effective tobacco control movements are built on teamwork and a diverse range of skills. There is room for everyone who is concerned about any aspect of tobacco use. The movement is not a private club reserved exclusively for activists. The different values, interests, concerns and commitment of its members must be respected. When it functions properly, the movement adds up to more than the sum of its parts and gives everyone a sense of participation in the process.

Coalitions of NGOs

Leadership of the movement is usually provided by a few NGOs working together as a coalition. Coalitions have the great advantage of avoiding duplication of effort, increasing geographical reach by linking people nationwide, multiplying resources through sharing, and presenting a single coherent strategy for change.

In Canada, a broad coalition of over 200 organizations with a tight inner core of five committed organizations sustained the campaign. Similarly, in South Africa, the campaign for legislation was led by a group of three NGOs representing cancer, heart and tobacco control associations, which in turn drew in shifting groups of allies for specific campaigns.

The advantages of coalitions are clear, but in practice there are also risks inherent in the process. There may be conflicts over funds or public credit for coalition activities. This can create envy and distrust. More time may be spent on administration of the coalition than on its campaigns. Members may shift all the responsibility for tobacco control activities to the coalition and reduce their own independent activities. Coalitions can also be slow in taking decisions because of their bureaucracies.

These pitfalls can be avoided if some basic rules are adopted:

- The leaders of the coalition must be deeply committed to tobacco control and be willing to subordinate their narrow self-interest to the overall goals of the cause.

- The objectives of the coalition must be clearly stated so that members fully understand the nature of their commitment.
- The decision-making structure must permit prompt and flexible action. Member organizations must empower their representatives to make binding commitments on their behalf.
- No decision of the coalition is binding on members unless everyone agrees to it. Each organization should remain free to speak and act for itself outside the coalition.
- Its members should support the coalition financially through an agreed-upon formula. Ideally, the coalition should not compete with its members for outside funding.
- The coalition should communicate regularly with all its members, to keep them involved and informed, and to integrate tobacco control programmes into their routine activities.

Resources for tobacco control

In many lower-income countries tobacco control is the part-time occupation of a few dedicated individuals. It is an activity conducted by concerned health professionals – and, more recently, lawyers and consumer activists – as a small, voluntary component of their work. Although individual initiative rather than organized coalitions drives the process, the networks thus established have been highly effective in putting tobacco control on the political agenda. Their efforts would benefit immensely from increased resources.

There are several possible sources of funding for NGOs, including government, international organizations and business. In countries such as Australia, South Africa, Sweden and the United Kingdom, the government has contracted NGOs to provide smoking cessation programmes; it may even directly fund them, as in the case of Action on Smoking and Health (United Kingdom).

Several international development agencies, trusts and foundations also fund NGO activities. Most recently, Cancer Research (United Kingdom), the American Cancer Society and the International Union Against Cancer have launched a fund to support human capacity development in tobacco control.

Businesses give to charities for two reasons: basic philanthropy and commercial interest. Philanthropic aid is usually a donation, which the NGO can use as it sees fit. In deals struck for commercial reasons, the money is more likely to be given for designated purposes. Companies have found that linking their brand name to a popular charity can serve their commercial interests as powerfully as conventional marketing – and it is cheaper. People buy their product in the belief that they are supporting a worthy cause. When cause-related marketing works, everybody feels good and everybody wins – the company, its staff, its customers and the users of the charity's services. The problem is that, most of the time, not everybody wins. Companies only fund charities and activities that have massive public relation potential, and there is no money for causes that are not 'attractive' or well known.

Alternatively, businesses will fund NGOs with whom they share common interests. Pharmaceutical companies that sell smoking cessation products recognize that a strong tobacco control environment is likely to encourage more smokers to quit, increasing their potential customer base. These companies have, therefore, an interest in supporting tobacco control and smoking cessation in particular.

However, many health advocates refuse to work with transnational pharmaceutical companies, citing concerns about the abuse of their patents on medicines to maintain high prices for essential drugs in poor countries. Further, the main purpose of these companies is to sell smoking cessation therapies, and advocates are concerned that the companies may shift the agenda away from policy advocacy to an excessive focus on cessation services. These companies are also subject to pressure and the threat of reprisals from the tobacco industry, which may be in the market for other pharmaceutical products.

Though controversial, several NGOs have overcome their inhibitions and cooperate with business.

A healthy business–NGO relationship

A healthy relationship is only conceivable when the parties have shared objectives. If business commitment to tobacco control legislation is weak, NGOs will find dialogue and collaboration frustrating or even counterproductive. Likewise, if NGO strategies are too radical, business might be concerned about adverse publicity and even possible litigation.

Where business has a positive social agenda and where NGOs are effective and accountable, there is the potential for a strong, collaborative relationship. This does not mean placid NGOs and radical companies, but a genuine partnership between NGOs and business based on mutual respect, acceptance of autonomy, independence and pluralism of NGO opinions and positions.

The most important questions must be asked at the outset. Is collaboration with business the right choice for that particular organization or cause? What goals will it set for itself? What tactics and methods of work will it adopt? How will it resolve differences of opinion? What are the potential conflicts of interest? The outcome will largely depend on how those questions are answered in the first place. A private–public partnership should therefore undergo the same scrutiny as any other strategy or tactic.

The private sector can be a useful partner for NGOs, if properly handled; what it can never be is their master. Public service also means serving the public, not the interest of those who provide the service. Perhaps the best long-term solution to the resource quandary is using part of the revenues from tobacco taxes to fund tobacco control programmes.

References

1. Environics Research Group Limited. *Public support for international efforts to control tobacco. A survey in five countries.* Toronto, Canada. 2001.

2. Roemer R. *Legislative action to combat the world tobacco epidemic, 2nd ed.* Geneva, World Health Organization, 1993.

3. World Health Organization. *Guidelines for controlling and monitoring the tobacco epidemic.* World Health Organization, Geneva, 1997.

4. Jha, P, Chaloupka, FJ. *Curbing the epidemic: governments and the economics of tobacco control.* Washington, DC, The World Bank Development in Practice series, 1999 (http://www1.worldbank.org/tobacco/reports.asp).

5. Action on Smoking and Health–UK. *Tobacco explained: the truth about the tobacco industry …in its own words.* London, ASH–UK, 1998.

6. The Democracy Center. *The Democracy Owners Manual.* The Democracy Center – Citizen Action Series, San Francisco, 2002 (www.democracyctr.org).

7. Pertschuk M. *Smoke Signals: The smoking control media handbook.* American Cancer Society, Atlanta, 1986 (www.strategyguides.globalink.org/guide10.htm).

15

Monitoring, surveillance, evaluation and reporting

What gets measured, gets done.
— Paul Esposito

INTRODUCTION AND DEFINITIONS

A comprehensive surveillance and evaluation system should be an integral and major element of all tobacco control policies and programmes. Empirical evidence shows that the most successful national tobacco control policies are supported by an effective surveillance and evaluation system. The development of a surveillance and evaluation system is an obligation for the Parties that adopt and ratify the WHO FCTC. Their obligations in terms of reporting and exchange of information (Art. 21) are subject to the establishment of:

> programmes for national, regional and global surveillance of the magnitude, patterns, determinants and consequences of tobacco consumption and exposure to tobacco smoke. Towards this end, the Parties should integrate tobacco surveillance programmes into national, regional and global health surveillance programmes, so that data are comparable and can be analysed at the regional and international levels, as appropriate (Art. 20 §2).

Surveillance is the monitoring of tobacco use, its health and economic consequences, the sociocultural factors that underlie it, and the tobacco control policy responses at regular intervals of time. Surveillance should be designed to ensure adequate information support throughout the evaluation process. *Evaluation* is a systematic way of learning from experience in order to improve, revise and adapt tobacco control policies and programmes. *Reporting* is the preparation and dissemination of evaluation reports on national or local tobacco control programmes at periodic intervals of time.

This chapter will cover some of the fundamental issues involved in effective tobacco control surveillance, highlighting the existing global surveillance mechanisms for youth (WHO–CDC GYTS, http://www.cdc.gov/tobacco/global/GYTS.htm) and adults (WHO STEPwise approach to surveillance of tobacco use, or STEPS, http://www.who.int/ncd_surveillance/steps/en). It also introduces key concepts in monitoring, evaluating and reporting on tobacco control programmes, so as to enhance and improve these programmes over time.

SURVEILLANCE

Tobacco use surveillance among youth – GYTS

In December 1998, WHO/TFI convened a meeting in Geneva with CDC, UNICEF, the World Bank and representatives from countries in each of the six WHO regions to discuss the need for standardized mechanisms to collect youth tobacco use information on a global basis. The outcome of this meeting was the development by WHO and CDC of a Global Tobacco Surveillance System, which uses the GYTS as its data collection mechanism. GYTS is a school-based survey designed to enhance the capacity of countries to monitor tobacco use among youth and to guide the implementation and evaluation of tobacco prevention and control programmes. GYTS uses a standard methodology for constructing the sampling frame, selecting schools and classes, preparing questionnaires, following consistent field procedures and using consistent data management procedures for data processing and analysis. The information generated from GYTS can be used to stimulate the development of tobacco control programmes and can serve as a means to assess progress in meeting programme goals. In addition, GYTS data can be used to monitor seven Articles in the WHO FCTC.

GYTS organizational structure – partners and roles

GYTS is a multi-partner project representing global, regional and national partners. Its purpose is to assist countries in assessing and responding to their country situation and needs in relation to the tobacco epidemic. Countries should utilize GYTS to guide the development, implementation and evaluation of their tobacco control programmes as part of their national capacity-building process. At the global and regional levels, WHO (headquarters and its six regional offices) and CDC are the lead agencies that jointly manage GYTS, consistent with their respective policies and procedures. A Management Committee comprised of members from both lead agencies, is responsible for the operational management of GYTS, consistent with the Terms of Reference agreed to by the lead agencies. At the national level, GYTS is managed through the governments, as defined by the countries' policies and procedures and their contracts with global partners. CDC's role is predominantly technical, while WHO is primarily responsible for GYTS management and implementation.

GYTS essential indicators

GYTS is composed of 56 'core' questions designed to gather data on seven domains: prevalence, knowledge and attitudes, media and advertising, access, school curricula, environmental tobacco smoke (ETS) and cessation. The questionnaire also allows countries to insert their own country-specific questions. The following is a brief summary of each domain relative to the GYTS questions.

Prevalence of cigarette smoking and other tobacco use among young people

The core GYTS questions in this section measure smoking experimentation, current smoking patterns, age of initiation and other tobacco use. These questions assess:
- how many young people have experimented with smoking cigarettes or use other forms of tobacco products;
- the age at which young people begin cigarette smoking;
- what brand of cigarettes young people smoke;
- where young people usually smoke.

Knowledge and attitudes of young people towards cigarette smoking

These questions measure general knowledge, attitudes and intentions that research has linked to the risk of smoking initiation and transitions toward more regular smoking. Several concepts are specifically addressed including susceptibility to smoking, which is a measure of how firm a never-smoker is regarding the intention to remain a non-smoker. Parental involvement, attitudes toward the perceived social benefits of smoking, knowledge and attitudes toward risks of tobacco use, and impact of peer pressure to use tobacco are also specifically addressed. The questions delineate:

- the strength of intention to remain non-smokers among young people who never smoked (index of susceptibility);
- what young people perceive as the social benefits and the health risks of smoking cigarettes;
- the extent of peer pressure on young people to begin cigarette smoking.

Role of the media and advertising in young people's use of cigarettes

These questions measure the exposure of young people to both pro- and anti-tobacco use messages in the mass media.

Pro-use messages: These are messages that promote tobacco use. Children buy the most heavily advertised brands and are much more affected by advertising than are adults. The average youth already has been exposed to billions of dollars in imagery advertising and promotions creating a 'friendly familiarity' for tobacco products – an environment in which smoking is seen as glamorous, social and normative. Young people are able to recall virtually no anti-smoking messages on television or in the movies, yet they are able to recall specific movies that portray smoking and are able to identify actors and actresses who smoke in their entertainment roles.

Anti-use messages: An intensive mass media campaign can produce significant declines in both adult and youth smoking. It demonstrates that comprehensive education efforts, combining media, school-based and community-based activities can postpone or prevent smoking onset in adolescents.

The questions under this domain look at:

- how receptive young people are to cigarette advertising and other activities that promote cigarette use;
- how aware and exposed young people are to anti-smoking messages.

Access to cigarettes

Many countries have passed laws banning the sale of cigarettes to young people below certain ages (15 and 18 are the most common). These questions measure the extent to which young people are able to purchase cigarettes in stores and whether they are asked to show proof of age. In addition, a series of questions have been added to determine the per cent of disposable income available to young people that is spent on cigarettes. The questions in this series explore:

- where young people usually get their cigarettes;
- whether sellers refuse to sell young people cigarettes because of their age;
- how much money young people spend on cigarettes.

Tobacco-related school curriculum

These questions measure student perception of tobacco-use prevention education. Schools are an ideal setting in which to provide this kind of education. School-based tobacco prevention education programmes that focus on skills training have proven effective in reducing the onset of smoking. The questions under this topic look at:

- what young people are taught in school about tobacco;
- young people's perceptions of their school's programmes to prevent cigarette use.

ETS

These questions measure exposure to second-hand tobacco smoke or ETS. Since ETS is a significant risk factor for lung cancer, heart disease, asthma exacerbation and induction, respiratory infections, and adverse reproductive outcomes, it is important to assess exposure in youth. The questions in this section measure exposure during the preceding 7 days and assess general knowledge or attitude about the harmful effects of ETS, including:

- the extent of young people's exposure to smoking at home and in public places;
- young people's perceptions of the harmful effects of ETS.

Cessation of cigarette smoking

Many smokers, including youth, are addicted to nicotine and need assistance in quitting. Recently, there has been an increased demand for cessation programmes for youth. A primary reason for this increased demand is the recognition that many young tobacco users are interested in quitting and that they frequently try to quit but are mostly unsuccessful. To monitor the potential impact of tobacco control policies and diversion and cessation programmes it is important to measure the short- and long-term likelihood that young cigarette smokers will quit.

GYTS sample selection

The quality and usefulness of results from GYTS depends largely on the procedures used to select the participating schools, classes (sections) and students. Because surveying every student is impossible, impractical and unnecessary, a sample of the population is selected. The results from a good sample can be generalized to the entire student population from which the sample is drawn. The results from a poor sample only refer to students who participate.

The following describes the two-stage sample design used for GYTS.

STAGE 1: Selection of schools

The target population for GYTS is youth in grades associated with ages 13–15 years. Each country compiles a list of schools, which includes grades (forms, levels, secondary[ies], or standards) associated with these ages. The schools are selected with probability proportional to enrolment size (PPE). This means that large schools are more likely to be selected than small schools.

The number of schools to select is dependent on both statistical and practical considerations. Statistically, the number of schools selected can affect the precision of the estimates. Given the same sample size of students, selecting a large number of schools, generally, yields more precise estimates than a sample of fewer schools. With the larger number of schools the average number of students selected per school is reduced, thus reducing the school 'cluster' effect.

Most countries implementing GYTS select 25, 50 or 100 schools, depending on the statistical precision required, time frame for the fieldwork and resources available for conducting the survey.

STAGE 2: Selection of classes (sections) and students

Classes (sections) are randomly chosen from the selected schools. All students in the selected classes (sections) are eligible for participation in the survey. The number of students interviewed in most GYTSs is between 1500 to 2000 students per sample site. Statistically a sample of 1500 students will yield representative estimates at a fairly precise level (± 5%) for any population enrolment size.

Once the sample size is set, the following process is followed. For a student sample of 1500 completed student interviews with an expected 80% student response rate, a sample of 1875 students is required. If 50 schools are selected at 80% participation, then 40 will agree to participate. Thus, 1875/40 = 47 students (on average) will be selected per school. This probably means one or two classes (sections) per school. Decreasing the number of schools to select will require selection of more classes per school. Increasing the sample size of students has the same effect of increasing the number of classes per school.

Conducting the survey: practical considerations

Timing of the survey

GYTS is now being conducted year-round in countries situated in both the northern and southern hemispheres. Determining the 'best' time of year for conducting GYTS will vary by country, because the start and end dates for school differ. It is recommended that GYTS be conducted during the middle of the morning. The early part of the school day should be avoided because it could eliminate those students who arrive at school late. Lunchtime should be avoided. Later times of the day become poorer choices as students may leave school early.

Manpower resources

Because fieldwork should last less than 2 months, the number of available field staff will help determine how many schools can be selected

Other resources

The larger the sample size, the greater the cost in terms of printing of questionnaires and other supplies

NO replacement or substitution is allowed for schools that do not agree to participate!

Data collection and processing

Data collection

Before initiating the collection of data, countries must participate in a workshop to train their research coordinators (RCs) in GYTS standard methodology and procedures. This assures continuity across the regions, consistency in sample design and selection procedures and questionnaire development (ensuring the core remains intact), and uniformity in field procedures for data collection.

Once the training workshop is over, RCs return to their respective countries and conduct the survey among students in selected schools. Each student completes a questionnaire with responses coded as filled in bubbles on answer sheets. After completing the data collection of GYTS, the RCs send the survey forms (answer and header sheets and school and classroom level forms) to CDC for data processing.

Data processing

Answer sheets received by CDC are scanned using optical scanning hardware. Scanned data files proceed through a data cleaning process that includes matching record length to scanned format, reviewing non-responses (out of range and missing) and logic editing. Each data record is weight-adjusted for school, class and student non-participation. Finally, all records are adjusted for grade and gender stratification. There is continuing interaction between CDC staff and the RC and regional office while cleaning and editing the data file.

Data analysis

Once the data has been collected and processed, WHO and CDC, in collaboration with associate partners, conduct data analysis workshops to provide hands-on training to the country RCs for an in-depth analysis of their data sets. Analysis workshops include training in the use of EpiInfo (free software that encompasses procedures for analysing complex survey data) and country report writing.

Data reporting

Once the data file is finalized, CDC produces 100+ Weighted Frequency Tables and 100+ Preferred Tables. CDC prepares a draft one-page fact sheet highlighting the main GYTS findings. The final data file, tables and the fact sheet are sent to the corresponding regional office via e-mail and hard copy.

Tabulated data: The raw data are used in calculations for tabulated data. As part of the data processing for GYTS, CDC prepares two types of tables, Weighted Frequency and Preferred Tables. The Weighted Frequency Tables are produced as separate tables for each question in the country questionnaires. Tabulations are given for 'total', by gender and by grade. A set of Preferred Tables is produced by CDC, which translates each core question, based on historical classification and including cross comparisons, into variables that are utilized as indicators to monitor tobacco activity within the country.

Country fact sheet: The country fact sheet contains highlights from the country's data. The purpose of the fact sheet is to provide the country with data in a one-page format that can be used for quick response to inquiries about GYTS and/or for initial data release. Data from all students who participate in a country's GYTS are included in the fact sheet.

Country report: The purpose of the country report is to promote the development of a country's tobacco control programme, which draws its evidence base from GYTS. This report should prove most useful as it relates to policy and programme development in the country.

Current status and preliminary findings

GYTS was developed to provide systematic global surveillance of youth tobacco use. GYTS provides data that can be used by countries to: (a) evaluate their country-specific tobacco control programme; (b) monitor trends in global youth tobacco use; and (c) compare tobacco use among countries and regions. As of January 2004, a total of 120 countries representing all six WHO regions have participated in GYTS (see Table 1). In addition, repeat GYTS have been completed in 14 countries, 10 are in the field, and 11 are preparing for the field.

For the first time, GYTS has documented in a systematic way a global problem in youth tobacco use. The problem is of equal concern in developed and developing countries. Of the 120 countries/regions that have completed GYTS, not a single site had a prevalence rate of current 'any tobacco use', 'current smoking', or 'other tobacco use' equal to zero. In addition, almost one in four students who ever smoked cigarettes smoked their first cigarette before the age of 10 *(1)*. Thus, future health consequences of tobacco use and dependency on tobacco appear to be a significant problem facing countries throughout the world. These findings suggest that immediate attention needs to be given to developing both global and country-specific tobacco control programmes to reduce tobacco use among young people.

Tobacco use surveillance among adults – the WHO STEPwise approach

STEPS is the surveillance tool for adults recommended by WHO, covering all risk factors contributing to NCDs, including tobacco use. The objective is to unify all WHO approaches to defining core variables for population-based surveys, surveillance and monitoring instruments to achieve data comparability over time and between countries.

STEPS is based on the concept that surveillance systems require standardized data collection as well as sufficient flexibility to be appropriate in a variety of country situations and settings. The STEP approach incorporates mechanisms for developing an increasingly comprehensive and complex surveillance system, depending on local needs and resources. The degree of complexity refers to whether questionnaires alone are used, physical measures are collected or blood collections/analysis are undertaken.

The STEPS process

STEPS is a sequential process, starting with gathering information on key risk factors by the use of questionnaires (Step 1), then moving to simple physical measurements (Step 2), and only then recommending the collection of blood samples for biochemical assessment (Step 3) (see Figure 1). Within each step, core, expanded and optional

Table 1. Number of countries participating in GYTS by WHO region

WHO regions	Number of countries			
	Completed	In field	Preparing for field	Training planned
Regional Office for Africa	27	2	3	14
Regional Office for the Americas	36	1	1	0
Regional Office for the Eastern Mediterranean	17	4	1	0
Regional Office for Europe	19	7	3	0
Regional Office for South-East Asia	6	2	0	2
Regional Office for the Western Pacific	15	2	1	10
Total	**120**	**18**	**9**	**26**

Source: CDC personal communication

information can be collected. At a minimum, core information provides the basic, comparable variables to describe prevalence and trends in the most common risk factors.

Expanded modules provide more detailed – though still standardized – information on the major risk factors. Optional modules can be added to provide data on risk factors not included in the standard STEPS approach, to obtain country or culturally specific information.

The risk factors of choice used in the STEP approach to NCD risk factors are those that respond to the following criteria:
• they make the greatest contribution to mortality and morbidity from chronic disease;
• they can be changed through primary intervention;
• they are easily measured in populations.

Tobacco use is one of the eight risk factors that fit these criteria. Others are alcohol consumption, low fruit/vegetable intake, physical inactivity, obesity, blood pressure, cholesterol and diabetes. The STEPS instrument including Step 1, Step 2 and Step 3 can be viewed in Annex 1.

The tobacco questions have been extracted from the STEPS instrument and the rationale for each question is explained below. Question-by-question specifications relevant to the tobacco questions can be viewed in Annex 2; these explain what is intended by each question.

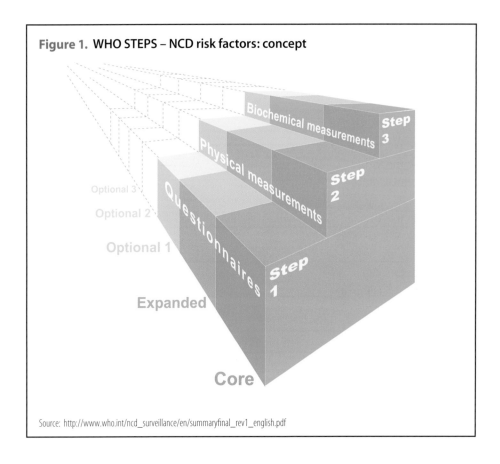

Figure 1. WHO STEPS – NCD risk factors: concept

Source: http://www.who.int/ncd_surveillance/en/summaryfinal_rev1_english.pdf

Rationale for tobacco questions

Tobacco use in communities can be measured through population surveys and/or by examining government data on apparent consumption of tobacco products calculated from cigarette production and import/export data.

All definitions used in STEPS, regarding smoking status are recommended by the WHO publication *Guidelines for controlling and monitoring the tobacco epidemic (2)*. According to these guidelines any population can be divided into two categories, smokers and non-smokers.

A smoker is someone who at the time of the survey smokes any tobacco product either daily or occasionally. Smokers may be further subdivided into two categories:

* a daily smoker is someone who smokes any tobacco product at least once a day;
* an occasional smoker (non-daily smoker) is someone who smokes, but not every day.

A non-smoker is someone who, at the time of the survey, does not smoke at all. Non-smokers can be divided into three categories:

* ex-smokers are people who were formerly daily smokers but currently do not smoke at all;
* never smokers are those who either have never smoked at all or have never been daily smokers and have smoked less than 100 cigarettes in their lifetime;

- ex-occasional smokers are those who were formerly occasional (but never daily) smokers and who smoked 100 or more cigarettes (or the equivalent amount of tobacco) in their lifetime.

STEPS Questionnaire: Tobacco section

Core questions: WHO suggests some core questions to establish the smoking status of each adult individual in the sample to determine the prevalence of tobacco use in the adult population.

1a. Do you currently smoke any tobacco products, such as cigarettes, cigars or pipes?
1b. If yes, do you currently smoke tobacco products daily?

These two questions permit the estimation of the main categories of current smoking status, which is the most important estimation in large health surveys. If there is an opportunity for more questions, it is highly recommended to use questions about previous history of tobacco use (see below-expanded questions).

2a. How old were you when you first started smoking daily?
2b. Do you remember how long ago it was?

The WHO guidelines actually recommend asking about number of years that a person smoked daily. This way it is possible not to count the time period when the person was not smoking. However, by asking the question in two different ways, controlling for recall error is possible. Age at onset is especially important in assessing the smoking status in adolescents, since adults are more likely to quit but young people are in the process of smoking initiation.

3. On average, how many of the following do you smoke each day? (e.g. manufactured cigarettes, hand-rolled cigarettes, pipes full of tobacco, cigars, cheroots, cigarillos)

This is an additional question about daily consumption and is also used for assessing the prevalence of tobacco use. The list of items should be modified to suit local tobacco use patterns.

Expanded questions: Whenever possible, the survey should contain expanded questions for determining the history of smoking status and use of smokeless tobacco.
4. In the past, did you ever smoke daily?
5a. If yes, how old were you when you stopped smoking daily?
5b. How long ago did you stop smoking daily?

If there is an opportunity for more questions, the questions on past consumption of tobacco are crucial. By combining the questions of current and previous use of tobacco, it is possible to determine the prevalence of all major categories of smoking status *(2)*.

6. Do you currently use any smokeless tobacco such as (snuff, chewing tobacco, betel)?

6b. If yes, do you currently use smokeless tobacco products daily?

7. On average, how many times a day do you use…

(record for each type)

Because tobacco is used in a variety of forms, it is essential to assess the use of smokeless tobacco particularly in settings where smokeless tobacco is preferred to smoked tobacco. In some countries of the African and Eastern Mediterranean Regions, the use of tobacco products such as chewing tobacco, water pipes, *narguileh* or *sheesha* often surpass cigarette smoking.

STEPS implementation at country level

The ultimate goal of the STEPS approach is to increase a country's capacity to develop a sustainable infrastructure for NCD surveillance *(3)*. To achieve this, strategic alliances are necessary at the global, regional and country level (see Figure 2). WHO headquarters provides global coordination for implementing STEPS across the WHO regions. WHO headquarters, in collaboration with the WHO regional offices, provides STEPS training to STEPS focal points by region and country.

WHO STEPS training utilizes a TOT approach, ensuring that knowledge transfer and capacity is improved and maintained at the country level. Training covers all aspects of the planning, implementation, data collection, analysis and dissemination of the results of a STEPS survey within the context of an integrated surveillance system. WHO regional offices implement the programmes within countries and organize the training workshops.

Current status

Currently, STEPS is being carried out in four WHO regions, namely the WHO African Region, the WHO Eastern Mediterranean Region, the WHO South-East Asia Region and the WHO Western Pacific Region, and covers over 35 countries. Over 50 countries have been trained in regional training workshops as well as national workshops.

Practical considerations

- Each WHO Member State implementing STEPS is advised to convene a group or a committee, which works as the equivalent of national interagency coordinating committee (see Figure 2). This committee should oversee the practical and logistic issues relating to the overall country level implementation of STEPS, as well as providing assistance in translating data into policy and programmes.
- The data collected must be relevant for the development of public health interventions.
- The collection and analysis of good quality data are not enough to inform policy in an environment in which the health agenda is subject to competing priorities. Therefore, it is necessary to further provide policy-makers with accurate, useful and easily interpreted results. The STEPS approach was designed with this fact in mind

Figure 2. Summary schema Global Strategy of NCD Surveillance

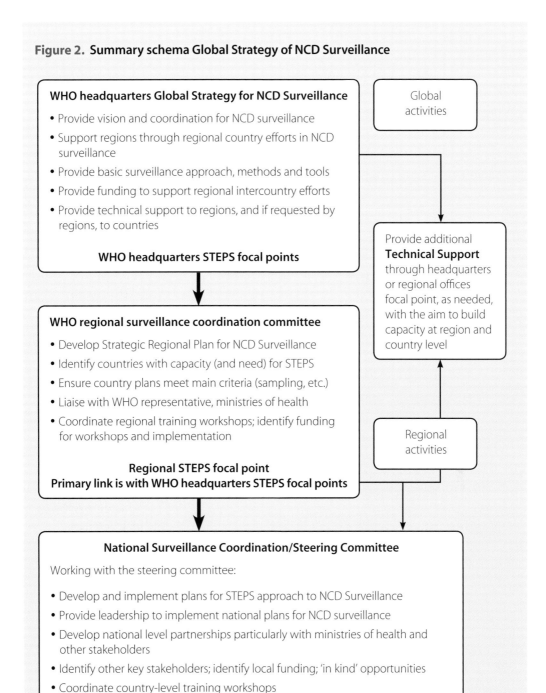

Source: http://www.who.int/ncd_surveillance/steps/en/planningmanualaugust03.pdf

and countries are assisted in preparing reports designed to capture the attention of public health policy-makers.

- The success of ongoing surveillance in developing countries depends on the commitment of governments and other partner organizations. Developing mechanisms to ensure sustainability is essential to achieving the goal of increasing a country's capacity for effective surveillance. Such surveillance will provide the essential information to formulate sound polices, which will lead to reducing the burden of tobacco-related disease.

MONITORING

Selecting essential indicators for monitoring the tobacco epidemic at the national level

Comprehensive and multisectoral tobacco control policies and activities control have social, psychological, political and economic dimensions. It is therefore often difficult to determine if outcomes are mainly due to the specific action undertaken or to other independent factors. It may be difficult to identify the effects immediately of each separate policy, and a considerable amount of time may be needed before any change is reflected in the final health indicators. Selecting intermediate outcomes is thus necessary as they can address:

- changes in tobacco use rates;
- changes in knowledge, attitudes and opinions;
- changes in the number and kind of policy measures;
- changes in economic outcomes such as costs of medical care;
- changes in tobacco-related mortality and morbidity.

Evaluation at the national level should utilize a few essential indicators to measure adequately all areas covered by a national programme that will enable comparisons with local jurisdictions and other countries. These areas are: tobacco consumption, tobacco prevalence, exposure to tobacco-smoke, tobacco-related mortality and changes in tobacco-control policy. Additional indicators could be incorporated into the surveillance system. While not essential, they facilitate a more detailed analysis of the programme's impact.

Tips:

- It is strongly recommended that national monitoring for tobacco control be aligned with STEPS and GYTS.
- Information should be obtained by reliable methods in accordance with appropriate standardized procedures and at regular intervals of time.
- When establishing a monitoring and evaluation system, review the available information resources to improve data exchange, procedures and methodologies, and data utilization.

Tobacco consumption

The amount of tobacco consumed in a population is one important measure of the magnitude of the tobacco problem. Moreover, monitoring the tobacco epidemic through the use of consumption estimates is a relatively inexpensive procedure, and provides a useful estimate of the severity of the tobacco problem in countries without prevalence data.

Practical considerations:

- Tobacco consumption is generally estimated indirectly from data on the sale, manufacture, trade and taxation of tobacco products. Government statistical offices collect and publish these data.
- For different reasons, these data do not always represent what has really being consumed (illegal trade, changes in the weight of tobacco per cigarettes, changes in smoking habits, etc.). Consequently, tobacco consumption should be supplemented by an estimate of the number of tobacco users, whenever possible.
- In most countries, tobacco use is synonymous with cigarette smoking. However, in many parts of the world, tobacco is used in a variety of other forms. Thus, when estimating consumption, it is essential to specify the type of tobacco used. At minimum, consumption should be estimated separately for two categories: smoking and smokeless tobacco use.
- This information should be monitored at least every 2 years once a national policy or programme has been launched. When possible, series going back some 20 years should be established (see Figure 3).

Prevalence of tobacco use

Accurate data on the prevalence of tobacco use in the total population, among men and women, and among specific subgroups are the most important and useful measures of the tobacco epidemic in a given population. High-risk groups can be identified and interventions targeting these groups developed. Gaps in tobacco control policy can be highlighted, guiding advocacy efforts. Periodic prevalence data also form the backbone for evaluating the effectiveness of programme and policy interventions within a given population.

Practical considerations:

- Prevalence estimates should always be calculated for males and females separately.
- Prevalence should also be calculated separately for different subgroups of the population according to age, sex and other relevant sociodemographic characteristics as ethnicity, educational level and linguistic groups (see Table 2).
- While cigarette smoking is the most common type of tobacco use, in countries where different types of tobacco use are present, the prevalence of different methods of tobacco consumption should be obtained.

In most of the countries only sample surveys can provide estimates of the prevalence of smoking among the adults and youth populations. Probability sampling is the only scientifically valid procedure for estimating prevalence in a population. Sample selec-

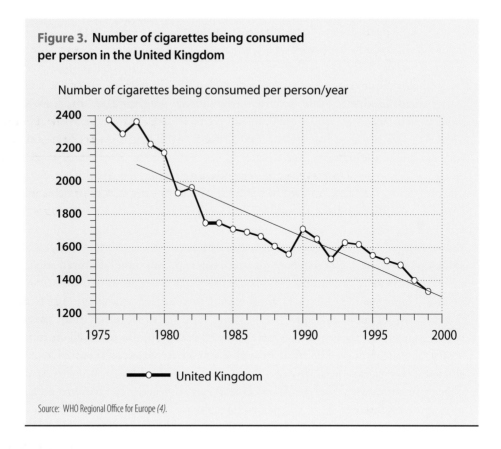

Figure 3. Number of cigarettes being consumed per person in the United Kingdom

Number of cigarettes being consumed per person/year

United Kingdom

Source: WHO Regional Office for Europe *(4)*.

tion, data collection, analysis and presentation are discussed in greater detail in the WHO publication *Guidelines for controlling and monitoring the tobacco epidemic*. This publication also provides templates for questionnaires to obtain prevalence data.

The estimate of tobacco use among young people requires surveys covering sufficiently narrow age groups. The indicators selected for monitoring tobacco use among young people are the same as for adults but specific questions about initiation should be asked. The GYTS provides a template for doing a school-based survey of tobacco use among young people aged 13–15.

Prevalence surveys should be repeated at least every 5 years, and, if possible, annually, to monitor trends in tobacco-use behaviour.

Exposure to tobacco smoke

Exposure to tobacco smoke among adults and young people is an essential indicator for evaluating tobacco control policies and activities for protection from second-hand smoke in indoor workplaces, public transport, indoor public places and other public places.

Practical considerations:

- In most countries only sample surveys can provide estimates of the exposure to tobacco smoke.
- Two main measurement approaches are possible: questionnaires inquiring about exposure to smoking by others in different settings, and surveys that test for biochemical markers of inhaled smoke (saliva and urinary cotinine concentrations). Both approaches are complementary, but cotinine assays are relatively expensive and require the use of laboratory resources. Therefore, in many countries, the questionnaire method is generally adopted.
- Again, data on second-hand smoke exposure should be broken down by smoking status, sex, age and socio-occupational category or socioeconomic status.

Tobacco-related mortality

Most countries have some system for collecting and analysing health information. The coverage and reliability of these data vary widely according to the country's level of health development. Developed countries have national vital registration systems, which are complete and reliable, while in developing countries the availability of data on mortality and morbidity is much less uniform. Thus, there are great differences in countries' capacities to monitor tobacco-related deaths and diseases. The challenge is how best to use available data to maximize their utility for tobacco control purposes.

Practical considerations:

- Only vital registration or sentinel surveillance sites of known reliability and completeness are likely to be useful for monitoring mortality rates for tobacco-associated diseases.
- The mortality rates by sex and age per 100 000 inhabitants should be monitored for the following causes of death according to the International Classification of Diseases (ICD-9/ICD-10 revisions):
  - malignant neoplasm of trachea, bronchus and lung (162/C33, C34)
  - chronic obstructive pulmonary disease (490–2, 494–6/J40–J44, J47)

Table 2. Smoking status and average number of cigarettes smoked per day, by age group and sex, age 15+, Canada 2001

Sex	Age group (years)	Pop. estimate ('000)	Smokers and ex-smokers				Never smoker (%)	Average cigarettes smoked per day
			Smokers (%)	Regular (%)	Occasional (%)	Ex-smoker (%)		
Total	All age groups	24 916	21.7	18.1	3.7	23.8	54.4	16.2
Male		12 270	23.9	20.3	3.7	27.3	48.8	17.1
Female		12 646	19.6	15.9	3.8	20.5	59.9	15.0

Source: Canadian Tobacco Use Monitoring Survey, 2001 *(5)*

- ischaemic heart disease (410–414/I20–I25)
- cerebrovascular disease (430–438/I60–I69) (see Figure 4)
- For each of these causes of death, series going back to 20–30 years should be established, if possible, to allow trend analyses.

Technical issues related to the assessment of health effects of tobacco can be reviewed in greater detail in the WHO publication *Guidelines for controlling and monitoring the tobacco epidemic*.

Tobacco control policies

Monitoring should capture the status and effectiveness of the different components of a comprehensive and multisectoral tobacco control policy, which include:
- legislation;
- taxation and economics measures;
- other non-price measures;
- training and education;
- cessation interventions;
- research.

Practical considerations
- For each of these domains, collect data on the acceptance of the measure, on the adequacy of its substance and, eventually, on compliance with its requirements.
  - Acceptance is mainly related to an appropriate and continuous public information process developed in order to obtain popular support.
  - Adequacy implies that the instruments for implementation are adequately established and that the planning, responsibilities and resources for enforcement are correctly identified (see Figure 4).
  - Compliance is mainly related to the legislative domain and to the respect of the law. Often compliance depends on how effective dissuasive civil or criminal penalties are imposed.

2. To monitor commitments by the Parties having ratified the WHO FCTC, it will be desirable to report on key tobacco control measures recommended by it.

Methodology and tools for monitoring the tobacco epidemic at country level

In most countries, sample surveys can provide estimates of the prevalence of tobacco use. Probability sample surveys are beyond doubt the most valuable tool for planning and evaluating tobacco control activities, enabling periodic reporting and cross-country comparisons. Compared with population surveys, they are relatively cheap and rapid. Since the observations to be made are few in number, they can be verified, reducing errors of observation. Finally, sample surveys make it possible to measure several factors in each member of the sample. The quality of the data produced

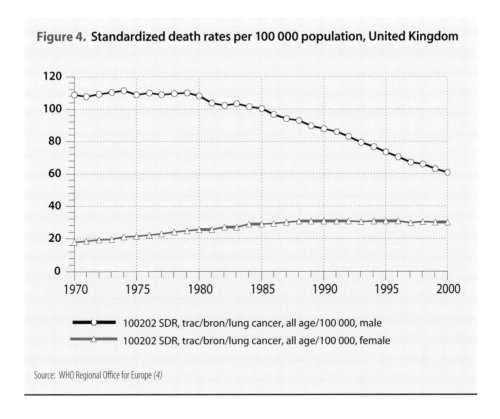

Figure 4. Standardized death rates per 100 000 population, United Kingdom

Legend:
- 100202 SDR, trac/bron/lung cancer, all age/100 000, male
- 100202 SDR, trac/bron/lung cancer, all age/100 000, female

Source: WHO Regional Office for Europe *(4)*

depends mainly on the quality of the observations made on each of the people questioned and secondarily on the way in which the sample is selected.

Populations groups to be studied

The adult population

Surveys of representative samples of the adult population provide a glimpse of the smoking problem's magnitude in the country and make it possible to estimate the prevalence of smoking in relation to certain attributes sex, age, socioeconomic or socio-occupational category. The WHO STEP targets adults.

Young people

The definition of 'young people' may vary from one country to another. The upper limit generally adopted is the legal age. To evaluate tobacco use among young people adequately, surveys covering sufficiently narrow age groups and questionnaires that ask about initiation are needed. GYTS provides a sampling methodology and questionnaire for a school-based survey of young people aged 13–15.

Health professionals and educators

Because health professionals are key to advancing tobacco control policies, their behaviour, knowledge, practice and opinions related to tobacco use are important. Surveys of health professionals should contain standard questions on smoking and tobacco use. They should also include questions on knowledge about the health effects of tobacco and current practice and knowledge about counselling patients on cessation.

Women of reproductive age and pregnant women

Because there are additional risks of smoking unique to women of reproductive age and pregnant women, there is a need for more detailed knowledge of tobacco use patterns among these groups. Questions on tobacco use prevalence can be incorporated into the monitoring of national programmes such as Making pregnancy safer.

Selecting a sample

There are numerous ways of selecting samples representative of the population. Random techniques (each member of the represented population has a well defined probability to be part of the sample) or empirical techniques, such as the quota method may be used. (In the quota method the individuals are not selected according a given probability but by their belonging to a specific quota of population, usually defined by sex, age, occupation and residence.) The technique chosen will depend on national resources and conditions, but the choice must be made in close collaboration with a statistician to ensure validity and reliability.

International standard instruments are available to obtain country health information and facilitate international comparisons. GYTS and the STEPS should be used to monitor prevalence at low cost and in a relevant and reliable manner. The World Health Survey (WHS) is a global instrument involving functioning, disability and health interventions. It includes questions on risks factors for disability, and tobacco use is part of its coverage (http://www3.who.int/whs/).

Monitoring health systems

WHO developed the World Health Survey (WHS) to provide low-cost, valid, reliable and comparable information, to build the evidence base to monitor health systems and to provide policy-makers with the necessary evidence to adjust their strategies and policies. The programme will be developed in individual countries through consultation with policy-makers and in collaboration with the people involved in routine Health Information Systems (HIS). It will be complementary to their efforts, to ensure periodic data input in a cost-effective way so that important gaps in health information are covered. It will also establish a baseline for efforts to scale up health activities. At present there are more than 73 countries active in WHS.

Sample size

The most important factor in establishing the reliability of estimated prevalence is the size of the sample. The larger the sample, the more precise the estimated prevalence, provided that the sample is a probability sample. The reliability of the prevalence estimate in a simple random sample is proportional to the square root of the sample. Therefore, reliability increases somewhat slowly with an increase in sample size.

 Tip:

In general, the reliability of the sample estimate of prevalence should be within 5 percentage points of the true prevalence figure. A sample size of less than 1000 could yield unreliable estimates, especially if subgroup estimates are required.

Questionnaires

The number and wording of questions in any given survey should be selected carefully, because the accuracy, completeness and usefulness of the data are largely dependent on the questionnaire. In addition, there are logistic considerations – cost, time constraints, etc. – that need to be considered.

Practical Considerations

- Define questions precisely and operationally, and specify exact criteria whenever necessary.
- The use of close-ended questions is strongly recommended.
- Pretesting is vital to discover potential problems or identify questions that may be misinterpreted, so that the questionnaire can be revised before it is administered to the larger population.
- If the questionnaire is to be administered by interviewers, they must all be trained to ensure uniformity. A detailed instruction manual for every interviewer is a must.
- Finally, plan data analysis beforehand, to ensure that adequate information is collected properly.

 Tip:

Smoking status of adolescents should never be assessed by proxy reports because parents, who are likely to provide answers, are often unaware or unwilling to accept that their children smoke.

Attitudes and opinions

The questions related to attitudes and opinions are of a facultative nature. They should be defined and tested in line with national or local context. What questions are asked will depend on the national tobacco control objectives, targets, resources and the probable frequency of the surveys.

Questions might be asked concerning:

- awareness of and support for government tobacco control policies;
- tobacco use – with information on the interest and pressure to quit, exposure to second-hand smoke, brands of cigarettes favoured, and indicators for nicotine dependence;
- health knowledge – awareness of tobacco-related diseases, the probability of contracting these diseases, the prognosis, and the benefits of quitting;
- social norms – prevailing attitudes about the acceptability of tobacco use.

Reporting survey data

Tobacco consumption data can be presented in various ways, provided that the average number of cigarettes smoked per day and the distribution of smokers by sex and level of consumption are shown.

Practical considerations

- The categories for average number of cigarettes smoked per day (<4, 5–14, 15–24, 25 and over) or (1–7, 8–12, 13–17, 18–22, 23–27, 28 and over) are suggested to avoid a 'digit preference' among smokers, who tend to report consumption in multiples of 5 or 10.
- For presenting age-segregated population data, 10-year age groups starting with 15–24 years should be sufficient. Broader age ranges could also be used, especially when the sample size is small.
- Reporting results of adolescent surveys requires a different approach because rates of tobacco use change rapidly during adolescence. Ideally, data should be reported for single years of age for each year from 10 to 19, with summary reports for the groups 10–14 and 15–19. If this is not feasible, statistically reliable information should be obtained and reported for the age groups 10–14 and 15–19. In every case, the age in question is the age at last birthday on the day of interview.
- In some countries, the data obtained from probability samples are used to estimate the number of people in the entire population who use tobacco. Whether using weighted or unweighted data, consult a statistician to ensure that the procedures used are valid. Results relating to estimates of prevalence should include the calculation of a 95% confidence interval if the sampling procedure allows it.

Refer to statistical textbooks for a more detailed discussion of this topic.

Qualitative studies

Qualitative, psychosocial or motivational studies aim to systematically analyse the reasons that impel individuals or groups to adopt or reject, consciously or unconsciously, a particular type of opinion, attitude or behaviour. Studies of this type are based on the technique of non-structured interviews, supplemented where necessary by semi-structured or group interviews. During these interviews, conducted by specially trained psychologists, the individuals are invited to express themselves freely and at length on the subject at hand.

Analysis of 50 or so in-depth interviews is enough to determine most of the attitudes and motivations that could be encountered among the population with regard to the subject concerned. Unlike opinion polls, the purpose is not to measure and establish percentages but to produce a typology of the different kinds of behaviours and attitudes existing among the study population, and to shed light on the principal mechanisms underlying and linking them.

Most of the qualitative studies have shown that side by side with a domain of rational knowledge there is a non-rational domain that is often more extensive. The non-rational domain results from people's personal histories from experiences since childhood and from the social and cultural values of the society to which they belong. The tobacco industry has extensively used these kinds of studies to develop sophisticated marketing strategies to expand and maintain their customer base.

One of the main reasons for the comparative ineffectiveness of information and education campaigns lies in the misunderstanding of the social and psychological mechanisms underlying the promoted behaviour.

When launching the pilot stage of a surveillance and evaluation system, a small number of in-depth interviews and a few group discussions with key population subgroups – opinion leaders, health professionals, journalists, etc. – could contribute to the assessment of a national tobacco problem in order to facilitate the build-up of policies and strategies.

SURVEILLANCE AND EVALUATION MANAGEMENT

The surveillance and evaluation system of a NTCP relies on the organization of regular data collection and on ad hoc studies. A distinction has to be made between the management of information gathering and the management of information evaluation. Information gathering has to be managed according the national health information strategy. Ideally, it should be coordinated with the various national health-related information systems with a view to:

- reviewing available information resources;
- improving the use of existing knowledge;
- integrating data gathering for tobacco control into existing data collection systems;
- standardizing and developing methodology for improving data reliability and quality.

The establishment of a national database or a national clearinghouse or both on tobacco control can mobilize collaboration and create synergies between relevant institutions, ministerial departments and even among the different programme areas of the heath ministry. Ensuring that the collection and processing of tobacco control data are well integrated into existing long-term health information systems is an effective way to facilitate regular data collection for monitoring.

Once a tobacco control policy or programme has been launched on the basis of a thorough assessment of the situation, the evaluation process will consist mainly of assessing its relevance and adequacy, reviewing progress in implementation and assessing impact and effectiveness for the reorientation and formulation of relevant policies and activities. Surveillance and evaluation play a major role in documenting tobacco control policy accountability for policy-makers, health managers and professionals, and for the general public.

The evaluation of a national tobacco control policy should be managed under the aegis of the health ministry. It can involve others ministries such as those of finance, trade, education and justice in order to ensure that the recommendations are relevant, constructive and applicable.

There are two different ways to evaluate a national tobacco control programme. Internally, evaluation should be integrated as a component of the programme, meaning that those who develop and implement the programme are also responsible for its evaluation. An alternative option is to ask a group of external experts to evaluate the programme independently. In many countries internal evaluation is part of the self-managerial process of the national tobacco control programmes while external evaluation is conducted periodically by the parliament or services of the chief of government.

References

1. The Global Youth Tobacco Survey Collaborative Group. United States Centers for Disease Control and Prevention. Atlanta, World Health Organization, Canadian Public Health Association, United States National Cancer Institute. Tobacco use among youth: a cross-country comparison. *Tobacco Control*, 2002, 11:252–270.

2. *Guidelines for controlling and monitoring the tobacco epidemic*. Geneva, World Health Organization, 1998.

3. Armstrong T, Bonita R. Capacity-building for an integrated noncommunicable disease risk factor surveillance system in developing countries. *Ethnicity and Disease,* 2003, 13(s): 2–13.

4. WHO Regional Office for Europe. European Health for All database available on http://hfadb.who.dk/hfa/.

5. Canadian Tobacco Use Monitoring Survey, 2001. Ottawa, Health Canada (http://www.hc-sc.gc.ca/hecs-sesc/tobacco/pdf/annual2001_supptables_eng.pdf).

Bibliography

Guidelines for controlling and monitoring the tobacco epidemic. Geneva, World Health Organization, 1998.

Evaluating tobacco control activities: experiences and guiding principles. Geneva, World Health Organization, 1996.

Health interview surveys. Copenhagen, WHO Regional Office for Europe, 1996.

The evaluation and monitoring of public action on tobacco. Copenhagen, WHO Regional Office for Europe, 1988.

Best Practices for Comprehensive Tobacco Control Programs. United States Centers for Disease Control and Prevention, Atlanta, 1999.

Tools for advancing tobacco control in the 21st century. The surveillance and monitoring of tobacco control in South Africa. (Surveillance and Monitoring) Geneva, World Health Organization, 2003 (WHO/NMH/TFI/FTC/03.7).

ANNEX 1

**STEPS Instrument for NCD Risk Factors
(Core and Expanded Version 1.4)**

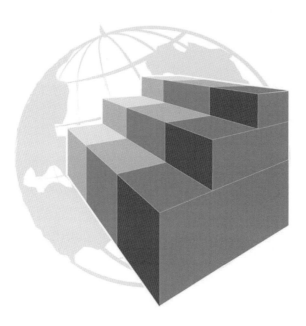

**The WHO STEPwise approach to Surveillance of
noncommunicable diseases (STEPS)**

STEPS Instrument (V1.4)

- This is the generic template which countries use to develop their own Instrument. It contains the CORE (unshaded and in double lined boxes) and EXPANDED items (shaded and in single lined boxes) and response options for Step 1, Step 2 and Step 3.

- The introductory statements, questions and response options should be translated and adapted where necessary to suit local conditions. *Italic typeface indicates where local examples should be inserted.*

- All CORE items should be included in the country-specific STEPS Instrument. Wording and response options for CORE questions should not be changed.

- Some countries may wish to expand the CORE questions. Recommendations for EXPANDED questions for the key risk factors are included in the shaded areas. These items may be modified but it is preferable to use them where possible.

- Additional questions can be added as OPTIONAL items to meet local needs. For example, questions asked in previous surveys could be added to link to previous data.

- The use of the coding column (as is used in this Instrument) facilitates easy, fast and accurate manual data entry. Using this approach does not replace the need for double data entry for maximum quality control (see data coding manual).

- Relevant skip patterns are shown on the right hand side of the coding column. They should be carefully reviewed. Modifications to the skip patterns will be needed according to the final items included.

EXAMPLE- for a current smoker who eats eight servings of fruit on a typical day

		Response		Coding column	Skip
S 1a	Do you currently smoke any **tobacco products**, such as cigarettes, cigars or pipes?	Yes 1 No 2 Don't know 7		1	*If No, go to Next Section*
D 1b	How many **servings** of fruit do you eat on one of those days? USE SHOWCARD	Number of servings Don't know 77		0 8	

- "Do not know", "Don't remember", "Not applicable", "Refuse" are all response options but should be used only as a last resort. In such cases, the first two categories and the last two categories are coded as "7", "77" or "777" and as "8", "88", or "888", respectively depending on the number of numerals in the other response options. Missing responses should be entered as "9", "99" or "999" at time of data entry.

- Interviewer training is essential to develop thorough knowledge of the instrument format, introductory statements, questions, skip patterns, response options, use of show cards and prompts (where needed). The STEPS Field Manual is a guide and resource for training sessions.

- Undertaking pilot work with the draft country-specific STEPS instrument is essential.

- Each country will need to prepare a list of the question numbers (e.g. D1a) and response code cross-referenced with the standard numbers and codes used in this generic template. This cross-referencing will facilitate communication and comparison.

This document is available electronically on the NCD Surveillance web site:
http://www.who.int/ncd_surveillance
Other documents cross-referenced in above are available by contacting *ncd_surveillance@who.int*

Respondent Identification Number ☐☐ ☐☐ ☐☐

Identification Information:

This is a draft cover page. Each country will adapt this page to suit their local needs. The exact details to be collected in each country–specific STEPS instrument will vary depending on the survey design and implementation procedures. However, regardless of how the interview is administered (e.g., household, clinic or other) a process by which the cover page containing personal identifying information is stored should be carefully designed and must meet recommended ethical standards. Clear instructions on handling and storage of the cover sheets must be provided to the interviewers.

I 1	Country/district code	☐☐
I 2	Centre (Village name):	☐☐☐☐☐☐☐
I 3	Centre (Village code): (SEE NOTE BELOW)	☐☐☐
I 4	Interviewer code	☐☐☐
I 5	Date of completion of the questionnaire	☐☐/☐☐/☐☐☐☐ Day Month Year

---

Respondent ID number ☐☐☐☐☐☐

	Consent			
I 6	Consent has been read out to respondent	Yes 1 No 2	☐	If NO, read consent
I 7	Consent has been obtained (verbal or written)	Yes 1 No 2	☐	If NO, END
I 8	Interview Language [*Insert Language*]	English 1 [Add others] 2	☐	
I 9	Time of interview (24 hour clock)		☐☐ : ☐☐	
I 10	Family Name			
I 11	First Name			

Additional Information that may be helpful

I 12	Contact phone number where possible			
I 13	Specify whose phone	Work 1 Home 2 Neighbour 3 Other (specify) 4	☐	

Note: Identification information I6 to I13 should be stored separately from the questionnaire because it contains confidential information. Please note: village code (or household code) is required as part of main instrument for data analyses.
Date of interview is required to calculate age.

Respondent Identification Number ☐☐ ☐☐ ☐☐

Step 1   Core demographic Information

			Coding Column
C1	Sex *(record Male / Female as observed)*	Male 1 Female 2	☐
C2	What is your date of birth? *If Don't Know, See Note* below and Go to C3*	Day ☐☐ Month ☐☐ Year ☐☐☐☐	
C3	How old are you?	Years	☐☐
C4	In total, how many years have you spent at school or in full-time study (excluding pre-school)?	Years	☐☐

EXPANDED: Demographic Information			
C5	What is your *[insert relevant ethnic group / racial group / cultural subgroup / others]* <u>background</u>?	*[Defined according to local demographic needs]*	☐☐
C6	What is the highest level of education you have completed? *[INSERT COUNTRY-SPECIFIC CATEGORIES]*	No formal schooling 0 1 Less than primary school 0 2 Primary school completed 0 3 Secondary school completed 0 4 High school completed 0 5 College/University completed 0 6 Post graduate degree 0 7	☐☐
C7	Which of the following best describes your <u>main</u> work status over the last 12 months? *[INSERT COUNTRY-SPECIFIC CATEGORIES]* USE SHOWCARD	Government employee 0 1 Non-government employee 0 2 Self-employed 0 3 Non-paid 0 4 Student 0 5 Homemaker 0 6 Retired 0 7 Unemployed (able to work) 0 8 Unemployed (unable to work) 0 9	☐☐
C8	How many people older than 18 years, including yourself, live in your household?	Number of people	☐☐
C9	Taking **the past year**, can you tell me what the average earnings of the household have been?	Per week	☐☐☐☐☐☐
		OR per month	☐☐☐☐☐☐
		OR per year	☐☐☐☐☐☐☐
		Go to Next Section	
		Refused 8	☐ *If Refused Go to C10*
C10	If you don't know the amount, can you give an **estimate** of the annual household income if I read some options to you? Is it *[READ OPTIONS]* *[INSERT QUINTILE VALUES]*	≤ Quintile (Q) 1 1 More than Q 1, ≤ Q 2 2 More than Q 2, ≤ Q 3 3 More than Q 3, ≤ Q 4 4 More than Q 4 5 Refused 8	☐

---

*<u>Note</u>: Coding Rule: Code "Don't Know" 7 (or 77 or 777 as appropriate).

Respondent Identification Number ☐☐ ☐☐ ☐☐

Step 1 Core Behavioural Measures

CORE Tobacco Use (Section S)

Now I am going to ask you some questions about various health behaviours. This includes things like smoking, drinking alcohol, eating fruits and vegetables and physical activity. Let's start with smoking.

		Response		Coding Column	
S 1a	Do you currently smoke any **tobacco products**, such as cigarettes, cigars or pipes?	Yes No	1 2	☐	*If No, go to Next Section**
S 1b	**If Yes,** Do you currently smoke tobacco products **daily**?	Yes No	1 2	☐	*If No, go to Next Section**
S 2a	How old were you when you **first started** smoking daily?	Age (years) Don't remember	 7 7	☐☐	*If Known, go to S 3*
S 2b	Do you remember how long ago it was? (CODE 77 FOR DON'T REMEMBER)	In Years OR in Months OR in Weeks	Years ☐☐ Months ☐☐ Weeks ☐☐		
S 3	On average, **how many** of the following do you smoke each day? (RECORD FOR EACH TYPE) (CODE 88 FOR NOT APPLICABLE) ☐☐☐☐☐☐☐☐	Manufactured cigarettes Hand-rolled cigarettes Pipes full of tobacco Cigars, cheroots, cigarillos ◄— Other (please specify):		☐☐ ☐☐ ☐☐ ☐☐ ☐☐	

EXPANDED: Tobacco Use

S 4	In the past, did you **ever** smoke **daily**?	Yes No	1 2	☐	*If No, go to S 6a*
S 5a	**If Yes,** How old were you when you **stopped** smoking **daily**?	Age (years) Don't remember	 7 7	☐☐	*If Known, go to S 6a If 7 7, go to S 5b*
S 5b	How **long ago** did you stop smoking daily?	Years ago OR Months ago OR Weeks ago	Years ☐☐ Months ☐☐ Weeks ☐☐		
S 6a	Do you **currently use** any **smokeless tobacco** such as [snuff, chewing tobacco, betel] ?	Yes No	1 2	☐	*If No, go to S 8*
S 6b	**If Yes,** Do you **currently use smokeless tobacco** products **daily**?	Yes No	1 2	☐	*If No, go to S 8*

---

* Amend skip instructions if EXPANDED or OPTIONAL items are added to the Tobacco section
* Amend skip instructions if EXPANDED or OPTIONAL items are added to the Tobacco section

Respondent Identification Number ☐☐ ☐☐ ☐☐

S 7	On average, how many **times a day** do you use …. *(RECORD FOR EACH TYPE)*	Snuff, by mouth	☐☐
		Snuff, by nose	☐☐
		Chewing tobacco	☐☐
		Betel, quid	☐☐
	☐☐☐☐☐☐☐ ←	Other (specify)	☐☐
S 8	In the past, did you **ever use** smokeless tobacco such as [*snuff, chewing tobacco, or betel*] **daily**?	Yes 1 No 2	☐

CORE   Alcohol Consumption (Section A)

The next questions ask about the consumption of alcohol.

		Response	**Coding Column**	
A 1a	Have you **ever consumed** a drink that contains alcohol such as beer, wine, spirit, fermented cider *or [add other local examples]* ? USE SHOWCARD or SHOW EXAMPLES	Yes 1 No 2	☐	*If No, Go to Next Section**
A 1b	Have you consumed alcohol within the **past 12 months**?	Yes 1 No 2	☐	*If No, Go to Next Section**
A 2	In the past 12 months, **how frequently** have you had at least one drink? *(READ RESPONSES)* *USE SHOWCARD*	5 or more days a week 1 1-4 days per week 2 1-3 days a month 3 Less than once a month 4	☐	
A 3	When you drink alcohol, **on average**, how many drinks do you have during one day?	Number Don't know 7 7	☐☐	
A 4	During each of the **past 7 days**, how many standard drinks of any alcoholic drink did you have each day? *(RECORD FOR EACH DAY* *USE SHOWCARD)*	Monday	☐☐	
		Tuesday	☐☐	
		Wednesday	☐☐	
		Thursday	☐☐	
		Friday	☐☐	
		Saturday	☐☐	
		Sunday	☐☐	

EXPANDED : Alcohol			
A 5	In the past 12 months, what was the **largest number** of drinks you had on a single occasion, counting all types of standard drinks together?	Largest number	☐☐
A 6a	**For men only:** In the past 12 months, on how many days did you have **five or more** standard drinks in a single day?	Number of days	☐☐☐
A 6b	**For women only:** In the past 12 months, on how many days did you have **four or more** standard drinks in a single day?	Number of days	☐☐☐

---

* Amend skip instructions if EXPANDED or OPTIONAL items are added to the Alcohol section

Respondent Identification Number ☐☐ ☐☐ ☐☐

CORE   Diet   (Section D)

The next questions ask about the fruits and vegetables that you usually eat. I have a nutrition card here that shows you some examples of local fruits and vegetables. Each picture represents the size of a serving. As you answer these questions please think of a typical week in the last year.

D 1a	In a typical week, on how many days do you **eat fruit**? *USE SHOWCARD*	Number of days	☐☐	*If Zero days, go to D 2a*
D 1b	How many **servings** of fruit do you eat on **one** of those days? *USE SHOWCARD*	Number of servings	☐☐	
D 2a	In a typical week, on how many days do you **eat vegetables**? *USE SHOWCARD*	Number of days	☐☐	*If Zero days, go to Section P*
D 2b	How many **servings** of vegetables do you eat on one of those days? *USE SHOWCARD*	Number of servings	☐☐	

EXPANDED: Diet

D 3	What type of **oil or fat is most often** used for meal preparation in your household? *USE SHOWCARD* *SELECT ONLY ONE* ☐☐☐☐☐☐☐	Vegetable oil — 0 1 Lard or suet — 0 2 Butter or ghee — 0 3 Margarine — 0 4 ◄—— Other — 0 5 None in particular — 0 6 None used — 0 7 Don't know — 7 7	☐☐	

Respondent Identification Number

CORE   Physical Activity (Section P)

Next I am going to ask you about the time you spend doing different types of physical activity. Please answer these questions even if you do not consider yourself to be an active person.

Think first about the time you spend doing work. Think of work as the things that you have to do such as paid or unpaid work, household chores, harvesting food, fishing or hunting for food, seeking employment. *[Insert other examples if needed]*

P 1	Does your work involve mostly sitting or standing, with walking for no more than 10 minutes at a time?	Yes 1 No 2		☐	*If Yes, go to P6*
P 2	Does your work involve vigorous activity, like *[heavy lifting, digging or construction work]* for at least 10 minutes at a time? *INSERT EXAMPLES & USE SHOWCARD*	Yes 1 No 2		☐	*If No, go to P4*
P 3a	In a typical week, on how many days do you do vigorous activities as part of your work?	Days a week		☐☐	
P 3b	On a typical day on which you do vigorous activity, how much time do you spend doing such work?	In hours and minutes hrs ☐☐ : mins ☐☐ OR in Minutes only or minutes ☐☐☐			
P 4	Does your work involve moderate-intensity activity, like brisk walking *[or carrying light loads]* for at least 10 minutes at a time? *INSERT EXAMPLES & USE SHOWCARD*	Yes 1 No 2		☐	*If No, go to P6*
P 5a	In a typical week, on how many days do you do moderate-intensity activities as part of your work?	Days a week		☐☐	
P 5b	On a typical day on which you did moderate-intensity activities, how much time do you spend doing such work?	In hours and minutes hrs ☐☐ : mins ☐☐ OR in Minutes only or minutes ☐☐☐			
P 6	How long is your typical work day?	Number of hours hrs ☐☐			

Other than activities that you've already mentioned, I would like to ask you about the way you travel to and from places. For example to work, for shopping, to market, to church. *[insert other examples if needed]*

P 7	Do you walk or use a bicycle (*pedal cycle*) for at least 10 minutes continuously to get to and from places?	Yes 1 No 2		☐	*If No, go to P9*
P 8a	In a typical week, on how many days do you walk or bicycle for at least 10 minutes to get to and from places?	Days a week		☐☐	
P 8b	How much time would you spend walking or bicycling for travel on a typical day?	In hours and minutes hrs ☐☐ : mins ☐☐ OR in Minutes only or minutes ☐☐☐			

The next questions ask about activities you do in your leisure time. Think about activities you do for recreation, fitness or sports *[insert relevant terms]*.   Do not include the physical activities you do at work or for travel mentioned already.

P 9	Does your *[recreation, sport or leisure time]* involve mostly sitting, reclining, or standing, with no physical activity lasting more than 10 minutes at a time?	Yes 1 No 2		☐	*If Yes, go to P 14*
P 10	In your *[leisure time]*, do you do any vigorous activities like *[running or strenuous sports, weight lifting]* for at least 10 minutes at a time? *INSERT EXAMPLES & USE SHOWCARD*	Yes 1 No 2		☐	*If No, go to P 12*
P 11a	If Yes, In a typical week, on how many days do you do vigorous activities as part of your *[leisure time]*?	Days a week		☐☐	
P 11b	How much time do you spend doing this on a typical day?	In hours and minutes hrs ☐☐ : mins ☐☐ OR in Minutes only or minutes ☐☐☐			

Respondent Identification Number ☐☐ ☐☐ ☐☐

P 12	In your [*leisure time*], do you do any moderate-intensity activities like brisk walking,[*cycling or swimming*] for at least 10 minutes at a time? *INSERT EXAMPLES & USE SHOWCARD*	Yes 1 No 2	☐	*If No, go to P 14*
P 13a	<u>If Yes</u> In a typical week, on how many days do you do moderate-intensity activities as part of [*leisure time*]?	Days a week	☐☐	
P 13b	How much time do you spend doing this on a typical day?	In hours and minutes OR in Minutes only	hrs ☐☐ : mins ☐☐ or minutes ☐☐☐	

The following question is about sitting or reclining. Think back over the past 7 days, to time spent at work, at home, in [*leisure*], including time spent sitting at a desk, visiting friends, reading, or watching television, but do not include time spent sleeping.

P 14	Over the past 7 days, how much time did you spend sitting or reclining on a typical day?	In hours and minutes OR in Minutes only	hrs ☐☐ : mins ☐☐ or minutes ☐☐☐	

Respondent Identification Number ☐☐ ☐☐ ☐☐

EXPANDED : History of High Blood Pressure

H 1	When was your blood pressure last measured by a health professional?	Within past 12 months — 1 1-5 years ago — 2 Not within past 5 yrs — 3	☐	
H 2	During the past 12 months have you been told by a doctor or other health worker that you have elevated blood pressure or hypertension?	Yes — 1 No — 2	☐	*If No, skip to Next Section*
H 3	Are you currently receiving any of the following treatments for high blood pressure prescribed by a doctor or other health worker?			
H 3a	Drugs (medication) that you have taken in the last 2 weeks	Yes — 1 No — 2	☐	
H 3b	Special prescribed diet	Yes — 1 No — 2	☐	
H 3c	Advice or treatment to lose weight	Yes — 1 No — 2	☐	
H 3d	Advice or treatment to stop smoking	Yes — 1 No — 2	☐	
H 3e	Advice to start or do more exercise	Yes — 1 No — 2	☐	
H 4	During the past 12 months have you seen a traditional healer for elevated blood pressure or hypertension	Yes — 1 No — 2	☐	
H 5	Are you currently taking any herbal or traditional remedy for your high blood pressure?	Yes — 1 No — 2	☐	

EXPANDED : History of Diabetes

H 6	Have you had your blood sugar measured in the last 12 months?	Yes — 1 No — 2	☐	
H 7	During the past 12 months, have you ever been told by a doctor or other health worker that you have diabetes?	Yes — 1 No — 2	☐	*If No, skip to Next Section*
H 8	Are you currently receiving any of the following treatments for diabetes prescribed by a doctor or other health worker?			
H 8a	Insulin	Yes — 1 No — 2	☐	
H 8b	Oral drug (medication that you have taken in the last 2 weeks	Yes — 1 No — 2	☐	
H 8c	Special prescribed diet	Yes — 1 No — 2	☐	
H 8d	Advice or treatment to lose weight	Yes — 1 No — 2	☐	
H 8e	Advice or treatment to stop smoking	Yes — 1 No — 2	☐	
H 8f	Advice to start or do more exercise	Yes — 1 No — 2	☐	
H 9	During the past 12 months have you seen a traditional healer for diabetes?	Yes — 1 No — 2	☐	
H 10	Are you currently taking any herbal or traditional remedy for your diabetes?	Yes — 1 No — 2	☐	

Respondent Identification Number ☐☐ ☐☐ ☐☐

Step 2   Physical Measurements

Height and weight | Coding Column

M 1	Technician ID Code		☐☐☐
M 2a & 2b	Device IDs for height and weight	(2a) height ☐☐ (2b) weight ☐☐	
M 3	Height	(in Centimetres)	☐☐☐.☐
M 4	Weight *If too large for scale, code 666.6*	(in Kilograms)	☐☐☐.☐
M 5	*(For women)* Are you pregnant?	Yes 1 No 2	☐ *If Yes, Skip Waist*

Waist

M 6	Technician ID		☐☐☐
M 7	Device ID for waist		☐☐
M 8	Waist circumference	(in Centimetres)	☐☐☐.☐

Blood pressure | Coding Column

M 9	Technician ID			☐☐☐
M 10	Device ID for blood pressure			☐☐
M 11	Cuff size used	Small 1 Normal 2 Large 3		☐
M 12a	Reading 1	**Systolic BP**	Systolic mmHg	☐☐☐
M 12b		**Diastolic BP**	Diastolic mmHg	☐☐☐
M 13a	Reading 2	**Systolic BP**	Systolic mmHg	☐☐☐
M 13b		**Diastolic BP**	Diastolic mmHg	☐☐☐
M 14a	Reading 3	**Systolic BP**	Systolic mmHg	☐☐☐
M 14b		**Diastolic BP**	Diastolic mmHg	☐☐☐
M 15	During the past two weeks, have you been treated for high blood pressure with drugs (medication) prescribed by a doctor or other health worker ?	Yes 1 No 2		☐

SELECTED EXPANDED ITEMS

M 16	Hip circumference	(in Centimetres)	☐☐☐.☐

Heart Rate (Record if automatic blood pressure device is used)

M 17a	Reading 1	Beats per minute:	☐☐☐
M 17b	Reading 2	Beats per minute:	☐☐☐
M 17c	Reading 3	Beats per minute:	☐☐☐

Respondent Identification Number □□ □□ □□

Step 3   Biochemical Measurements

CORE	Blood glucose		Coding Column
B 1	During the last 12 hours have you had anything to eat or drink, other than water?	Yes 1 No 2	□
B 2	Technician ID Code		□□□
B 3	Device ID code		□□
B 4	Time of day blood specimen taken (24 hour clock)		hrs □□ : mins □□
B 5	Blood glucose		mmol/l □□.□
		Low 1 High 2 Unable to assess 3	□

CORE	Blood Lipids		
B 6	Technician ID Code		□□□
B 7	Device ID code		□□
B 8	Total cholesterol		mmol/l □□.□□
		Low 1 High 2 Unable to assess 3	□

SELECTED EXPANDED ITEMS			
B 9	Technician ID Code		□□□
B 10	Device ID code		□□
B 11	Triglycerides		mmol/l □□.□□
		Low 1 High 2 Unable to assess 3	□
B 12	Technician ID Code		□□□
B 13	Device ID code		□□
B 14	HDL Cholesterol		mmol/l □.□□
		Low 1 High 2 Unable to assess 3	□

ANNEX 2

Question-by-question instruction guide for tobacco section

1.1 Step 1 – Questionnaire (self-reporting)

> The purpose of the question-by-question instruction guide is to provide background information to the interviewers as to what is intended by each question.
>
> Interviewers can use this information when respondents request clarification about specific questions and they do not know the answer. Interviewers and supervisors should refrain from offering their own interpretations.
>
> Questions are in bold. Responses to both the core and expanded questions are provided.

1.1.1 CORE – Tobacco use

Smoking is the main way tobacco is used worldwide and the manufactured, filter-tipped cigarette is becoming increasingly dominant as the major tobacco product. Other forms of smoked tobacco are potentially as dangerous, although the adverse consequences of some of them are more limited because the smoke is not usually inhaled. In certain cultures tobacco is chewed, sucked or inhaled with significant adverse effects on the local tissues. Nonetheless, because of the major health effects associated with the smoking of tobacco, only this form of tobacco use is included in the core questionnaire.

The smoking-related questions recommended for the STEPS approach are based on the WHO definition found in *Guidelines for controlling and monitoring the tobacco epidemic (2).*

The questions below ask about current smoking or use of any tobacco products, as well as with duration and quantity of daily smoking.

S 1a **Do you currently smoke any tobacco products, such as cigarettes, cigars or pipes?**
Think of any tobacco products the respondent is smoking and/or using currently. Each country will have updated Annex 1, Section S, by adding the tobacco products that are specific to that country.

S 1b <u>If Yes,</u> **Do you currently smoke tobacco products daily?**
This question is for daily smokers/users of tobacco products only.

S 2a **How old were you when you first started smoking daily?**
This question is for daily smokers/users of tobacco products only.

Think of the time when the respondent started to smoke or use any tobacco products daily.

S 2b Do you remember how long ago it was?

This question is for daily smokers/users of tobacco products only. If the respondent does not remember his/her age, then record the time duration in weeks, months or years as appropriate.

S 3 On average, how many of the following do you smoke each day?

Use tobacco products listed in Section S page 25 and specify the number of each tobacco product the respondent is smoking and/or using each day.

Specify zero if no products were used in each category instead of leaving categories blank.

1.1.2 Expanded – Tobacco use

S 4 In the past, did you ever smoke daily?

Think of the time when the respondent may have been smoking and/or using tobacco products on a daily basis.

S 5a <u>If Yes,</u>

How old were you when you stopped smoking daily?

Think of the time when the respondent stopped smoking or used any tobacco products on a daily basis.

S 5b How long ago did you stop smoking daily?

If the respondent does not remember his/her age, then record the time duration in weeks, months or years as appropriate.

S 6a Do you currently use any smokeless tobacco such as [snuff, chewing tobacco, betel]?

Smokeless tobacco occurs in some cultures.

S 6b <u>If Yes,</u>

Do you currently use smokeless tobacco products daily?

This question is for daily users of smokeless tobacco products only.

S 7 On average, how many times a day do you use…

Record for each type of smokeless tobacco products.

S8 In the past, did you ever use smokeless tobacco such as [snuff, chewing tobacco, or betel] daily?

Record the appropriate response.

1.1.3 List of tobacco products*

Section S; Q S1a to S8 (including core and expanded)

- Cigarettes
- Cigarillos
- Cigars
- Cheroots
- Chuttas
- Bidis
- Goza / Hookah
- Local tobacco products (each country to add to the list)
- Local tobacco products (each country to add to the list)
- Local tobacco products (each country to add to the list)

* Countries can add photos and illustrations as appropriate

16

Research and exchange of information

As a general rule, the most successful man in life is the man who has the best information.
—Benjamin Disraeli

INTRODUCTION

Today, there is general and scientific agreement that tobacco use is dangerous to human health. Despite this consensus, tobacco use remains socially acceptable in many parts of the world, highlighting the tobacco industry's success in promoting a hazardous product. The ability to reduce the global burden of mortality and morbidity from tobacco-related illnesses necessitates that every person recognizes the hazards of tobacco use and the deceptive nature of the tobacco industry. This requires the application of a systematic means of gathering information on the harms of tobacco and the tobacco industry's strategies to promote a dangerous product. It also demands a strategic use of mechanisms to disseminate scientific information to the general public.

FROM HYPOTHESIS TO POLICY

Lessons learned from the history of tobacco control

Carrying out systematic research and translating the information gathered into public information is essential to convince individuals, communities and governments to take action to reduce tobacco consumption. A mechanism to communicate the evidence for tobacco control will help facilitate the movement to control the tobacco epidemic.

Sound public health policies often arise in response to health hazards uncovered by research. To illustrate, how did an early hypothesis that smoking caused lung cancer lead to the creation of a policy that required the tobacco industry to include a health warning on all cigarette packs in the United States by 1967? In 1939, less than

---

Box 1. Lung cancer research and tobacco control policy

1939 Franz Muller observes dose–response relationship between smoking and the development of lung cancer.

Early 1950s Morton Levin publishes a study in the *Journal of the American Medical Association* linking smoking and cancer; Ernst L Wynder and Evarts A Graham also publish a study in the Journal of the American Medical Association showing that 96.5% of lung cancer patients interviewed were smokers.

1954 Sir Richard Doll and Bradford Hill publish their finding in *The British Medical Journal* that heavy smokers are 50 times more likely to get lung cancer.

1964 The United States Surgeon General's Report concludes that smoking is a health hazard requiring action.

1967 The first tobacco control policies in the United States are established, based on the strength of the evidence from the above studies.

30 years before the policy was made, health warnings on tobacco and cancer were published in the book *The Nazi War on Cancer (1)*.

In it Franz Hermann Muller of Germany observed a strong dose–response relationship between smoking and lung cancer. The 'hypothesis' was further supported by three key case control studies in the 1950s. Two studies were published in the *Journal of the American Medical Association*; one by Morton Levin linking smoking and cancer and the other by Ernst L Wynder and Evarts A Graham showing that 96.5% of lung cancer patients interviewed were smokers *(2, 3)*. In 1954, more evidence appeared when Sir Richard Doll and Bradford Hill published in *The British Medical Journal* their finding that heavy smokers are 50 times more likely to get lung cancer *(4)*. In 1964, after evaluating the existing evidence, the United States Surgeon General's Report, concluded that cigarette smoking is:

- a cause of lung cancer and laryngeal cancer in men;
- a probable cause of lung cancer in women;
- the most important cause of chronic bronchitis;
- a health hazard of sufficient importance to warrant appropriate remedial action.

This pivotal Surgeon General's Report provided the data on which the first public health policies were based to address tobacco use in the United States. It illustrated how a hypothesis supported by scientific research, and strengthened by publication and information dissemi-

> *"...I am going to start by asking you to face certain facts, certain vital statistics... The vital statistics I would like you to bear in mind are 7, 57, 139 and 227... They are the death rates per 100,000 per year from cancer of the lung of men who were non-smokers (they are the 7), men who smoked 1–14 cigarettes daily (they are the 57), men who smoked 15–24 cigarettes daily (they are the 139) and men who smoked 25 or more cigarettes daily (they are the 227)... Those vital statistics are basically the reason why we are here tonight... These vital statistics are really vital. They threaten the life of the tobacco industry in every country of the world."*
>
> —Confidential Philip Morris memo, 1969
> The Present Position: Main Evidence Against Smoking

Box 2. The case against second-hand smoke

1986   The National Research Council of the United States publishes a key report on the hazards from second-hand smoke entitled *Environmental Tobacco Smoke: Measuring Exposures and Assessing Health Effects*.

1986   IARC publishes *Evaluation of Carcinogenic Risks of Chemical Smoke: Tobacco Smoking (Vol. 38)*, reinforcing the case against second-hand smoke.

1993   The United States Environmental Protection Agency classifies second-hand smoke as a 'Class A', or definite human, carcinogen.

late 1990s   The first public policy banning smoking in public places goes into effect in several states of the United States.

"• **Delay the progress and/or release of the study.**

• **Affect the wording of its conclusions and official statement of results.**

• **Neutralize possible negative results of the study, particularly as a regulatory tool.**

• **Counteract the potential impact of the study on governmental policy, public opinion, and actions by private employers and proprietors.**"

—From a Philip Morris memo in 1993, identifying the aims of a multi-million dollar campaign to undermine the IARC study on second-hand smoke. Campaign for Tobacco-Free Kids, *Trust Us We're the Tobacco Industry*, 2001. Bates No. 2501341817-23

nation can drive policy-makers into action (this example is summarized in Box 1) *(5)*.

How did the cigarette industry react to the mounting evidence against smoking? A confidential Philip Morris Memo showed that as early as 1969 the industry recognized the power of research.

A second example of how research can drive public policy involves second-hand smoke (summarized in Box 2). In 1986, the National Research Council of the United States published a key report on the hazards from second-hand smoke entitled *Environmental Tobacco Smoke: Measuring Exposures and Assessing Health Effects (6)*.

The evidence against second-hand smoke was reinforced in the IARC monograph, *Evaluation of Carcinogenic Risk of Chemical Smoke: Tobacco Smoking.* In 1993, the United States Environmental Protection Agency (EPA) classified second-hand smoke as a 'Class A', or a definite human carcinogen. As a result of these and other similar studies, several governments established legislation to ban smoking in public places to protect non-smokers from the deleterious effects of second-hand smoke.

In response, the tobacco industry launched a systematic effort to discredit scientific information on second-hand smoke. Tobacco control researchers concluded that the effort launched across the tobacco industry against one scientific study – the largest European study by IARC showing a 16% increase in the point estimate of risk for lung cancer for non-smokers – was "massive" and "remarkable" *(7)*. Today, the industry continues to conduct a sophisticated campaign against studies that conclude that second-hand smoke causes lung cancer and other diseases in non-smokers, to subvert the normal scientific process and to retard or prevent effective tobacco control policies from being developed and implemented in countries *(8)*.

RESEARCH AND INFORMATION EXCHANGE FOR TOBACCO CONTROL AND THE WHO FCTC

The WHO FCTC provides guidance on surveillance, research and exchange of information on tobacco control. It encourages countries to direct attention towards:

• establishing a national system for the epidemiological surveillance of tobacco consumption, periodically updating economic and health indicators to monitor the evolution of the problem and the impact of tobacco control;

- facilitating regional and global tobacco surveillance and exchange of information on tobacco control indicators by:
  - initiating and cooperating directly, or through competent international bodies, in the conduct of research and of scientific assessment;
  - promoting, supporting and encouraging research that contributes to reducing tobacco consumption and harm from tobacco use, particularly in developing countries.
- facilitating the full, open and prompt exchange of scientific, technical, socioeconomic, commercial and legal information, as well as information on practices of the tobacco industry, by:
  - compiling and maintaining a database of national and subnational laws and regulations on tobacco control and enforcement, and cooperating in developing complementary programmes for national, regional and global tobacco control;
  - compiling and maintaining a central database of information from national surveillance programmes;
  - strengthening training and support for all those engaged in tobacco control activities, including research, implementation and evaluation.

The global agenda for tobacco control research

Back in 1999, researchers and policy-makers from developing countries, international donors, and research bodies with global mandates recognized the need for a global agenda for tobacco control research. Participants gathered at the meeting on Global Research Priorities for Tobacco Control, co-hosted by Research for International Tobacco Control (RITC) and WHO in Washington, DC, in March 1999, and at the Global Forum for Health Research in Geneva, Switzerland, in June 1999.

At these two meetings, experts in tobacco control research agreed that tobacco control policies and programmes must be based on strong scientific evidence to achieve progress in controlling the tobacco epidemic. They concluded that a serious and concerted effort to strengthen tobacco control research is urgently needed. This would require:
- advocacy for investment in research;
- building sustainable capacity in developing countries;
- targeting select priority themes;
- establishing appropriate institutional arrangements to move research forward.

The priority themes were identified and are listed in Boxes 4 and 5 (see also Box 3 for information on work done by RITC/IDRC and WHO in the area of tobacco control research). These form the core of the global research agenda recommended by WHO and its partners. Some of the themes relate to country- and region-specific issues, while others are broader in scope and have the potential to affect international policies and practices. The development of common research instruments and methodologies would facilitate data-gathering and allow for cross-country comparisons.

**Box 3. WHO and Research for International Tobacco Control/
International Development Research Centre (RITC/IDRC)**

In 1998–1999, Research for International Tobacco Control (RITC), a multidonor Secretariat housed at the International Development Research Centre (IDRC) in Ottawa, Canada, conducted a series of regional consultations to guide the formulation of tobacco control research agendas in developing countries. The meetings involved participants from Latin America and the Caribbean, South and South-East Asia, and eastern, central and southern Africa.

Following these regional meetings, RITC was asked to act as a convener in preparing a draft document outlining global tobacco control research priorities. The resulting document was endorsed by the Global Forum for Health Research in June 1999 and published jointly by RITC and the WHO Tobacco Free Initiative under the title *Confronting the epidemic: a global agenda for tobacco control research.*

The research priorities identified in the global agenda parallel many of the provisions of WHO FCTC and, as such, establish a framework for an evidence base to support signature, ratification and implementation of the global treaty. Research needs to address both demand for and supply of tobacco are outlined. The need for country-specific research that is compelling and relevant to legislators in individual countries is specified.

The global agenda also identifies dissemination as a key aspect of tobacco control research. Tobacco control research in developing countries is critical as the evidence base for the development of sound policies and programmes. RITC-funded projects are required to include a dissemination component that outlines strategies for knowledge transfer within the scientific community, and also considers the preparation of policy briefs and other modalities to inform decision-makers and media or advocacy strategies to improve public awareness of issues related to tobacco control. Effective knowledge transfer requires an understanding of the political processes that shape policy decisions and the interplay of various stakeholders in influencing the legislative agenda. *Tobacco Control Policy: Strategies, Successes and Setbacks (9),* contains narratives from six countries around the world: Bangladesh, Brazil, Canada, Poland, South Africa and Thailand. Each country has successfully introduced tobacco control legislation. The strategies and struggles that led to the passage of legislation are documented in order to inform and inspire other countries.

Box 4. Global Agenda for Tobacco Control Research: critical themes

Country-specific research

The lack of standardized and comparable data is a recurrent theme. Surveillance systems should capture country and regional data on:

- tobacco use prevalence and consumption patterns (particularly among young people and health professionals);
- trends in tobacco-attributable morbidity and mortality;
- awareness levels of the health risks associated with tobacco use among different segments of the population;
- pricing policies, backed by country and segment-specific elasticity studies to determine the impact of taxation on tobacco control;
- behaviours and attitudes related to tobacco control measures, to understand how social norms are formed and transmitted and to allow cross-cultural comparisons of regional and cultural differences in the acceptability of tobacco use.

Policy interventions

Research is crucial to determine the impact of tobacco control policies objectively, such as raising prices through increased taxation, instituting policies for smoke-free public places, restricting tobacco marketing, advertising and promotion, and restricting young people's access to tobacco. Specific research areas include:

- Economic research
- elasticity-of-demand studies to determine optimal levels of taxation according to social class, age and geographical conditions;
- the determinants, process and impact of illegal trafficking, and the influence of smuggling on tobacco use;
- opportunities for and barriers to the harmonization of prices at regional level.

- Legislative research
- effect of international trade agreements on production, trade and marketing of tobacco products;
- empirical and theoretical research to assist in drafting, implementing and evaluating policies, including advertising bans.

Programme interventions

The global research agenda should be grounded in a comprehensive public health model of nicotine addiction that encompasses environment, agent, host and vector. Areas that require scientific scrutiny include:

- opportunities for and barriers to tobacco control;
- optimal components (programmes and policies) of a comprehensive tobacco control strategy;
- communications research on the development of effective messages to counter tobacco industry promotions;
- behavioural research to evaluate the efficacy of prevention and treatment programmes;
- sociocultural studies to determine the cultural acceptability of specific interventions and to elucidate differences in responsiveness among ethnic and cultural groups;
- development and evaluation of novel approaches to preventing tobacco use, especially among populations at disproportionate risk;
- assessment of the relative effectiveness and consequences of prevention interventions that employ single-risk strategies versus multiple-risk strategies.

Treatment of tobacco dependence

Two broad research fields are of particular importance:

- examination of a range of approaches to increase cessation rates in different populations;
- evaluation of new pharmaceutical interventions and delivery mechanisms, their costeffectiveness, and their impact in diverse sociocultural, physiological and genetic subgroups.

Tobacco product design and regulation

Product modification (in nicotine/tar content, delivery system, additives, taste, size, etc.) to change use patterns and/or reduce harm among various subgroups is another potential research area. The following components are

Continues...

Continued from previous page…

possible research topics:
- the biology of tobacco addiction;
- characterization of additives to tobacco products;
- assessment of alternative labelling for tobacco products;
- evaluation of the public's expectations about tobacco products and people's behaviour with respect to new products;
- formulation of an objective basis for future decisions about nicotine and tar content derived from public health findings.

Tobacco industry analysis

While some research on the tobacco industry will be country-specific, research on the international role of the transnational tobacco companies (TTCs) will also be important:
- characterizing the ownership, corporate structure and regulation of the tobacco industry at both the local and international level, including dominant industry forces, manufacturing practices, alliances and trends in relative market share;
- tobacco and cigarette production as an international and regional trade issue in terms of foreign exchange earnings, employment, country imports and exports, and trafficking;
- political mapping of tobacco industry relationships with governments (including lobbying activities);
- tobacco industry involvement in smuggling activities;
- tobacco industry advertising, marketing and promotion efforts (particularly with respect to women, youth and other high-risk groups), the impact of changes in advertising on consumption, and public perceptions of advertising and promotion by TTCs;
- industry influence on issues related to smoking and addiction (including their influence on the content and direction of research).

Tobacco farming

Many aspects of tobacco cultivation are poorly understood, including occupational hazards, the environmental impact, economic benefits and sociocultural impact (particularly for women and children). Important research topics include:
- the relationship of tobacco production to the destruction of the ecosystem, particularly concerning deforestation, pesticides and degradation of soil nutrients;
- attitudes, beliefs and practices of tobacco farmers and the underlying historical/cultural context;
- the economic impact of tobacco control on developing countries that grow and manufacture tobacco or tobacco products for domestic or foreign markets;
- opportunities for alternative crops and alternative livelihoods: information on crop options for farmers and on employment outside tobacco growing for their children;
- cultivation and curing practices at the country and subnational level;
- occupational health hazards related to cultivating, curing and handling tobacco, including the use of pesticides, herbicides and fertilizers;
- the impact of tobacco cultivation on women and children;
- the feasibility of diversification in countries heavily dependent on tobacco farming and tobacco manufacturing, and mechanisms for supporting these countries in their diversification efforts.

WHO FCTC

Research data from the global agenda outlined above was pivotal in providing technical assistance for the development and implementation of the WHO FCTC. In addition, research is needed for the ratification and implementation of, as well as monitoring and compliance with WHO FCTC. Key areas of study include:
- global political support: mechanisms to secure ratification and implementation;
- structure and design of monitoring mechanisms to be established by the WHO FCTC and related protocols;
- verification of the effectiveness of the Convention.

Box 5. Global Agenda for Tobacco Control Research: cross-cutting themes

Cross-cutting research themes include a number of issues that will need to be taken into consideration in all thematic areas.

High-risk populations (e.g. youth, women, indigenous populations)

- there is a need to identify high-risk segments of the population, e.g. those with high or escalating rates of prevalence, youth as an entry point to tobacco use, others targeted by industry promotions;
- basic biologic and behavioural research needs to be done to understand the sociocultural, psychological, physiological and genetic factors that influence the initiation of tobacco use, progression to nicotine addiction, and smoking cessation among high-risk segments of the population;
- studies should be conducted on the influence of tobacco advertising and promotion, especially in high-risk groups and
- research needs to be done to determine why some high-risk groups are resistant to interventions.

Country readiness

- qualitative and quantitative research should be conducted to assess each region's/country's readiness for tobacco control measures as evidenced by indicators such as knowledge of health effects of tobacco use, support for interventions, and priority given to tobacco control by key opinion leaders, including politicians and health professionals.

Dissemination

- research should be carried out to provide a better understanding of how to translate knowledge into effective practice, particularly in policy development (the research should include knowledge synthesis as well as methods for ensuring the dissemination, adoption, implementation and maintenance of strategies known to be effective);
- mechanisms should be developed for optimal dissemination of proven prevention and treatment interventions through different delivery channels at the local and national level;
- there should be a means of dissemination of the results of research to policy-makers.

Capacity development

- the capacity for tobacco control (including research) should be assessed, especially in areas not directly related to health such as economics and policy analysis;
- researchers and research institutions currently (or with the potential to become) involved in tobacco control research should be identified as well as the needs and activities of current stakeholders in tobacco control initiatives, in order to relate research to policy, programme and practice needs.

Mobilization of human and financial resources

- there should be a concerted mobilization of human and financial resources to implement a comprehensive research agenda, build partnerships and stimulate comparative research and analysis.

CHALLENGES TO EFFECTIVE TOBACCO CONTROL RESEARCH

While research plays a critical role in guiding public policy to control tobacco use, it remains an underdeveloped area in some countries. Capacity and resources remain limited, and are often concentrated within some developed countries and selected developing countries – such as China, India, South Africa and Thailand – that are already advancing faster than the rest of the global community with regards to tobacco control policies and programmes. In 1990, it was estimated that approximately US$ 148–164 million were allocated to global tobacco control research and development. This represented an expenditure of only US$ 4.31 per disability adjusted life year lost *(10)*. Most of this funding supported research activities predominantly in developed countries, making the findings and recommendations only partially relevant to the socioeconomic and political climate in many developing countries. Furthermore, the majority of global funding is directed toward health-related research rather than multidisciplinary, policy-oriented tobacco control research that is crucial for developing effective interventions to curb tobacco use.

Four major challenges to effective tobacco control research in developing countries were identified during the series of meetings conducted by RITC/IDRC and WHO in 1999 *(11)*.

1. The lack of standardized and comparable data. There is a clear need for regional surveillance systems and research to provide comparable baseline data on: the prevalence of tobacco use; consumption patterns and trends; patterns of and trends in tobacco-attributable morbidity and mortality; existing policies and programmes; and ongoing and completed research initiatives. While a certain amount of material exists, databases of this nature are costly to maintain. What is especially needed is detailed information broken down by sex, age group, populations at risk and regions and provinces.

2. The absence of a network for communication of information, data and best practices. While many of the electronic networks have contributed positively to the discussion of tobacco control, they are not universally accessible in the developing world. Having accessible communications networks would promote the efficient dissemination of research findings, and assist in harmonizing research efforts by facilitating collaboration and partnership across countries and regions.

3. Lack of adequate capacity for tobacco control research, especially in non-health-related areas such as economics and policy analysis. The current and potential socioeconomic burden of tobacco production and consumption underscores the need to bolster research capacity in developing countries. A scarcity of skills and competence for multidisciplinary and policy research is compounded by the failure of donor agencies to be proactive in funding research on evolving issues.

4. A need for concerted mobilization of human and financial resources in order to implement a comprehensive research agenda, build partnerships and stimulate comparative research and analysis. This is recognized under the WHO FCTC, which calls for countries to work together to augment the resources for tobacco control research and information exchange.

A practical approach to research for developing countries

Establishing a strong research agenda requires strategic planning and commitment. While investments in capacity-building and infrastructure are needed, the costs need not be prohibitive. A pragmatic approach and priority setting are essential. The following guidelines should be given serious consideration.

- Assess current research resources, needs and gaps. If data exist, there may not be a need to spend time and money in developing a new survey or study. Instead, resources should be directed towards locating, collating and analysing existing data to address the needs of the tobacco control programme.

- Set research priorities based on policy needs. Effective research should support and direct the development of public health policy. When choosing research priorities, select areas that address gaps in policy and advocacy. Avoid doing research for research's sake. Because resources are limited, all tobacco control research should lead to improvements in policies or programmes to reduce tobacco consumption. Using this criterion should assist you in eliminating research projects that are redundant, unnecessary or superfluous.

- Partner with scientific and academic institutions. Most countries, no matter how small or underdeveloped, will likely harbour research capacity in the academic setting. By building relationships with these institutions, it is possible to identify local researchers who can assist in developing, implementing and evaluating research projects. Moreover, the equipment and technology needed for research, such as statistical software and other computer applications are usually available in universities and other institutions of higher learning, as well as within the scientific community.

- Integrate a research agenda into the national plan of action. The research agenda should address those areas of the plan of action that require supporting evidence.

- Be quick to identify potential opportunities for collaborative research. Tobacco control cuts across many programme areas in public health as well as other sectors of government. There may be opportunities to 'piggyback' tobacco control research projects into the research agendas of these programmes and sectors. For instance, revenue and tax departments may have the resources to evaluate the impact of cigarette smuggling on the national economy. Research on lifestyle interventions to reduce the mortality from non-communicable diseases could include a component on the cost effectiveness of smoking cessation. Actively search for these potential opportunities to collaborate in generating data for the tobacco control programme.

- Participate in intercountry collaborative research projects. There are also opportunities for collaborative tobacco control research among countries. For example, the South-East Asian Alliance for Tobacco Control and the London School of Tropical Medicine and Hygiene are currently supporting several South-East Asian countries in conducting research on the tobacco industry documents that affect the region.

- When creating the national research agenda, be guided by the Global Agenda for Tobacco Control Research developed under the auspices of WHO and IDRC.

- Integrate research into surveillance and monitoring systems. Most of the data generated by periodic surveillance can be used to answer specific research questions.
- Include a dissemination strategy when planning the research agenda. Information generated by research must be shared and disseminated to the general public for maximum impact. Most researchers frequently neglect this critical aspect. Information that is not made public is often useless, and cannot drive public policy.
- When planning the research agenda:
  - Consider multisectoral areas of research. Include the systematic evaluation and study of economic, media, sociological, cultural and legislative aspects of tobacco control.
  - Make use of all opportunities to obtain data. For instance, obtain data on smoking status during all clinical encounters.
  - Be creative. For example, use village health care workers to obtain data from the field.
  - Use both qualitative and quantitative methods to generate information.
  - Build local capacity.
  - Constantly search for funding opportunities.
  - Link research to the evaluation process.

RESEARCH FOR ADVOCACY

The previous chapter covers the major issues related to establishing surveillance systems to capture fundamental information about tobacco production, consumption and health impacts. However, in addition to these technical research areas, NTCPs also need to carry out research to support advocacy for tobacco control. This is particularly important in developing countries where scarce resources must be utilized efficiently to produce tangible results.

Research for advocacy in tobacco control aims to establish data that will lead to introducing or strengthening laws and policies to reduce tobacco consumption. The research is conducted as part of a comprehensive strategy to establish effective tobacco control interventions. Unlike epidemiological studies or randomized clinical trials, research for advocacy can take several creative forms *(12)*.

- Opinion polls or surveys. These are useful as evidence to policy-makers that the general public supports tobacco control measures. Opinion polls can also identify areas where greater public education and tobacco control advocacy are needed.
- Economics research. The World Bank's publications *Curbing the Epidemic: Governments and the Economics of Tobacco Control (13)* and *Tobacco Control in Developing Countries (14)* provide concrete ideas about economic issues relevant to tobacco control. Local data that demonstrate how tobacco control interventions will not harm a country's revenues, but could, in fact, be beneficial to the economy and underscore the costs of tobacco use to a nation's economy, can persuade politicians to support tobacco control policies and laws.

- Country-specific review of the internal tobacco industry documents. This was discussed in Chapter 13.
- Qualitative research. This type of research uses personal stories and quotes to give a human face to the tobacco epidemic. If used strategically and communicated effectively, information from this type of research can be extremely powerful.

The following are tips and suggestions for developing and conducting tobacco control research for advocacy. Refer to the publication *Low Cost Research for Advocacy* for a more detailed discussion of the topic *(12)*.

- Plan ahead. Develop a research agenda that complements and is consistent with the aims and objectives of your national plan of action for tobacco control. Base specific research activities according to your national needs. In addition, determine how you will use the information gathered by the research activities to achieve the expected outcomes of the national plan of action. In particular, have a strategy for disseminating the results of research activities to the appropriate target audiences.
- Obtain the appropriate technical expertise when designing and conducting policy-oriented research projects. Depending on the nature of the research activity, you may need to consult experts in quantitative or qualitative study design and statistics. Seek the assistance of experts outside of the health sciences, particularly when doing qualitative studies. Colleagues in the social sciences, marketing research and anthropology may be particularly helpful.
- Be guided by previous work, if at all possible. There is a growing body of published and online research for tobacco control done in both developed and developing countries that provides information and tips on research topics and methodologies. Furthermore, research techniques used in marketing may be applicable for advocacy-related tobacco control studies. Avoid reinventing the wheel and adapt existing data, methods and research instruments, if at all possible. This saves resources, time and effort.
- Communicate results strategically. Findings should be framed to address the policy issue driving the research directly. When presenting the results of your research, keep your message focused on the relevant issues and ensure that you reach your intended target audiences directly, usually the media and political decision-makers. (See Chapter 8 for tips on effective communication.)
- Use the information to pursue specific policy initiatives. The ultimate gauge of success in research for advocacy is whether or not the findings contributed to a definitive change in the policy or legislative environment for tobacco control.

UNDERSTANDING THE MECHANISMS
FOR INFORMATION EXCHANGE

The timely exchange of information is a vital component of an effective research strategy for policy change. In countries where the tobacco control programme is newly established, understanding the evidence related to tobacco control and linking the evidence to the formulation of effective policies will depend largely on access to information from local, regional and global counterparts. In general, published articles represent the tip of the information triangle (see Figure 1). This means that those interested in tobacco control, including NTCP, must have access to journals or databases. In some developing countries where resources are limited, access to subscriptions may be costly. However, some journals, such as *Tobacco Control*, provide free electronic access to journal articles for citizens of developing countries *(15)*. The broad base of the triangle may include important research information or databases that have not been published. This creates an important need for developing a registry of tobacco research to provide easily accessible information and feedback.

The following are possible barriers to tobacco information exchange in developing countries that may contribute to the paucity of published research:

- Research
  - lack of funding
  - limited technical support and available training
  - few tutors or mentors
- Publication
  - English language may be an obstacle for some

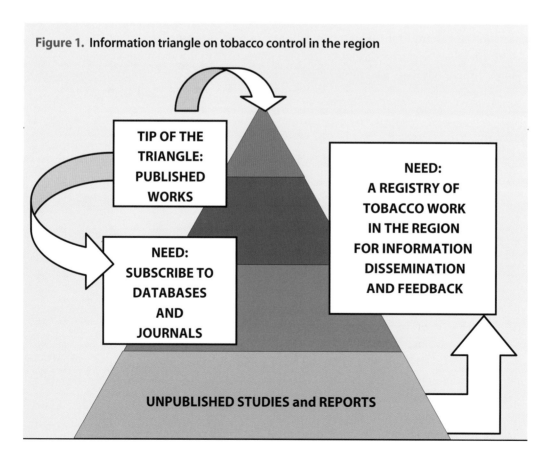

Figure 1. Information triangle on tobacco control in the region

TIP OF THE TRIANGLE: PUBLISHED WORKS

NEED: A REGISTRY OF TOBACCO WORK IN THE REGION FOR INFORMATION DISSEMINATION AND FEEDBACK

NEED: SUBSCRIBE TO DATABASES AND JOURNALS

UNPUBLISHED STUDIES and REPORTS

– uncertainty about journal options
 – other needs/advocacy concerns compete for writing time
- Information access
 – poor working facilities
 – erratic communication
 – no Internet access
- Political constraints
 – government-supported tobacco industries
 – desire to deflate/inflate statistics showing tobacco toll
 – competing health priorities.

Access to tobacco control information is vital to support existing tobacco control programmes. Information empowers; ideally, there must be a flow of information between developed and developing countries to ensure a better future for tobacco control research, and to enhance the probability that scientific information will lead to beneficial health policies. Electronic media may help to narrow the information gap between developed and developing countries, even if building up information communication technology (ICT) of lower-income countries may be slow at the beginning. There is reason to expect that access to the World Wide Web will increase tremendously in the next few years. Ideally, information must flow both ways, because there are insights and lessons to be learned from the experience in the developing world. Tapping the Internet may improve information flow in all directions as countries and regions are establishing free networks for the exchange of tobacco control information.

Models for research and information exchange

There are several online discussion groups, mail and news groups and information clearinghouses that national tobacco control officers can join, provided that they have the equipment and Internet access. Three examples are highlighted in Boxes 6, 7 and 8.

Setting up a clearinghouse for tobacco control information

Countries in other parts of the world that share geopolitical boundaries and/or cultural traditions may want to set up a clearinghouse for tobacco information that specifically addresses their needs. Provided the technical expertise and financial resources are sufficient, it is possible to accomplish this. The basic steps for creating an online clearinghouse for tobacco control are listed in Box 9.

 The clearinghouse should use reference sources classified as preprimary, primary, secondary and tertiary. Human resources may include people from government, NGOs, academic institutions and private organizations. A system must be developed for indexing, cataloguing and tagging of available resources. A clear description of

Box 6. GLOBALink

Perhaps the best known of the current online tobacco control communities is the International Union Against Cancer's (UICC) GLOBALink *(16)*. GLOBALink serves over 3900 members in 133 countries around the world (as of December 2003). The site provides tobacco control professionals – including advocates, educators, lawyers, policy-makers, researchers, smoking-cessation specialists – opportunities to network, to exchange ideas and obtain information.

GLOBALink allows its members to search for the latest, most accurate information and analysis on tobacco control, by enabling them to exchange information with top tobacco control professionals and to access specific research including publications, guidelines and reports.

In addition to providing information and network facilitation, GLOBALink offers a wide range of additional services:

- petitions, campaign coordination (petitions.globalink.org);
- calendars, directories, databases;
- access to other tobacco control links (www.tobaccopedia.org);
- custom search-engines for tobacco industry documents;
- free web hosting (www.localink.org) – GLOBALink currently hosts more than 150 tobacco-control web sites including the well-known site Tob*Info* (www.tobinfo.org) for countries in central and eastern Europe and newly independent states (in English and Russian);
- distance learning (www.tobaccoAcademy.org).

GLOBALink is evolving with the needs of its membership. Because there is a real need for partnerships in the tobacco control scientific community, *GLOBALink Research* was launched in early 2003. *GLOBALink Research* provides research information and discussion groups and will be serving as the core system for the Global Tobacco Research Network, a project of Johns Hopkins University.

GLOBALink's efforts to bring together tobacco control communities earned it several awards, including the prestigious Luther Terry Award in the category of Outstanding Tobacco Control Organization (2003), and the WHO Tobacco or Health Medal (1997).

Source: *(17)*

Box 7. International Agency on Tobacco or Health (IATH)

IATH is a unique public health charity registered in the United Kingdom, dedicated to supporting tobacco control advocates in countries with fewer resources. For most of the organizations that IATH serves, lack of funds, especially hard currency, prohibits access to vital communications taken for granted by colleagues in the industrialized world: international conferences, computer access to the Internet and e-mail, even subscriptions to scientific journals, are simply beyond their means. IATH's monthly mailing – its news bulletin and other useful materials – ensures that they are up-to-date on all major areas of tobacco control, and its ad hoc advice service helps them with specific problems. IATH also carries out a range of other work aimed at reducing the burden of disease caused by tobacco, including policy consultancy, training, lecturing and writing.

The core of IATH's information service is a monthly mailing to all its contacts. The main item in the mailing is a news bulletin covering scientific developments, news of the latest tobacco control legislation, new marketing tactics by the industry, legal initiatives, cessation developments and other important news from all over the world.

Continues…

Continued from previous page…

In addition to the bulletin, the mailing includes various materials of significant value to national tobacco control agencies: e.g. fact sheets on tobacco and specific diseases; policy notes on individual aspects of tobacco control policy; cessation notes; and tobacco control literature, posters and other educational materials.

IATH also provides an ad hoc advice service for its contacts. Typical requests concern local opportunities for legislation and other policy changes; and how to counter specific marketing ploys and lobbying tactics of the tobacco industry. In responding to such requests, IATH is able to draw on a wide range of information and an extensive network of colleagues around the world to provide practical help and advice.

IATH provides its main services free of charge to selected contact agencies. These include government health agencies, NGOs such as cancer, heart and chest disease societies and consumer organizations, as well as dedicated anti-tobacco groups. As of August 2003, IATH was serving 265 contact agencies in 118 countries.

Source: *(18)*

Box 8. The Clearinghouse for Tobacco Control

The Clearinghouse for Tobacco (C-TOB), developed with a grant from the Rockefeller Foundation by the National Poison Centre, Universiti Sains Malaysia (USM), is an Internet web site *(19)* that makes evidence-based tobacco literature and related abstract, summary and comparison materials widely available to healthcare professionals, NTCP officers, tobacco control advocates and the public. C-TOB hopes to provide services in different languages to facilitate information exchange with provisions for interactive communication and learning.

C-TOB provides the following services:

- It distributes free or low-cost anti-tobacco materials from a systematic collection of available items on anti-tobacco materials;
- It collects culturally diverse prevention, intervention and treatment resources tailored for use by parents, teachers, youth, communities and prevention/treatment professionals, in a systematic manner;
- It customizes searches in the form of annotated bibliographies from drug and tobacco databases;
- It provides a system of electronic tobacco information exchange among South-East Asian countries in particular and the rest of the world in general;
- It develops and implements an electronic content management system for handling tobacco-related information materials, including fact sheets, brochures, pamphlets, monographs, posters and videotapes;
- It publishes an electronic newsletter providing up-to-date tobacco control literature with articles of particular relevance to developing countries;
- It has established a network of experts and related organizations to support the creation of a systematic data and information centre on tobacco-related activities and research;
- It provides technical support to countries in conceptualizing, planning and implementing tobacco control programmes tailored to their particular needs and situation;
- It coordinates fellowship training programmes in the tobacco control information management.

Box 9. Steps for creating a web-based clearinghouse for tobacco control information

1. Set up a panel of reviewers – local, regional and international:
   - search for relevant documents
   - compile the documents
   - review the documents
   - summarize the contents
   - disseminate the information.
2. Create web-based tobacco research database.
3. Require registration of users with user names and log in passwords.
4. Categorize users:
   - receive queries
   - provide literature retrieval service.
5. Establish and support the virtual community.

---

the form in which they are available (i.e. videotape, audio and text) should be made. Finally, after a systematic review of the material, the information may be released as approved to the target users.

COMMUNICATING THE EVIDENCE FOR TOBACCO CONTROL

Research on tobacco control must communicate the evidence for action to major stakeholders. A mechanism to promote the exchange of tobacco control information to effect change is necessary. There are several venues that can be utilized to ensure that new tobacco-related data are communicated in a timely and effective way to critical audiences. These are discussed in greater detail in Chapter 8.

As an example, C-TOB, together with South-east Asia Tobacco Control Alliance, hosted a workshop entitled Communicating the Evidence for Tobacco Control (20). The workshop provided an avenue for discussion where stakeholders in tobacco control learned about ways that evidence from research can be used to support and promote bans on tobacco marketing. Through the workshop, researchers and tobacco control advocates were trained to communicate research evidence more effectively to policy-makers, the public and civil society. At the same time, policy-makers were introduced to the available evidence and experience in countries with successful tobacco control strategies.

CONCLUSION

For more than three decades, WHO and the Surgeon General of the United States Public Health Service have released reports on the adverse impact of tobacco use on health. The tone and content of these reports have changed over the years. Early on, there was a need for critical review of the epidemiological and biological aspects of tobacco use. Today, the deleterious effects are well documented, and the reports have begun to investigate the social, economic and cultural consequences of these effects and what needs to be done to address them. However, the formidable task of curbing the tobacco epidemic still needs utmost attention and global cooperation. Hopefully, translating research into policy and creating mechanisms for the exchange of information will lessen the guesswork for those who are just beginning their efforts for tobacco control while strengthening the work of those who started much earlier. Despite the obstacles, optimism and persistence must prevail, because the costs of the tobacco epidemic are too high if not addressed.

References

1. Micozzi MS. Book Review on: The Nazi war on cancer. *New England Journal of Medicine*, 1999, 341:380–381.

2. Levin M, Goldstein H, Gerhardt PR. Cancer and Tobacco Smoking. *Journal of the American Medical Association,* 27 May 1950, 336–338.

3. Wynder EL, Graham EA. Tobacco Smoking as a Possible Etiologic Factor in Bronchiogenic Carcinoma: A Study of 684 Proved Cases. *Journal of the American Medical Association.* 27 May 1950, 143:539–542.

4. Doll R, Hill AB. The mortality of doctors in relation to their smoking habits. A preliminary report. *British Medical Journal,* 1954, 228(i):1451–55.

5. *Smoking and Health.* Report of the Advisory Committee to the Surgeon General of the Public Health Service, US Department of Health, Education and Welfare. Public Health Service Publication no. 1103. Washington, DC, 1964.

6. National Research Council. *Environmental Tobacco Smoke: measuring exposures and health effects.* Washington, DC, National Research Council, 1986.

7. International Agency for Research on Cancer. *Passive smoking and lung cancer in Europe.* Lyon: IARC, 1998.

8. Ong EK, Glantz SA. Tobacco industry efforts subverting International Agency for Cancer's second-hand smoke study. *Lancet,* 2000, 355 (9211):1253–1259.

9. Research for International Tobacco Control, *Tobacco control policy: strategies, successes and setbacks.* Washington, DC, The World Bank, 2003.

10. *Investing in health research and development. Report of the ad hoc committee on health research relating to future intervention options.* Geneva, World Health Organization, 1996.

11. Baris E et al. Research priorities for tobacco control in developing countries: a regional approach to a global consultative process. *Tobacco Control,* 2000, 9:217–223.

12. Efroymson D. *PATH Canada Guide: low cost research for advocacy.* Dhaka, Bangladesh, PATH Canada, August 2002 (http://wbb.globalink.org/public/Eng_res_Guide.pdf).

13. *Curbing the epidemic: governments and the economics of tobacco control,* The World Bank Development in Practice series, 1999.

14. Jha P, Chaloupka FJ. *Tobacco Control in Developing Countries.* Oxford, Oxford University Press, 2000.

15. Written communication, Mr Simon Chapman, Editor of *Tobacco Control*, 20 December 2003.

16. Globalink (http://www.globalink.org/).

17. Written communication, Mr Ruben Israel, Globalink, 7 January 2004.

18. Written communication, Mr. David Simpson, Director, International Agency on Tobacco or Health, 7 January 2004.

19. Clearing house for tobacco control. National Poison Centre, Universiti Sains Malaysia, Malaysia (http://www.prn2.usm.my/main.asp).

20. *Communicating the evidence for tobacco control myths and facts 2002.* Clearing house for tobacco control, Universiti Sains Malaysia, Malaysia, 2002.